*Un*Broken

RECLAIM YOUR WHOLENESS

A manifesto to healing in a world that keeps us sick, suffering, and stuck.

Karyn Shanks MD

With life-changing guided practices to invigorate and sustain resilience.

Cover design and graphics by Robin Deutschendorf
Brown Wing Studio, Iowa City, IA.

Print ISBN: 978-1-7339176-5-0
E-Book ISBN: 978-1-7339176-6-7
Audiobook ISBN: 978-1-7339176-7-4
Amazon ISBN: 978-1-7339176-8-1

Heal Literary Press

Heal Literary Press
Middleton, WI
HealLiteraryPress.com
First Edition

For Brian, Sean, and Aidan, loves of my life.

*Un*Broken

Ungebrocen (Old English), c. 1300:
whole, unviolated, uninterrupted, untamed.

Not perfect.

Not unscathed by life.

Not without scars or suffering.

But real. Fully lived. Unbroken. Holy.

A life made more beautiful and whole by braving, living, and nourishing an authentic life.

— Karyn Shanks MD, from *Heal: A Nine-Stage Roadmap to Recover Energy, Reverse Chronic Illness, and Claim the Potential of a Vibrant New You.*

CONTENTS

Author's Note.

I remember it vividly. Gnawing fear in the pit of my gut, bordering on ... what? Trepidation, disappointment, but also something more powerful. It was a dawning confusion my body understood long before my mind could make sense of it.

I was a second-year medical student, and I had just completed my study of the human sciences—biochemistry, cell biology, anatomy, physiology— gorgeous understanding of the inner workings of the human organism. A harmony of knowledge passed through generations of seekers, thinkers, and healers. I couldn't wait for what I was certain came next: how to apply this knowledge to human beings. How to *help* people with it, to show them how to heal. This was the sacred purpose for why I was here. This was it. This was what I'd been preparing for through years as a nurse, a pre-med student, and my first grueling year as a medical student.

Instead, where I landed was in a foreign world of isolated facts, of how to name and classify things. We left behind the integrated, dynamic, and highly nuanced human systems biology and never looked back. All that beauty lost. Although I couldn't articulate it at the time, it felt like the incredible soaring symphony I was immersed in during my first year of medical school simply stopped. With no warning, no preparation, and no explanation, complete silence. Instead, I learned: What do we call this disease? What does it look like under the microscope? What drug best treats this disease? What is the list of most likely diseases given the signs and symptoms of the patient and what is the treatment protocol for each one of them? We moved into a world of memorized "facts" that was largely disconnected from those sacred sciences I'd believed were cornerstones to *healing*.

I felt like I was being catapulted far from where I believed I was going, far from where I was *meant* to go. How could I have gotten it so wrong? But it was true. I lost the beautiful medicine I'd believed in, the medicine I knew in my bones had been calling to me for so long, bringing me to exactly where I was in that moment. Only the moment stopped making sense. I no longer trusted what I'd once known for sure. More than confused, I became unmoored.

What I felt in my body was grief. Grief for the disconnect from what I thought medicine was. Grief for the loss of the richly nuanced context of the unique human people behind the names we learned to give their problems. Behind the drugs we used to manage their suffering. I continued to grieve as I dutifully memorized textbooks filled with the taxonomy of medicine, as I spit this knowledge out at the bedsides of my patients. I grieved as I was rewarded for mastering the names for their 'many parts, many problems,' the diagnoses they were reduced to. How we talked about them as if they were the labels themselves, often in front of them: "the diabetic," "the alcoholic liver disease patient with massive ascites," "the DSM-3 code major depressive disorder patient." I grieved as I was discouraged from using the wisdom of my heart and my evolving understanding of the beauty, complexity, and mystery of humans, what led me to medicine in the first place. I grieved as I was taught suffering people were broken and needed to be fixed.

Though completely disillusioned, something guided me onward, and I completed my medical school and residency training to become a full-fledged doctor of the western biomedical paradigm. Was it faith that pushed me? Faith that I'd one day reclaim that symphony I once clearly heard and believed in? As I became a practicing doc, I listened closely to my clients' stories. I heard their hopes and dreams and what they were truly seeking from medicine. In those stories, I detected the quiet strains of the symphony I had lost. They helped me recover from the limited approach to healing and distorted view of people my medical training taught me. By showing me who they were and telling me what they needed, they guided me back to what medicine really is, what it should be, what it *had* to be: grounded in real people with real experiences that defy simple names and one-size-fits-all fixes. They helped me become a better doctor.

As I learned from my clients, I saw how they grieved too. Some of them could name what they grieved for. Others felt it but couldn't find words to explain it. But they all grieved the same losses of the larger context of our humanity I did—how they got lost in the 'many parts, many problems,' and the fixes of the medicine they'd put their trust in. All that grief—my grief as a medical trainee and later as a practicing physician and patient, myself, my clients' grief, and the grief of a suffering world—ties into a larger story that explains how we got here. We do not think of ourselves as 'many parts, many problems' for no reason. We see the world this way because of cultural stories passed to us through many generations that have engendered our science, our medicine, and our community and familial belief systems. Stories that separate us into parts. That separate us from ourselves. That see us as "broken" when we're sick or suffering—disconnected from our own wholeness and the sacred wisdom within us—in need of the standard "fixes" of medicine we're taught will put us back together again.

My disappointment as a second-year medical student began one of the most important odysseys of discovery of my life. I learned the disconnected, one-size-fits-all medicine I was indoctrinated into, taught to all of us as "fact," is a story. And why wouldn't it be? Everything we think we know is a story. It's *all* story. We're storytelling creatures after all, weaving together "the facts" to make sense of things and to keep us safe. Even when the stories aren't true or are too oversimplified to do us good. Even when we get lost in our stories, or are neglected by others' stories in crucial ways, no longer seen or known for who we are.

But as you'll see, as we take this journey together, we get to not just scrutinize but *redefine* those stories. We get to scrutinize every story we've ever been told, including—*especially*—those so powerful and all-pervasive, we may not realize they're stories at all.

What my clients have shown me with absolute certainty is how the truest stories are the ones that understand their suffering for what it is: wisdom. That guide them toward what they seek in the relief of their suffering: wholeness. My clients are simply asking medicine to see them. To see how they and their lives matter. How everything they lose beneath the gaze of a medical paradigm that reduces them to broken parts is essential wisdom they need to reclaim.

All this is to say—what my journey of reckoning with the paradigm of medicine I was trained in has shown me—we need a new story of medicine that sees us as already whole, already capable of healing, defying easy descriptions. Not 'many parts, many problems.' Not a collection of broken pieces, but an unbroken whole.

This book celebrates the revelatory and evolutionary potential of human beings. It's a story of hope, of expansion into new possibilities of what healing is, of what our lives can be, of how our medicine can better serve our lives, and of how we can better serve ourselves. But to understand the truth of this, which I do in my bones, I had to face the shattering of my worldview as a young medical trainee and the trajectory as a doctor I thought I was on. The profound disillusionment I experienced, led me to ask big questions, like: What the hell are we doing? Is *this* healing? How are we serving peoples' true needs? How can *I* do better? These anguish-driven questions asked countless times, sometimes directly to my clients, helped me learn what true healing is for real people and to radically change my course: as a doctor in meaningful helping relationships, and as a teacher who deeply explores the larger context of why we suffer and how we can heal.

I wrote this book to honor our collective grief over having lost parts of the sacred knowledge of our wholeness—in ourselves and our medicine. To make sense of the grief and explore how this happened—how and why did we learn to think of ourselves as broken in our suffering? And to propose a more expansive approach to healing that reclaims who we are and have been all along: Unbroken. Wise. Already whole.

Every page of this book was written as a devotional expression of gratitude for all my clients who taught me what healing is and must be for them, and for the many mentors whose wisdom inspired me and widened my perspective. *UnBroken* contains all the wisdom of my heart and brain and the knowledge I've acquired so far in the realm of my greatest passion—of human healing and our vast potential for resilience no matter our current circumstances—crystalized into the lessons and practices on these pages.

I promise you two things. First, I'll respect you as the wise person you are, even as you suffer, even as you seek fresh perspectives about your healing, knowing you can parse through the ideas to find what you need. I'll tell you the truth as best I know it, always acknowledging it's the best story I can tell today, though it will change and evolve as I do. Second, and this is the most important: I promise that *your* truth, *your* wisdom is right there inside you, even if you don't always feel it or know it's there. I promise to help you tap into that wisdom more deeply and to trust it beyond all else. *This* is the medicine I believe in, that best serves our potential as people, because it knows us as we are: Unbroken. Wise. Already whole.

With Love,
Karyn Shanks MD

Wise words to the wise (because the wisdom is in you).

Y ou are sacred. Your body is sacred. Reclaiming the sacred wisdom that is in you—that *is* you—will heal you. Will heal our planet.

But let's not get ahead of ourselves.

We're here because we're sick and suffering. Or maybe we just feel stuck. Chronic illness. Burnout. Low energy. Overwhelm. Confusion.

Where did our vitality go? Our sense of purpose? Our *selves*?

This is what's at stake when we are ill and suffering, isn't it? We lose our sense of connection to what matters most. We lose *ourselves.* Our joy, our enthusiasm for life, and our vision for our futures.

We think of ourselves as broken. We've spent endless hours, days, even years looking for our fix. The elusive perfect treatment, person, or piece of knowledge that puts us back together again. That helps us find the selves we've lost.

Some of you lucky folks may have found that fix. You feel better. Your life feels back in your hands. You're flowing again.

But what about the rest of us? Or those of us who found our flow only to lose it again?

Where have we gone wrong? Why do we feel stuck in our suffering? Why do we lose our hope? Why do we start to feel better only to feel worse again? Why are there answers for everyone else but not for us? Sometimes it seems that way, doesn't it? And why is there an epidemic of countless people sick and suffering just as we are?

What if I told you we've been barking up the wrong tree?

The problem isn't *us*. The problem is how we've been taught to *think about ourselves* when we're sick, suffering, or stuck:

- We believe our bodies are wrong, that we're broken and need to be fixed. Rather than: *our bodies are wise and fully capable of change, with healing potential built right in.*
- We believe our suffering can be reduced to something easily defined—a "disease" that comes from outside or "bad" genes that come from within—a commonplace condition that has a simple "cure." Rather than: *our gorgeous complexity and uniqueness provides a dynamic equilibrium of exquisite possibilities.*
- We believe the "experts" will fix us, distrusting our own wisdom, seeking answers outside ourselves. Rather than: *owning ourselves, directing our care, hiring "experts" for a job but not expecting them to have all our answers.*

This, my friends, is what keeps us stuck.

I know this so well. I was limited by these same disempowering beliefs, though I wouldn't have known how to put it into words when I was suffering and confused. For many years, beginning in my twenties, I struggled with intermittent fatigue that could be so debilitating I could barely get through some days. I had frequent injuries to joints and muscle attachments that seemed to come out of nowhere. At first all this seemed "normal." To be expected for a busy medical trainee, a new mom, and an active athlete. But it escalated as I grew into my thirties and forties. My docs and physical therapists treated each of my injuries as separate problems, without curiosity for why there were so many of them, why they recurred, and why they were often resistant to healing. And the exhaustion? Couldn't possibly be connected.

I felt broken. *Literally*.

I hit rock bottom after surgery to repair a torn tendon in my shoulder, just one more in a long series of injuries. I was completely sidelined from the activities I loved. No more yoga, workouts at the gym, or walks in the woods. I was relegated to lonely physical therapy sessions at home. Aside from the expected shoulder pain during my recovery—which was *awful*—I also experienced blowout exhaustion with nausea and a brain that felt scrambled. I struggled to stay upright. I barely made it through workdays, even with limited hours. Pain moved into my low back and hips. Simple tasks like unloading the dishwasher caused excruciating pain, as did walking. What the hell? How did I get from shoulder surgery to widespread pain and the worst fatigue I'd ever experienced? My doctors didn't have a clue. I felt useless, trapped, and confused.

This scary place of incapacity and despair drove me to seek answers in new places. I diagnosed my own low blood pressure after I checked it on a whim one day, seeing my husband's blood pressure device on the kitchen counter. My blood pressure was 80/50 in the sitting position, then dropped to 70/30 when I stood up, both extremely low. I was shocked. But it was also a *Eureka!* moment, when I began to understand what had happened to me. No wonder I was so exhausted and couldn't stay upright for very long with blood pressure that was not only quite low but dropped even lower when I stood up! And, *yah*, my brains were scrambled—there was very little oxygen getting to my head!

Then, through my own research, I put together how the years of injuries and fatigue were hallmarks of a hypermobility syndrome known as Ehlers Danlos syndrome (EDS), well recognized but often undiagnosed. I scored very high on the Beighton scoring system, a standardized nine-point scale used to help make the diagnosis of EDS that measures joint flexibility, such as being able to bend your pinky backward, touch your thumb to your forearm, and easily touch your palms to the floor, all which I had always been able to do quite easily.[1] All my problems finally made sense when understood in the context of unique connective tissue, stretchy ligaments, and lax joints.

I gradually learned what to do. I was able to normalize my blood pressure with simple strategies that I continue to use today, including vigilant hydration and electrolytes to keep my blood volume up. Sometimes I need to use more aggressive strategies to keep my blood pressure high enough to feel good. My fatigue completely resolved. My energy has been mostly excellent, with transient dips here and there, for over a decade.

In addition, my shoulder, back, and hips healed, and pain resolved. I keep my joints as strong and stable as possible through smart workouts, and I have a team of knowledgeable docs and therapists to help me when I need them. I've used savvy rehab approaches as well as injection therapies—prolotherapy and platelet-rich plasma (PRP)—to tighten ligaments and stabilize joints. I still

---

[1] Sound like you? Use the Beighton scoring system to do your own self-assessment. The Ehlers-Danlos Society. www.ehlers-danlos.com/assessing-joint-hypermobility/.

Karyn Shanks MD

get injured sometimes, and that can be frustrating, but now I know why it happened and what to do about it.

Most importantly, I've had to reset my mind and the way I used to think about myself as "broken," "unlucky," and "a problem needing to be fixed." I've had to teach myself that I'm safe. Even when I'm in pain or exhausted, I'm safe. And there will always be a solution.

Everything that happened to me made sense once the root causes were revealed. Rather than "broken," I'm complex. Rather than "unlucky," I'm unique. And rather than "a problem needing to be fixed," I'm a magnificent creature of exquisite possibilities whose needs must be understood. All my symptoms and problems were the wisdom of my uniquely hypermobile body. Once I understood that, I was able to shift myself and my body into an equilibrium of robustness. And most important? I learned to trust myself and my ability to figure things out even when my docs couldn't. I learned to use my agency with my healthcare providers to ask for what I need. I was able to step out of the framework my early docs used to look at me and my problems ('many parts, many problems') and acknowledge how limiting it was. I grew to understand and appreciate my completely miraculous human body.

See, when we're sick and suffering, we're not broken. We don't need to be "fixed."

We need to learn to trust ourselves and the exquisite sacred language of our bodies.

OUR FOUNDATIONAL GUIDING PREMISE.

Your body is all wise.

The story that we're broken when we're sick and suffering has huge consequences. "Broken" is derived from Old English "brecan": to divide solid matter violently into parts or fragments; to injure; to violate; to destroy; to curtail; to subdue; to tame. That's what happens to us when we're reduced to parts, when we equate suffering with being broken: we're not just violated, we're subdued. Like 'breaking in' a wild horse so it can be saddled. We're no longer seen as who we authentically are, who we *know* we are, untamed like the wild horse. In the face of that, we may even *forget* who we are. And in that forgetting, something sacred is lost.

In that spirit, the foundation to all we will explore and practice in this book is this: *Your body is all wise.*

Your pain, suffering, illness, and exhaustion are your body's wisdom.

Your body *is doing precisely what it was designed to do* given your present circumstances. It's not broken. *You're* not broken. You're not diseased or dysfunctional. You don't need to be fixed or drugged or silenced.

Just like mine was when it screamed its needs through exhaustion and pain, your body is calling to be understood. We need to learn to *decode* the exquisite language of your body as it tells us precisely what it needs to heal.

WHAT I'M ASKING YOU TO DO.

Throughout this book, we'll be listening carefully to our bodies' wisdom. We'll learn to understand what our bodies are asking for:

- What are your unmet needs? What resilience factors are necessary to deepen your healing?
- What stands in your way? What toxins, irritants, or disempowering stories keep you stuck in pain, suffering, illness, and exhaustion?
- Where does your body need energy and attention? Where do *you* need energy and attention?
- How can we better understand the unique terrain of your life and all that can help you thrive? What parts of this terrain are calling for your attention and action?

These are the essential questions to guide our healing, that lead inevitably to a powerful new story of our bodies' innate wisdom.

In this book, we'll explore our new story of healing. We'll break away from the common cultural notions about our bodies and the nature of illness and suffering.

We'll look closely at our systems of medicine and the ways they no longer provide the support we need. While we won't reject them outright, we'll realize what they're good at *and* how they are limited. We'll see how they can't support us at the deeper levels of healing and resilience we need most.

This is huge. We've placed a lot of trust in the old stories and the experts that uphold them. We've felt safe in these stories, even while we've suffered.

Karyn Shanks MD

And we *should* be able to trust our systems of medicine. I want you to know that. We're not wrong to expect the experts to help us the way they promise. What's *wrong* is the failure of our experts to adapt to the evolving nature of our complex needs. Of our personal, collective, and planetary needs. Somewhere along the line, medicine stopped growing, but our problems did not.

I want you to know it's okay. Your feelings are necessary. This shift is part of the work our bodies are asking us for.

Open your heart and soften your mind.

In that spirit, on this journey of healing, I'm asking, first and foremost, that you open your heart and soften your mind.

What do I mean?

Open your heart to yourself.

Don't make yourself wrong for suffering. Extend compassion to yourself for what you've been through and create a safe space for curiosity and further exploration. We'll be practicing this together throughout this book.

Soften your mind.

The mind wants more than anything to latch onto "the truth." We're heading into territory that may seem unfamiliar to you. Your mind, doing what all minds do, may resist at first. Especially because the promise in this new information is that you'll heal and feel better. You may not want to believe it. None of us wants to feel disappointed … *again*.

Don't make yourself wrong for what you feel. Notice your resistance, judgement, or fear—*whatever* arises for you.

Then, feel free to set down this book. It may not be the best information for you at this time. If this book is about anything, it's about trusting what you know to be your truth. But remember: all great journeys bring up all kinds of feelings, including fear and resistance. That's good. We're venturing into new territory. New territory is inherently *unknown* territory. But unknown territory also has the potential to release us from the constraints and suffering of our pasts, opening us to the promise and freedom of our vast, untapped potential.

Brave this journey with me right now.

WHAT TO DO WITH FEAR WHEN IT ARISES.

Fear is part of the sacred language of your body, a key theme of this book. Feeling fear is not wrong.

Fear, itself, *can* be scary. But see if you can soften your stories about it. Soften your mind. Stay curious about what scares you.

Your mind wants to make a big deal out of fear. As we work together, we'll explore how fear, and the stories we create about fear, have kept us alive throughout human history. It's powerful. And the stronger our biological expression of fear (anxiety, restlessness, racing heart, and so on), the more terrifying our stories.

Instead of protecting us as we hope they will, these stories can keep us suffering and stuck.

The fear that arises when we venture into unknown territory is mostly fear of uncertainty about the unknown (what will happen to us?) and fear of failure (what if we fall flat on our faces?).

If we're perfectly honest, we live with uncertainty and the unknown at every second of every day, we just don't let ourselves see it. Believing we know where we are and where we're going, well, that's a story too.

And failure? Total story one hundred percent of the time. Failure is just a perspective that casts us in the worst possible light. In truth, failure can be the time when we're most open to learning and discovering our better path.

Keep this in mind as we go. And if fear arises (it probably will), put the book down, sit quietly for a moment, and practice this sequence:

- Quietly settle into your body. Breathe. Close your eyes if it feels comfortable.
- Notice the fear and any other sensations or feelings in your body (discomfort, constrictions, anxiety, energy shifts, and so forth) without trying to change or fix them. See if you can witness them with curiosity, welcoming them as wisdom of your body. They may be uncomfortable, but they're not your enemy.
- Become aware of any stories—meaning you assign the fear (I don't feel safe, it's dangerous, I shouldn't be doing this, I might fail, I don't believe this).
- See if you can *allow* your stories to exist without censoring, silencing, or trying to fix them.

Karyn Shanks MD

- Hold all your sensations, feelings, and stories with compassion. Let them be safe with you. You're honoring the wisdom of your body and how stories—even the most uncomfortable ones—have kept you and your ancestors alive, even if they no longer serve you.

We honor the wisdom of our bodies based on their intrinsic knowledge, biology, and past experiences while at the same time embracing the possibilities of the future—of healing that is already ours.

We can only do this by holding it all at the same time.

While this may seem daunting, trust me, we were built for this.

We'll develop our practice of holding ourselves with compassion and reverence further as we move through the lessons in this book.

HOW TO USE THIS BOOK.

First and foremost, do it *your* way, in any order you choose.

That said, the three parts of this book, *We belong, We flow,* and *We rise,* present my thesis and the practice of this work in the order that makes the most sense to me. Let me briefly explain it to you, then you can decide how to dive in.

We belong takes us through the overarching premise of this book: that we're wired to belong. Belonging leads to safety, and safety is the foundational requirement for healing our pain, suffering, and chronic illness. We're living in an age of *lack* of safety. While our belonging, both individually and collectively, is in jeopardy for myriad reasons, none is as insidious or dangerous as a powerful cultural narrative that's disconnected us from ourselves, each other, and our planet Earth from the moment of our birth: the mind-body divide. Its deep imprint operates inside each one of us, dictating how we think about ourselves and what we can expect our potential to be. It's reinforced by our families, our communities, culture, science, and medicine.

We flow shows us our own gorgeous potential and the incredible possibilities that exist within each one of us. Already whole, we're exquisitely suited for healing our pain and all the problems that have kept us sick and stuck. We are introduced to the 21st century science of directable human potential { XE "directable human potential, science of" } —epigenetics, neuroplasticity, core functional systems biology, and transformational psychology. This body of science upends the outdated reductionistic narrative of 'many parts, many problems' and it shows us what's possible when we see ourselves as we are. We explore how this science gives rise to the dynamic principles of the human body that we can personally direct to our advantage. We explore the terrain of our healing, everything that makes us *us*, that becomes the roadmap we use to understand our needs for resources and energy to create the robustness and resilience we're capable of. For many of us, this means we can rise out of pain, suffering, and chronic illness.

Finally, in *We rise*, we get to work. We learn the nine *Unbroken* core resilience steppingstones. Through the series of short lessons and highly accessible micro-practices that we're encouraged to make our own, we'll activate our healing potential. We'll remember who we are. We'll reclaim our most gorgeous sparkly wholeness.

A WORD ABOUT PRACTICE.

Understand that practice is the only way to take in new knowledge, to learn deeply, to *unlearn* what no longer serves, and to grow and expand into your vast untapped potential. To help you, I've included 'Pause and breathe' practices throughout this book. Please pause your reading to do them. You'll find audio versions of all the practices in this book on my website, www.KarynShanksMD.com, so you can sit back, relax, and let me guide you through the practice. Extract what you need and keep practicing. That living, breathing, walking, embodied being of your own incredible wisdom I promised you'd be? Practice—*daily* practice—is how you get there.

One word of advice about practice. Approach it with a beginner's mind each time. That's often difficult. We're taught to be as exceptional as possible, and we feel we must become instant experts at everything. But what happens when we're exceptional, when we believe we already know all there is to know? That's right, *we stop learning*.

Practicing with a beginner's mind, giving up what we *think* we know, opens space for new knowledge, new learning, *un*learning, and the wisdom we forgot we had in us. Mistakes and missteps become portals to something new, perhaps the things we need most. Practice done with a beginner's mind helps us develop gorgeous new neural pathways to transport us gradually to our sparkly wholeness.

Karyn Shanks MD

LAST WORDS.

How did we forget our sacred wholeness and the vast well of wisdom inside us?

When did we become a culture of experts and exceptionalism that disempowers us to know ourselves, understand the language of our own bodies, and trust the healing power of nature is accessible to every single one of us (not just the exceptional few)?

These, my friend, are the questions we'll explore and answer in this book. By the time you finish, you'll bring forth yourself as a living, breathing, walking, embodied being of your own incredible wisdom. You'll remember who you are. Unbroken. Wise. Already whole.

You'll understand that the wisdom is in you. You'll use this wisdom to direct your healing life.

By now you've had a glimpse of what we'll learn and practice together on this journey.

More than promises, it's an embodied process of embracing and reclaiming our wholeness. Our bodies' language through sensations and feelings. Our stories and survival impulses. Our trauma. Our hopes and dreams and the vast potential within us. *All* of us.

We'll claim all this for ourselves through practice and experience and tapping into our wisdom (yes, *your* wisdom).

I'm so excited for you. And grateful to take this journey with you.

Love,
Karyn

SECTION ONE
We belong.

Even when we're not paying attention—living unconsciously, not knowing who we are—our lives are miraculous.
But knowing we are the Earth, understanding the genius of our bodies, realizing our incredible human potential, and claiming the laws that flow through our own veins—that's how we live amazing lives of wonder, purpose, endless growth, and love. That's how we heal.

CHAPTER ONE
Not just any belonging.

We belong.

We're made to belong. Countless natural processes, shaped by billions of years of evolution on this Earth, formed the web of life from which we emerged. We are designed to live and thrive in communities we call ecosystems. We shape and are shaped by these ecosystems. Humans. Plants. Animals. Microbes. On land, in the sky, in the oceans. Across the Earth, within our neighborhoods, our homes, and our bodies, we belong.

Full participation in this enormous and wondrous web of life is our birthright. We *flourish* in our unique communities and ecosystems. How we stand as individuals and together in this great web of life is the crux of everything that has ever mattered. How we love. How we heal. How we reach our life's potential. Belonging is *everything.*

It's not just that we depend on belonging to survive. Belonging nourishes us, making us the magnificent and beautiful creatures we are. It unleashes everything we've ever been capable of. It is our most essential and sacred need as humans—we belong to ourselves, to one another, to our families and communities, and to our planet Earth.

At its best, belonging holds us as the precious beings we are. Shows us our beauty and power. Affirms our authentic selves and bolsters our wholeness. Like the trees and grasses and flowers of our planet Earth, belonging grows our strong roots, activating the vast potential within us, so we bud and flower and bear fruit.

We know this.

Every one of us has been touched and sustained by belonging in countless ways, whether we've ever consciously noticed or thought about it precisely in this way. In how we're held and loved in the families we're born into or the families who adopt us. In the neighbors and communities that welcome us as one of them. Belonging is in the comradery of our friend groups from school, work, our sports teams, and shared interests. We belong to our gym buddies and yoga partners and to all the people who've held us when we've needed help—our caregivers, therapists, and support groups. We belong to our treasured pets and backyard visitors. And we belong to places—our homes, gardens, trees, and walking paths.

We belong to all the people and places who support us through the web of our communities, nations, and the world at large. The folks who run our grocery stores, grow our food, protect our neighborhoods, and build all the things we use every day. We belong to the artists, musicians, and actors who teach, entertain, and tell our stories. The list is endless.

We also belong to the Earth and all the layers of her rich and complicated biome. Every bit of belonging we experience is born from our evolutionary relationship to this planet. Earth's processes define us. Her laws permit what we can do. Her biome feeds and clothes and shelters us. We *are* the Earth and every bit as complex and magnificent and vulnerable as she is. Belonging to the Earth is the original belonging of our species and is foundational to all the rest.

What does belonging have to do with healing?

To activate the healing potential within us, we must know who we *truly* are. We must know the incredible, often unrealized, wisdom and healing capability we carry inside us. This is our birthright. This is the essence of our relationship to this Earth. How in all our connections, from parents to teachers to friends to the great web of life, we are shown who we are through belonging.

Furthermore, to heal, we must *feel safe* to be who we truly are.

What is safety? For humans, safety isn't just the absence of danger. Danger will always be there. Belonging not only nourishes and supports and shows us who we are, it's *the* essential condition to feeling safe. Belonging *is* safety. We're wired—genetically, biologically, emotionally, and psychologically—to seek safety through all our connections: to ourselves, our people, our Earth. Even when belonging leads to negative consequences, it helps us feel safe.

Karyn Shanks MD

That's what belonging is supposed to do, what it *can* do. But a lack of belonging, a lack of feeling safe is all too common. It's why we're sick, suffering, and stuck. This is what we'll unpack in this section of the book.

SAFETY IS OUR HIGHEST PRIORITY.

Safety is and *must* be our highest priority as humans.[2] Every aspect of us is dedicated to survival. All thirty trillion cells and the organelles they contain. All our organs, especially our brains, nervous systems, and immune systems. The vast terrain of our minds. All our most critical biological resources—the recruitment of energy, nutrients, attention, and behavior—are always directed toward safety before anything else.

Safety's importance is obvious—it keeps us alive. I mean this literally, but the need for safety goes far beyond protecting ourselves against predators and harsh conditions. Babies who are not held in the physical safety of a caregiver's touch will not develop physically, emotionally, or cognitively. They may die. Growing up in unsafe neighborhoods or disenfranchised social communities is associated with higher rates of chronic illness, mental illnesses, addiction, and early death. Loneliness is one of the greatest risks for despair, depression, and suicide.

Feeling safe removes some of the demands of the body's relentless survival impulses. Safety frees up precious resources, expanding our opportunities for growth and potential as humans. We can become more of who we're meant to be. Safety allows us to live fully and successfully as more our whole true selves, while healing our pain, suffering, and illness.

When we don't feel safe, the total focus of our entire organism shifts toward restoring safety.

When we're urgently threatened—say a semi cuts us off on the highway or our kid runs into the street—we enter full on survival mode with all our energy, attention, and resources laser focused on the task before us, whether swerving out of the way of the truck or leaping in front of our kid. We don't have to think, everything unfolds without our conscious awareness. Nothing else exists or matters in those moments. Large portions of our brains and an

---

[2] Stephen W Porges. Polyvagal Theory: A Science of Safety. 2022. We are elaborately wired for safety.

entire branch of our nervous system—the Autonomic Nervous System, famous for our "fight, flight, or freeze" responses to crisis—is dedicated to survival biology, the body processes that prioritize your urgent survival needs and restoring safety.

Beyond the emergencies of accidents and near misses, safety can also be threatened by problems in our relationships. The breakups, cold shoulders, unkind words, and breaches of trust—our lover tells us to take a hike, our best friend stops answering our texts—all the experiences that signal disconnection, often trigger the same urgent survival responses. If threats to our safety are less immediate but more persistent—say we live in an unsafe neighborhood or a chaotic neglectful family, we're continuously stressed at work, we're in a difficult relationship, or we're just trying to do too much without enough downtime—our internal resources shift to help us survive each day. But there's a cost. We're moved away from opportunities to learn, grow, and expand our potential because our limited resources are directed elsewhere. Without resolution, the cost of surviving the disconnection can mean exhaustion and lost potential.

The survival experiences of our ancestors are also part of our own survival biology. What happened to our parents and grandparents and great-grandparents resulted in adaptive changes in their genetic expression, which are passed on to us. This is an important part of how the traumatic experiences of our ancestors, what we call intergenerational trauma, continues to influence the lives of generations to come.

WITHOUT SAFETY, EVERYTHING FALLS APART.

No matter how you slice it, without belonging and all the experiences that signal belonging, we won't feel safe. And without safety, everything falls apart.

We don't just need literal, concrete safety, we also need the *perception* of safety. To appease human sensibilities and our human brains, it must *feel* safe. How something feels to us is highly nuanced to who we are, how we're uniquely wired, and what we've been through.

We all get this. We've all felt unsafe in circumstances that on the surface *appear* safe. At first, something doesn't feel right in the relationship or the environment we're in. Then, the lover breaks up with us. The best friend isn't our best friend anymore. Our friend group rejects us. It's not the right place for us. Or if we're young children, we may never know the facts, we just don't feel safe.

To feel safe in our belonging, it must do two things. First, it must literally keep us alive. We must be fed and sheltered and physically protected from harm. But that's not enough. It must also connect us in ways that help us meet our primary emotional needs as humans, nuanced to *us*, so we *feel* connected, *feel* nourished, *feel* comforted, *feel* cherished. If we don't feel all that, we won't feel safe. And all our survival impulses move us away from harm. If our perception that we're not safe persists, we move away from who we can be.

This is why so many of us have never felt like we belonged, even if it appears as though we should have. We were sheltered, clothed, fed, and part of a family, a pack, a community. But, regardless, we felt scared. We might have been physically safe, but we weren't emotionally safe, and we knew it. This is also something I know well. My parents did their best. My sister, brothers, and I were always taken care of physically when we were very young. But my parents began their family accidentally, as teenagers. They were immature— still children themselves—and unsupported in crucial ways that undermined their ability to take on parenthood and their own emotional growth at the same time. As a result, my home was chaotic and highly stressful, with unpredictable outbursts of anger and criticism, and long spells of silence and emotional distance. Our emotional needs were scarcely seen, much less met in those conditions. I did not feel safe. And while I don't believe it was my parents' intent, I did not learn all the beautiful things about myself then that belonging should have taught me.

Many of us have never felt like we belonged. Our families, communities, schools, and friend groups couldn't see us, meet our needs, or help us feel safe. Even if they loved us, as I believe my own parents did, we still didn't feel safe. We may have been highly sensitive or easily overwhelmed. Our needs were too much for the people who cared for us. We've felt vulnerable and scared our entire lives.

Even for those who have felt true belonging and safety, there are also times in life when belonging is *temporarily* interrupted, where essential connections are disrupted, and we may feel lonely or afraid. A trusted friend hurts our feelings, our children move out of the house, or we're injured and can't meet our walking buddies. Ideally, when things return to normal, we shake it off, the breach is repaired, the disrupted connection is restored, and we feel safe again. We may never *stop* feeling safe because we're able to see how the breach is temporary.

But when the breach is permanent? Say, our longtime lover breaks our heart when they leave us. We feel devastated. Our belonging to that person is severed and our safety feels deeply threatened. Hopefully, in our devastation, someone who loves us holds us in that suffering, helps us through all the feelings that arise, is fiercely compassionate as they tend to our needs and help us lick our wounds. We'll shift back into belonging and safety. We'll heal.

However, if our essential connections are interrupted when we're especially vulnerable—say, when we're very young and can't meet our own needs (our parents are too busy to notice our feelings or tempers fly without repair), or when we're sick, suffering, or completely overwhelmed and we're not held the way we need to feel safe—we may not be able to repair the breach on our own. The lack of belonging may *feel* permanent.

Breaches in safety, temporary or lifelong, for whatever reasons, may be amplified by our culture and families through disempowering messages about who we are and what we should be capable of, even when we don't feel safe, when we're alone, sick, suffering, or overwhelmed.

Hey, shake it off! Buck up! Just think positively. What's wrong with you? Count your blessings.

We might respond to those messages by wondering what's wrong with *us*. We may disconnect from *ourselves*. We may see ourselves as *defective and responsible* for feeling afraid, alone, and like we don't belong. We'll do whatever it takes to feel safe again, as we're wired to do.

As a highly sensitive child, scared and confused by the energy of my immature parents, I believed the problems in our household were about *me*. Often unhappy, I was frequently told I was "pouty." *Hey, why do you always have a frown on your face?* Rather than inquiring about the reason for the frown, *my* feelings were wrong. *I* was wrong.

If our disconnection to ourselves isn't healed, if we don't feel we belong, if we feel unsafe, regardless of the circumstances, we'll carry that with us. We'll define ourselves by it. We'll tell all our stories by it. We'll live our lives by those stories. We'll teach them to others.

It's not safe to be myself or to feel scared, lonely, sick, suffering, or overwhelmed. I am defective and responsible for feeling scared, lonely, sick, suffering, or overwhelmed. My body is wrong. My feelings are wrong. I am wrong.

Karyn Shanks MD

This lost sense of connection and safety shifts our genetic expression and biology.[3] It shifts our brains. It changes every aspect of who we are and who we can be. The trajectory of finding safety diverts us from our true potential. Our resources flow toward survival rather than thriving.

WE BELONG TO THE EARTH.

Beyond the physical and emotional belonging we need from other humans, we must also trust our belonging to the Earth. As we all know, this connection has been threatened. Not only have many of us forgotten our to the Earth, the Earth's biome and resources are shrinking. Our increasingly vulnerable Earth no longer supports us in all the robust ways it used to. Our minds may not fully comprehend that, but our bodies do. Neuroception, our intrinsic ability to 'read the room,' is always scanning the environment for the signals of safety understood by our nervous systems. Neuroception and savvy safety-oriented brains kept our ancestors alive in unforgiving environments. We're wired just the same. We *feel* what's at stake in our bodies even when we're not consciously thinking about it.

Without the safety of belonging, to ourselves, to each other, to our communities, to our planet Earth, we may not trust anything or anyone, including ourselves. This lost connection will be carried into the next generation. And the next.

BUT THAT'S NOT OUR DESTINY.

It's not supposed to be this way. This is not our destiny. It's not the Earth's destiny.

Yet, this is what's at stake right now. Our safety. Our belonging. Feeling disconnected and unsafe—and carrying it's genetic, biological, and emotional imprint within us—is a core part of why we're sick, suffering, and stuck.

This is what we're called to heal right now.

How?

---

[3] Rachel Yehuda and Amy Lehrner. Intergenerational transmission of trauma effects: putative role of epigenetic mechanisms. World Psychiatry. 2018.

First, we must reconnect to ourselves—to our wisdom, resources, and power. We must remember who we are, who we're meant to be. This is our only viable, sustainable recourse to healing ourselves. To creating safety. To belonging more deeply. It has never been more urgent.

THE STORY OF WHO WE WERE MEANT TO BE.

What would it feel like to fully belong to ourselves, our people, and our planet? To feel safe in that? What could that look like?

We're people. We're daughters, sons, mothers, fathers, and siblings. We're teachers, preachers, and healers. We're friends, neighbors, and citizens of our communities.

We're all that.

We also belong to the Earth. We are the Earth. Every molecule and sinew. Each breath.

Remember?

I mean, look at us. See how our bodies look just like her. How our bodies' form and function are so perfectly adapted to a human life. See how we emerge from mystery to be carved to her purpose—our purpose. How we live to move, laugh, play, breathe, sleep, love, and awaken to each new day.

We see all this in our children, who are gestated, birthed, and grown. Isn't it always miraculous? We're amazed by how they transform themselves through desire, insatiable curiosity, and how we hold them in absolute love.

And we see this in ourselves. How we protect, survive, and adapt in all of what we do. All of who we are. Taking it all in—nothing unnoticed. Everything accounted for. We see and feel the Earth's genius in us. We live our wholeness.

Notice how interconnected we are to the Earth's vast biome—the plants, microorganisms, animals, water, soil, and air. How they're essential to us, support and nourish us, become us, are made from us. The great web of life.

How we sparkle just like her. Ignited by her chemistry, shimmering as she dances through our bodies, sustaining us through our moments.

How we vibrate with her energy—the life force that literally makes us who we are.

How we flow. Rhythms and waves carrying this life force, landing us in our best possible outcomes, rippling with all our choices, experiences, and adaptations.

How we feel. Emotions inhabiting these bodies to attune with our environments, know what we know, guide us with their wisdom, and reach out to one another. Like every living creature on the planet.

How we connect. Together. In safety, community, and love.

See how Earth's wisdom—her laws, intelligence, and potential—are woven into us. How these laws for equilibrium, ecological balance, and resilience lead us toward the best possible version of our wholeness.

Then, appreciate how we rise when fully attuned to Earth's wisdom. Welcoming it as our own, we move toward the fullest expression of who we are and who we can be. We harness this wisdom to direct our lives to our best advantage, creating the most sustainable equilibrium and resilience. Elevating ourselves.

We belong to the Earth. We belong to each other. We belong to ourselves.

This is how we were created, how we're wired. We are meant to belong. To feel safe in that belonging. To realize our full potential as humans within the safety of that belonging. This is how it could be if we lived in full conscious connection to ourselves, one another, and our planet Earth. If we fully belonged to all living things. If we felt safe.

Though, where we land regardless is always miraculous if we stop to think about it. Even when we've become disconnected, living our lives unconsciously, not knowing who we are, our lives are miraculous.

But knowing we *are* the Earth, understanding the genius of our bodies and how they operate, realizing our incredible human potential, and *claiming the laws that flow through our own veins* ... well, that's how we reconnect. But not just that, it's how we live amazing lives of wonder, purpose, endless growth, and love. *That's how we heal.*

WHAT WENT WRONG.

If that is truly meant to be our story—*we are the Earth and her genius, we are part of the great web of life, we live in safety, connection, and love*—then what the hell happened?

Where did all that miraculousness go?

We're still of the Earth and the great web of life. We still *are* the Earth. Her laws still define and direct us. But it appears we've totally forgotten, doesn't it?

Something has gone terribly wrong. It appears we hold a different story of who we are.

We've never suffered more.

We're sicker than we've ever been, with a worldwide pandemic of chronic illness crippling our economies, crippling *us*, and befuddling our healthcare systems that don't know what to do with us. Long COVID, chronic fatigue, tick-born illness, environmental toxicity, heart disease, metabolic disorders, cancers, and so much more. Add to that the burnout, overwhelm, poverty, systemic racism, and all the forms of cultural overload and exhaustion that leaves none of us untouched.

It's clear how disconnected we've become. From ourselves, one another, our communities, and the Earth, herself. From our bodies, emotions, and our own intrinsic wisdom and power. We no longer feel safe. We no longer *are* safe.

It's nothing short of catastrophic.

SEE OUR EARTH.

We've disconnected from our precious Earth, the primary source that holds all our other connections.

Look at her. Look at what we've done to her. There's no turning a blind eye anymore. There's no unseeing or unknowing what we've done.

The destruction of Earth's ecosystems is so widespread, we've lost planetary *and human* health and resilience on a massive scale.[4]

For so many decades, the human ecological footprint has exceeded Earth's capacity for regeneration, which has led to unprecedented loss of Earth's biodiversity, resources, and resilience. The great web of life to which we belong is no longer robust or thriving.

Earth's growing toxicity and loss of protection of human communities has catapulted us into a global crisis of chronic disease and suffering.[5]

---

[4] WWF (World Wide Fund for Nature). Living Planet Report 2020—Bending the curve of biodiversity loss. 2020.

[5] Jeff Tollerfson. Why deforestation and extinctions make pandemics more likely. Nature. 2020.

Karyn Shanks MD

It's hard to see a way back to what we've lost.

Could this happen if we trusted our connection to planet Earth? Trusted our connection to ourselves? If we felt safe?

We feel all of this. Even if we don't know what to call it, our bodies know. We're intrinsically biologically connected to our planet Earth and her great web of life. When this connection is threatened, when her resources are threatened—*our* resources for survival—what happens to us?

Knowing what we know and seeing what we see, there's only one possible conclusion.

We don't feel like we belong. We're not safe.

PAUSE AND BREATHE.

Bleak, but true.

Yes, it's a bleak story. I'm so sorry, it is. Breathe.

Here's the thing. To heal, we *have* to face facts. We *have to* know where we stand *now* to make meaningful choices about where to step next.

That you've made it this far tells me you already know this. Thank you for your courage in taking this journey with me, for opening your eyes and hearts.

From this place of conscious awareness, we find our strength. One breath, one step, one small yet fierce choice at a time. We embrace the truth to heal.

Pause, breathe, and stay with me. We can do this. We can get through this. Wherever we're starting from, we *can* flourish.

CHAPTER TWO
Why it went wrong: core trauma.

There's only one way to look at this personal and global catastrophe of disconnection: *Trauma.*

WHAT IS TRAUMA?

Trauma is what happens inside us when our suffering isn't held—when *we're* not held—in fierce belonging and safety. When we feel abandoned—by our parents, our communities, our institutions, our culture, our planet— especially when we're the most vulnerable or hurt, we disconnect from ourselves and the truth of our experience.

When we're very young and not seen or heard, *that's* trauma. When we're suffering or sick and not seen or heard, *that's* trauma. When we learn our needs don't matter—when *we* don't matter—in any context, *that's* trauma. When there is chaos all around us and we believe we have no control, *that's* trauma. No matter what we've been through, it's the belonging and safety that protects us. Without them, trauma takes over.

We all have our stories of trauma, though we may not call it that. It can stem from growing up in emotional chaos, as I did. Or, for me and so many of my clients, trauma can be rooted in being sick and in pain for years and put in the wrong diagnostic-therapeutic box. While perhaps not the intent of our docs, they did not see or understand our needs. *That's* trauma.

Trauma can be intergenerational and cultural—suffering and disconnection is passed on to us through the narratives, behavior, and emotional signatures of danger and unprotected vulnerability. Our parents and caregivers bring their own trauma and disconnection into our relationships with them.

Trauma is also planetary. Through the process of neuroception, we react subconsciously to Earth's devastation, toxicity, and shrinking resources even when we're not aware of it. We don't feel safe, so we disconnect.

Gabor Maté MD, a man who has devoted his life to the study of trauma, puts it this way: "trauma results in a lasting rupture or split within the self, due to difficult or hurtful events."[6] These events can be bad things that happened to us (abuse, loss, disempowering stories about who we are) or good things that *did not happen but should have* (love, comfort, experiencing our beauty and goodness through the actions of our earliest caregivers). Perhaps most importantly, according to Dr. Maté, "trauma is not what happens *to* you but what happens *inside* you." So, often we *feel* the trauma in our bodies even if we don't remember, even if we were never aware of its source, even if what happened didn't fit common understanding of what trauma is.

Trauma leaves its imprint by hijacking all our resources toward creating safety—or at least the best version of safety we're capable of. The connection and safety we lack shows up in the disempowering stories we create to defend ourselves against hurt, unwanted parts of ourselves, and the very real threat of not surviving what happened to us. This becomes a barrier to emotional intelligence, healthy relationships, and personal growth. *These are the conditions for disconnection and chronic illness.*

What do we lose when we're persistently traumatized and feel unsafe? Beyond the energy and resources to support our healing, we lose ourselves. We lose our potential and possibilities. We may suffer from persistent fatigue, chronic illness, addictions, and mental illness, misconstruing them as "diseases" that happened to us because of unfortunate genetics or circumstances outside our control. The science is clear: all chronic human problems have their roots in trauma.[7]

My trauma tethered me to the revolving door of conventional medicine that kept me captive in a diagnostic box (many injuries, many parts, many problems) that didn't fit my actual circumstances (hypermobility leading to

---

[6] Gabor Maté. The Myth of Normal: Trauma, Illness, and Healing in a Toxic Culture. 2022.

[7] Gabor Maté. When the Body Says No: Exploring the Stress-Disease Connection. 2003.

many injuries) or my needs. My body knew. My caregivers did not. I trusted them because they were the "experts." I had to crash and burn before I searched elsewhere for answers, included turning to myself for insights, research, and new ways of looking at my circumstances. But not everyone is as lucky as me. They may remain stuck in the despair of feeling broken and unlucky.

Because our collective and individual trauma is so deep, so widespread, so catastrophic, and hits us at the most basic levels of our identities as humans, there's only one thing we can call it: *Core* trauma.

Core trauma keeps us sick, suffering, and stuck. It has made us forget who we are. The Earth, herself. Sparkling, vibrating, flowing, feeling, connected, rising, miraculous beings who know exactly who they are, tapping into the wisdom of the Earth and her nurturing resources to live, grow, heal, and thrive.

How do we call our potential back?

How do we feel safe again?

How do we reckon with our core trauma of disconnection to belong to ourselves, one another, and our precious Earth again? To feel whole? To heal our suffering?

You guessed it. We step up. To ourselves. To our safety. To who we were meant to be.

PAUSE AND BREATHE.

Create a safety circuit: Mind. Feet. Hands. Heart. Breath.

Let's bolster our safety. We need it, don't we?

While we depended on others for safety when we were young (though we may not have always gotten it) and have been taught in endless ways to seek it from sources outside ourselves (often unreliable, aren't they?), there's a lot we can do to help *ourselves* feel safe.

We can bolster all the layers of safety for ourselves—emotional, physical, energetic (we know what negative energy feels like, don't we?).

Let's begin with what we know.

Where do you feel most safe? Is it a place? With a particular person? A pet? Is it within you? Reading a particular book passage? In prayer or meditation?

What does it feel like to have that safety? Warm? Calm? Whatever it is, hold that.

If you don't know where you feel safe, please don't worry. We're about to activate a powerful internal safety circuit that you can turn to at any time.

Let's go there now.

Stand or sit with your feet against the ground. If you can, remove your shoes, wiggle your feet around, create sensation against the bottoms of your feet. Let your feet feel the ground beneath you. Activating the sensory receptors in your feet anchors you to the ground by providing important safety signals to your brain and nervous system.

Place your hands firmly over your heart, let your heart know you're there. This immediate physical connection between your hands and heart also teaches your body you're safe. It makes sense, doesn't it? When you hold a child with tenderness and fierce love, when you remind them you're there, they settle, knowing they are held in safety. And not just us, all species make this connection of safety through touch—look at dogs, elephants, and dolphins. So, tell your heart you're there.

With feet on the ground and hands over your heart, gently close your eyes or keep a soft gaze in front of you. Breathe, and rest here for a moment, without trying to fix or change anything.

Then, notice your breath: the cool air as it enters your nose, and the warmer air as you exhale. Conscious breathing through the nose activates the vagus nerve, a key player in the Autonomic Nervous System (ANS) safety-social connection circuit.

As you hold, imagine you are directing breath into your hands. Notice their temperature and pressure against your chest. Like your feet, activating sensation in your palms sends safety signals to your brain. You're anchored in your body and on the Earth.

Direct breath into your heart. Notice the beat of your heart and any sensations that arise in your chest.

Direct breath to your feet, noticing how they feel anchored to the ground.

Rest here as long as you'd like.

There. We've created an important safety circuit between your mind, breath, heart, feet, and hands.

Let's hold this circuit as we use our powerful words.

I forge a powerful bond of safety with myself by anchoring to the ground and connecting to my heart. I allow my attention and breath to complete and hold this circuit, to hold me in safety. Regardless of how it feels right now, the bond of safety is established.

With this connection between my mind, breath, feet, hands, and heart, I affirm my safety. I am safe. However I have known or felt safe in my life, I create it here within my own body. I give myself permission to settle into it with the utmost tenderness. With practice I will trust it.

Mind. Breath. Heart. Feet. Hands.

This is my safety circuit. I can come here whenever I need to. I can layer in images, sensations, and feelings of love, compassion, and safety from my memory banks. If I can't access these now, I can still complete the circuit. I am still safe.

CHAPTER THREE
Finding our way back to belonging.

To find our way back to belonging, we must understand what has happened inside us. How did we become disconnected? Why don't we feel safe in our bodies, in our relationships, in our communities and institutions, on our planet? What *is* our core trauma?

Where do we begin?

First and beyond all else, we must accept the assignment put before us. The assignment our bodies, communities, and our Earth crave. The assignment that is now so clear, so urgent. Accepting this assignment will ignite the process of restoring our connection and lead us back to safety and our potential as people.

OUR ASSIGNMENT IS TO HEAL.

There's only one access point to this assignment.

It must go through us. It can only be activated by each one of us.

Our only recourse to reconnect, restore our sense of safety, and reclaim the energy and potential that are our birthright, is for each one of us to step up to this assignment.

You. Me. Us.

Think of it this way:

We're always at the helm of our healing, whether we think we are or not. It's nature's law. We're there regardless. It's ours.

But we may not know it. We may be living our lives unconsciously, unaware of our own needs, giving our power and wisdom away by asking others to fix what's wrong with us (because whether we like it or not, that's what we've been taught to do). We feel unsafe, but we don't know why.

That doesn't mean healing isn't possible. It's still miraculous what a body can do without consciously directing it. Without knowing what we're truly capable of. Healing still takes place.

But that level of healing is not transformational in the way it *could be* when we are directed and focused on what we're doing. That would allow us to ascend out of suffering to step more fully into our gorgeous potential.

All that healing and potential is yours to not just have, but to direct to your own advantage. That's why we're here. That's what we'll explore throughout this book.

So, *this* is your assignment. *Our* assignment: to reclaim the remarkable wisdom, resources, and power that are ours when we connect to our whole selves and the legacy of human potential from planet Earth.

This is where we're going right now. Together.

PAUSE AND BREATHE.

I accept my beautiful assignment to heal.

Okay, I know that's a lot. It's liberating and challenging at the same time. We've *got to* breathe after all that, don't we?

Let's stop right here for a moment. Not to fix anything. Not to change anything. Not to create anything new just yet (we'll get there). But just to rest and breathe.

Let your eyes gently close. Place your hands over your heart. Let your heart know you're there. Be gentle with yourself. Rest and breathe.

See if you can tap into whatever feelings or sensations are there right now. There's no wrong answer. Just notice. See if you can welcome the sensations or feelings you find. Again, without trying to fix or change them.

What's there?

Tightness, anxiety, judgement?

Weariness, overwhelm, frustration, fear, confusion?

Excitement, inspiration, a sense of urgency?

Or some combination?

Whatever it is, I welcome all of you and everything you feel to take this journey with me.

I invite you to *consider that everything you feel is your inner wisdom and guidance.* Precisely what you need at this very moment. It doesn't need to be changed or fixed or silenced but allowed to carry the signature of your truest self.

Finally, let's use our powerful words together (feel free to use your own words if you choose):

I allow myself to feel whatever it is I feel right now. This is me. It's exactly right. There's nothing to change or fix.

I welcome all my feelings and sensations. I welcome myself with gentleness and curiosity. If I can't welcome them, I allow all my feelings and sensations to bring to my attention what I most need to heal. I can hold it all. It is all worthy of being held. So gently.

If I haven't before, I begin to understand my feelings and the sensations of my body as intrinsic wisdom.

I allow it all. I welcome it all. I honor it all.

This is where I begin.

This is how I can accept my beautiful assignment to heal. By accepting myself. By accepting my body, my sensations, my feelings, my thoughts, my stories. All my shit. All my glory. Because what we feel,

what we can look upon with grace and compassion and a measure of
reverence, we can heal.

ALL THINGS HEAL.

The primary urgeof all nature is to heal. *All things heal. Always.*
What does this mean?

All creatures and ecosystems of the Earth reach their best possible
equilibrium given present circumstances and resources, no matter how bleak
or disastrous they seem to be. Even when there's no consciously tended
activation of the healing, *the best equilibrium will occur*. Nature is never half-
assed.

We know this law of nature, don't we? We just didn't realize it applied to us.

We see it all around us in landscapes devastated by forest fires, hurricanes,
and tornadoes. How new trees and flowers emerge. How waters flow again,
the birds and animals return. A whole new landscape takes the place of what
once looked like total annihilation.

Inherently part of this natural world, we have the same potential for rebirth
into something we couldn't imagine before. Our own annihilation through
pain, suffering, and chronic illness can miraculously morph into new growth
and potential.

How it happens or the extent to which it takes us toward our true potential
is up to us.

We can *passively* accept our innate impulse to heal and fall short of our
desires and true potential. We can stay sick, suffering, and stuck. Or we can
learn to *actively direct* this process.

We can harness the gifts of nature, of our minds and our own biology, to
engage and support and elevate our *equilibrium of healing*—the dynamic
process within us that, like all of nature, achieves the very best balance given
the circumstances acting upon us.

Even the chronic illness or suffering many of us are experiencing at this very moment is *an equilibrium of healing*—the body is functioning at its highest level given present circumstances. Even as we hurt, every bit of our suffering is the exquisite language of our bodies articulating what they need, though perhaps in a language that's been lost to us, that we no longer trust.

We can change the equilibrium of chronic illness and suffering by harnessing this incredible energy for healing, the primary urge of all nature, and direct it to our own advantage. All the circumstances that determine what our equilibrium of healing can be are in our hands (energy, resources, experiences, and so forth). We'll dive more deeply into this equilibrium of healing, the science that explains it, and strategies we can use to unleash the potential within us in the next two sections of this book.

With this knowledge, we'll shift our circumstances in ways of our choosing, so we're not just blowing in the wind, passively accepting what comes (what we're told *will* come). We can change our brains, transform our stories, reclaim our personal agency, restore our connection and safety, and reactivate the healing potential within us. We can ease our suffering by addressing our needs at their root.

THEN, WE ACKNOWLEDGE OUR TRAUMA.

Okay—we've accepted our assignment to heal. We want to heal our pain and suffering, heal our chronic illness, heal feeling stuck and hopeless and not knowing what to do. We know the energy of healing is ours to direct to our own advantage.

What's our next step?

We've got to heal our core trauma to feel safe again.

How does that work? How do we know what our core trauma is?

We start by opening our eyes. We *acknowledge* our trauma, all the ways we suffer and feel stuck, understanding that only core trauma could disconnect us so profoundly from knowing what to do about it. From knowing our innate earthly beauty, power, and wisdom.

Even if we've never thought to call it trauma, we accept that we're hurt. We may be sick, suffering, and feel stuck. We accept this as the truth of where we are right now, acknowledging how uncomfortable it is, how disconnected and unsafe we feel. Not judging or making it wrong but allowing this exquisite language of our bodies to be seen and heard and held. *That's* our next step.

When we acknowledge the core trauma within us, we're letting how we feel—all the sensations, energy states, emotions, and symptoms of illness—*show us what happened.* Our trauma reveals itself through how we're sick, suffering, and feel stuck. These are our trauma signatures, the wisdom inside us, that show us what most needs our attention. Perhaps how we've been misunderstood and not had our needs met. We're holding all the ways we feel, all the sensations and experiences of being sick, suffering, and stuck, with the greatest reverence and compassion, without taming, sanitizing, or making any of it "acceptable" to others. By opening our eyes, we begin to reclaim all this magnificent truth about us. Even if it hurts, it's magnificent.

TELLING A NEW STORY.

But wait.

There's another part of healing our core trauma we must reclaim.

Our access to it.

It's not enough to be *told* who we are. It's not even enough to simply open our eyes, because we've been told countless untrue stories about what we're looking at. It's not even enough to see the science so our savvy intellects can scrutinize the new knowledge. We've got to *believe* it. We've got to believe who we are and what our true potential is. It must become our personal story. Sometimes our personal stories are so tenacious and unyielding, we won't believe another perspective even if it's true, even if it smacks us upside the head.

This will be our greatest challenge on this path to healing: changing our stories.

We know that to receive our legacy of potential from our planet Earth, we've got to reckon with our core trauma—the legacy of our culture that would disconnect us from the very essence of who we are: our intrinsic wisdom, resources, and power.

Here's my question though.

If we're so wise, resourceful, and powerful, so packed to the brim with beauty and potential, *how come we don't know it already?*

Why does it feel like we're hearing it for the first time? If it's true, wouldn't our parents have taught us? Our teachers? Our *doctors*? Wouldn't they want us to know?

Of course, they would.

Problem is, they don't know either.

The core trauma has landed in all of us. It operates unconsciously. It's hidden within all our stories—in what we "believe," what we "know for sure," and "the way things are." It operates within our cultural narratives about who we are, individually and collectively, as what's "normal" and "true."

And the more tightly we hold our truths? The more we let those truths define who we are? The more core trauma is operating, putting the brakes on all we can be.

To gain full access to the healing potential within us, the primary urge of all nature to heal, and to activate it within us, *we must tell a new story.*

One small glitch though.

We may not know we've been telling a "story."

A BRIEF WORD ABOUT STORIES.

This whole conversation about what keeps us sick, suffering, and stuck is about stories. Heck, "sick," "suffering," and "stuck" are stories, themselves, aren't they?

We're storytelling creatures. Stories are how our brains work to make sense of everything that happens to us. They're our neurological operating system and a core attribute of how we know ourselves.

Stories help keep us alive.

For our remote ancestors, survival depended on reading a complex, often harsh, environment. Was the rustling in the grass a tiger ready to pounce on them and their children? Did the withered crops signal a life-threatening drought?

Our survival stories look different today. When my children were small, if I lost sight of them for even a moment, I jumped into full panic mom-mode until I was one-hundred percent certain they were safe. Clearly my first story was, "oh shit, something terrible has happened!" We all have these stories.

Stories persist through the generations. We adopt them as our code of life. They become "the truth," "the facts," "how things are."

What happened to my parents and grandparents will happen to me. I've got to pull myself up by my bootstraps to become successful.

From this perspective, stories become our minds and our biology. They're what we do automatically to learn, create meaning, and stay safe.

We also tell stories as a culture. These are the narratives adopted by groups of people to explain their circumstances and stay safe. The most powerful stories reflect what the dominant people within a culture value most or believe the most strongly.

We're all prone to trusting these stories without question. I trusted the medicine I grew up with and trained in. I trusted the doctors, the "experts," to know what was best for me in my pain and fatigue. I had to unravel the tenacious cultural stories of the "all powerful" institution of medicine and the diagnoses it gave me to understand myself more deeply.

There are countless such cultural stories. We'll be exploring one of the big ones shortly.

Why do we need to know about stories?

Because stories are both our problem *and our solution.*

Stories are what make us feel unsafe *and* they are our path back to safety.

Stories disconnect us from ourselves and one another *and* help us navigate our way home.

Stories are what keep us sick, suffering, and stuck, we just may not know it because we believe we're operating with "the truth" and "the way things are."

I am all alone in my suffering. I have this disease. I am my pain, my fatigue, my diagnosis. I'm broken. I must wait for the experts to figure out how to fix me. My doctor knows me better than I do. I cannot control this. This is my destiny.

Our stories may be trauma-based, having kept us and our people alive. There is powerful survival biology behind these stories, locking us into the status quo even if they no longer serve.

Or they may be all-pervasive cultural narratives dictating "the truth," defining "experts," manipulating and disempowering us from our *own* truth.

But stories are also our gateway to opening our possibilities and potential.

We're also creatures of transformation. Our genetic expression is not fixed, and our brains can change and grow and heal. These are the keys behind the sciences of epigenetics and neuroplasticity, the engines of our capacity to change our genetic expression, our brain structure and function, and, you guessed it, our stories. (We'll explore epigenetics and neuroplasticity more in Part Two.)

Karyn Shanks MD

Someone near and dear to me learned he needed cardiac bypass surgery. At first, he felt ashamed—*how did I let this happen?* However, he took his initial sense of failure and transformed it into a new story. Rather than a story of disempowerment—"the heart patient waiting for the doc to fix things,"—he chose a new story, one that empowered him. He brought in others to help him create a story of transformation and opportunity for vibrant growth. Initially he worked on cardiac "pre-hab" focusing on getting his body into the best shape possible for surgery. With the help of his chosen team, his story expanded into an emotional and spiritual journey of getting him ready for a whole new start, a new chapter in his life.

Like this brave man, when we stop to think about what we truly want and need, rather than just what the "experts" tell us, we can look at, scrutinize, and reimagine our stories.

I invite you to keep all this in mind as we explore our personal and collective stories of suffering and healing. What comes up for you? Where do you feel most stuck or scared? Is there a better story to support you and your aspirations for healing? To help you feel safe? To empower you to create the changes you need and to see yourself and the world in more expansive, realistic, and hopeful ways?

Here's what I most want you to know.

Our stories, personal and collective, should strengthen us and open us to our highest possibilities, not disempower us. We should feel safe in them. Otherwise, what good are they?

We all know what these disempowering stories are, don't we? If not consciously, our bodies know. We know how they make us feel. We may not recognize them as stories. We may not have realized we have a say in whether to adopt these stories as our own or reject them, regardless of what our families and friends and institutions and all the masses are doing.

My story that my docs had all the answers, even when they weren't helping me, left me feeling disempowered and without recourse. How could they and their medicine be wrong? *I* was wrong. What was wrong with *me* that I kept getting injured? What was wrong with *me* that I was drop dead tired? I thought myself an oddball, an anomaly, *broken* because the all-knowing healers I turned to didn't know what to do with me.

Until I told a new story.

There was a core issue leading to hypermobile joints, extra-stretchy ligaments, and low blood pressure that my docs hadn't figured out. That core issue caused the recurrent injuries, pain, and severe fatigue I'd experienced for years. Once I'd put this together and could tell the new story of EDS hypermobility syndrome, many of the solutions to my problems fell into place. That made me realize there was a 'story behind the story' that I had to retell. Our doctors and their medicine are not omnipotent. And *I* am at the helm of my body. We'll dive more deeply into this in a bit.

Diagnoses are stories. Many of my clients come to me with a list of diagnoses and the treatments they've been offered. "This is my diagnosis," they might say. "This is what's wrong with me." "This is because of bad genes; my mother had it and so did her uncle." "These are the drugs I'm on to treat my diagnoses."

My job is to help them scrutinize the stories they've been told, the diagnoses. Do the stories fit, understand their suffering, and, most importantly, help them heal? Do they feel empowered? Or do the stories fall short, leaving them to see themselves as failures?

Diagnoses are stories. Stories are flexible. They must fit, empower, and tell our truth. They must unleash an equilibrium that unwinds our suffering. And they must always evolve as we learn more. Diagnoses may be helpful and lead to treatments that are spot on but they're still stories, they're not facts, they're stories.

PAUSE AND BREATHE.

How to deconstruct a medical story.

We've barely gotten started with this story business, so let's keep this simple.

You've been given a diagnosis or multiple diagnoses. You have a treatment plan. But you're not feeling better. Or you're feeling better

Karyn Shanks MD

but not as well as you'd like. Or you're feeling worse. Or you're not sure either way, but something doesn't feel right. There's friction.

So, what do you do?

Do you hang in there, trusting your doctors? Do you fully adopt their story about you and what they believe is best for you?

You can absolutely continue to trust your doctors. Many of our doctors are not only highly skilled, but wonderful people who have our best interests at heart.

However, always be careful about fully adopting any story at any time for any reason. Including diagnoses, the "facts" of medicine. Including those that come from people you trust. That doesn't mean they're wrong. It means we create space for an even better story to emerge. There's always more to know, right? The story is always evolving. It *should* evolve. And you have a hand in that. You *must* have a hand in it.

You can trust your advisors *and* scrutinize their stories at the very same time. Even your doctors. *Especially* your doctors.

I said we'd keep this simple. So, let's break this down into three easy steps for now. We'll pick up on this process to add in more complexity later.

- First, what's your story as you best know it right now? I have xyz diagnosis and am supposed to adhere to xyz treatment and it's not working. I don't feel better, I'm not myself, I still feel pain, something doesn't feel right. Tell it like it is to you. Blurt it out, don't self-censor.
- Second, breathe into the story you just told. Literally breathe. First into your body. Let your body soften on the exhale. Then, breathe into your story. No matter how certain you've been about your story or how certain your doctors have been about your story, use your breath to

soften its edges, to loosen its bindings, and to create space around it for something new to emerge. A new idea or direction? A new diagnosis or treatment? Or just space, just softening. Space is the first step to deconstructing the story that no longer serves. Space is also the first step to you accessing your inner wisdom to guide you.

- Third, place a question into that space you just created. *What's a better story? What else do I need to know? To do? What's my next step toward my healing?* Don't over-think this step. Don't feel like you have to know the answers. Just ask. Keep your questions simple, positive, and present tense. Then, let them go. You may get an immediate answer to your question that comes in as words or feelings, but you probably won't. Your answers will come in time and maybe in pieces. Stay alert and curious. And keep breathing, softening, and asking.

Finally, as you evaluate and question your stories for how they strengthen versus disempower you, *be so very gentle with yourself.* These are the questions of disrupters and troublemakers. Everyday people don't question their stories. But we do. And we're so needed. We're enlightened leaders. And we're called to be so brave.

Now, on our journey back to belonging and safety, let's peek at one of the most disempowering and disconnecting cultural stories ever told.

Karyn Shanks MD

CHAPTER FOUR
Born into a legacy of disconnection: the mind-body divide.

To tell our new story of healing it's crucial we understand an old one. A story that's central to how we understand ourselves as humans. Like all stories that take hold in our culture and in ourselves, it had great value at one time. But now? This story doesn't work, it holds us back, and it's stolen many lives that were packed to the brim with possibilities. It's a story that has disconnected us from who we are, landing us in core trauma.

You may not have heard this story in these words, but you'll recognize it all the same. You'll see how you've *lived* this story. We all have. It's been a cornerstone to all human life for centuries.

This is the story of the mind-body divide. It's the worldview that misconstrues us as being made up of unconnected parts. This story says our minds and bodies are separate. Mind does not affect body, and body does not affect mind. It's pervasive. It's in every bit of our suffering. And it rules our cultural institutions, from religion to politics to science and medicine. The story of the mind-body divide is the legacy of a culture that's forgotten who we are.

Following the dark ages of human history, knowledge and discourse expanded on a wide range of human subjects. In spreading this new knowledge, simplicity was prioritized over complexity, and certainty over ambiguity. Because humans and nature and the universe are complex, our forebearers chose stripped down, less sophisticated versions of these new stories, discarding old wisdom in favor of the new. They turned a blind eye to what was perhaps too mysterious to understand, like the powerful intangibles of the human mind, human emotions and feelings, human spiritual yearnings, human relationships, and the connection of humans to the Earth.

Expecting the world to fit into a simple, easy to understand framework can leave gaping holes in our understanding. The mind-body divide story oversimplifies what it means to be human. As such, it became a powerful engine of how we disconnect from ourselves from the moment we are born, never fully knowing how complete we already are.

MANY "PARTS."

We've come to think of ourselves as having all kinds of parts: bodies, minds, emotions, spirits, you name it. We might *say* they're all part of the same whole, but we have very different words for each, a clear signal we consider them separate. In the English language we have no words to merge these parts. A foundational premise of this book is that we are a composite of our wholeness: of body and its biology *with* mind, emotions, spirit, and all our human experiences. But we lack words to bring these ideas together more closely. The closest we come to a composite word to describe us is "self," though what self represents for each of us depends on the story we use to explain ourselves. For many of us, for instance, self is biased toward "mind" because we localize ourselves to our thoughts. Expressions of true mind-body-spirit holism require lists of words tagged with explanations for how they're integrated.

Even though current science and collective wisdom have been slowly leading us back to understanding ourselves as more of a unity of mind, body, and spirit, we're still profoundly influenced by the old story. We see it in how we're taught to value certain attributes of ourselves over others (rational thinking over feelings, for instance) and, as we'll see, how it's the guiding philosophical underpinning of science, the scientific method, and the dominant healing tradition of our world, western biomedicine. Likewise, we see its influence in Judeo-Christian religions that focus on morality and the condition of the human spirit, but don't concern themselves with teaching people how to take care of their bodies.

So where did the idea that the human mind and body are separate come from?

It's complicated. And, like everything, it's a story too.

Walk with me, as we explore three aspects of the mind-body divide origin story that I believe have made it so powerful and pervasive:

- The cultural scientific revolution that led to mind-body dualism in science and medicine.
- A male-dominated culture and the logical, rational, linear thinking style.
- The traumatized brain.

MIND-BODY DUALISM IN THE SCIENTIFIC REVOLUTION.

Mind-body dualism arose during the 16th and 17th centuries, a time known as the scientific revolution, during which there was an explosion of scientific knowledge, especially in mathematics and physics. This era brought people out of dark times of widespread fear by providing rational explanations for phenomena of the natural world they didn't understand (for instance, the sun doesn't literally "disappear" behind the clouds, nor is the earth flat).

Separation of mind and body is most closely associated with the highly influential 17th century philosopher-mathematician, René Descartes.[8] He asserted that the mind and body cannot possibly exist in a unified way, because the body is mechanical and subject to the mechanical laws of physics, while the mind is not. Therefore, he espoused, the mind and body must live in separate dimensions and operate by separate principles. In other words, body does not affect mind and mind does not affect body. This idea took hold of the culture and became a core part of the trajectory of science and medicine.

Mind-body dualism likely answered an important need during the 1600s. It freed people from suffering imposed by pre-Christian and Christian ideology that attributed illnesses to non-physical or supernatural forces, often punishing people for personal and collective wrongdoing or weakness. There were witches and bad spirits everywhere. If your crops failed, the Gods were angry.

During the scientific revolution, the body became the domain of science, while the mind followed the soul into the domain of religion. This gave science

---

[8] See Jonathan Westphal. Descartes and the Discovery of the Mind-Body Problem.

and religion their own separate turf. Once the human body became the domain of science, great advancements were achieved in the fields of human anatomy, physiology, and medicine. Powerful patrons of science could lay claim to the social capital of new discoveries. On the other hand, powerful religious leaders could exploit matters of the mind and soul to give them control through fear. Sound cynical? As you'll continue to see and surely won't be surprised, power and control are all over this story.

THE MIND-BODY DIVIDE IN SCIENCE AND MEDICINE.

Because mind-body dualism became a dominant cultural paradigm during a time of intense growth in science and medicine, it profoundly shaped how we investigate and understand human health and illness. The scientific method became the accepted approach for investigating not only the physical sciences but also all the biological sciences, including medicine. The biomedical model of disease, born from the scientific method, became the underpinning of western medicine, defining what constitutes human health, what makes people sick, and what the most "appropriate" prescriptions for healing should be. Though it played an important role in bringing us out of the dark ages, it also disconnected us from the intrinsic wisdom of our emotions, gut feelings, and spirituality—all parts of our wholeness and key aspects of our healing.

As you'll see, powerful as western biomedicine can be for specific health problems, it is limited. Our challenge is to help it evolve into an even more advanced, sophisticated, *and integrated* (body-mind-spirit) paradigm of healing. One that the world urgently needs right now.

THE SCIENTIFIC METHOD: HOW WE SCRUTINIZE "THE FACTS" TO CREATE "THE FACTS."

The scientific method is the widely accepted experimental approach used in all the sciences—chemistry, physics, biology, and medicine. It is considered the most objective process to understand the true nature of everything, including humans and how they function. As such, it underpins every assumption, disease theory, and treatment protocol of western biomedicine.

Karyn Shanks MD

The six steps of the scientific method.

- Make an observation: The grass is green.
- Turn your observation into a question: Why is the grass green?
- Form a hypothesis, a statement about your question, that can be tested: The grass is green because little green leprechauns paint it that color.
- Make a prediction based on your hypothesis: By observing, I will see the leprechauns.
- Test the prediction in a rigorous manner: Look for the leprechauns.
- Statistically analyze your results and use them to form theories as well as new hypotheses, predictions, and to ask new questions: No leprechauns, I wonder if it's the chlorophyl that makes grass green?

HOW WELL DO THE SMALLEST PARTS EXPLAIN THE WHOLE?

When utilizing the scientific method, it is generally agreed that the simplest question allowing for the smallest observation with the fewest variables will lead to the most uncomplicated *and accurate* understanding of the subject being investigated. This assumption is known as reductionism, the major philosophical underpinning of the scientific method.

At first glance, reductionism makes sense as a way to see and analyze and interpret the world with the most clarity. And in some respects, this is true. But there are key problems.

Reductionism falls apart when we attempt to extrapolate many small incremental findings to complex systems, like human beings. The premise of reductionism is that the smallest parts explain the whole. This may be true for a car engine or a rock formation. And we absolutely benefit from understanding how various molecules and chemicals and electrical charges operate within a human system. But does understanding the smallest parts of our physiology explain the whole of a human person? Do they explain the whole of a population of human persons?

No. Reducing a system as complex as a human being to its smallest parts does not reveal the needs of the whole.

Reductionism might size us up quite accurately if we were made from Legos. Take us apart and we're a pile of bricks of all shapes, sizes, and colors laying on the floor in your living room. Understanding each one of these Lego parts helps us put them back together to create, say, a dinosaur. They need to be selected by shape, size, and color to arrange in a way that looks like a dinosaur, and for the dinosaur to be stable and hold together.

But this process all falls apart when thinking about humans. We are, of course, infinitely more complex than a Lego dinosaur. There is no way to fully understand complex humans by simply understanding their parts. It just doesn't work that way.

You can see how trying to understand complex living organisms through the lens of the reductionistic scientific method falls short, right? Reductionism, itself, isn't wrong, it's our assumptions about what we learn from it that are wrong. The problem is in how we stick to the story derived from the reductionistic process that sees living things, like people, as simple machines. Sure, we can reduce humans to parts, we can study parts, we can draw conclusions from those studies about parts. But what happens after that? We believe we understand the whole when really, we only understand the parts.

Here's the problem. After studying the smallest parts of humans, we then fail to shift our gaze from those smallest parts back toward the whole and figure out how to study *that*. We forget we *need* to study the whole because we believe we already know what we need to know. Furthermore, the scientific method not only studies the smallest parts, it studies parts from *populations* of individuals, but doesn't leave much room to consider individuals, themselves. And no matter how hard we try to group people together who are similar in age, gender, and other key characteristics, individuals are *never* identical.

We need a lens that doesn't stay fixed, that can move in and out, that sees how the smallest parts relate to the whole and vis versa, helping us tell a better, more complete, and accurate story. Even if the story of being human is challenging. Even if the story of being human is largely mysterious, complex, and shifts in fundamental ways from individual to individual. Even if it leaves us with unanswered questions. Even if it makes us squirm to not know everything.

See? We're not Legos.

DOES THE SCRUTINY OF SCIENCE ADD CLARITY TO WHAT WE KNOW?

Karyn Shanks MD

Once the scientific investigation is complete and the results are analyzed by powerful and accurately applied statistical methods, conclusions are generated. These conclusions are intended to tell us whether the original hypothesis was correct or incorrect and lead to the next questions and hypotheses to test. Results are shared in the scientific community, so that collaborations of discovery are created and invigorated as new knowledge emerges. Publishing results keeps everyone in the loop about what's been investigated, stoking the fires for further investigation or suggesting new or improved treatments.

It is also important that new knowledge is scrutinized for its quality—the relevance of the questions and hypotheses, the rigor of the scientific investigation, the application of the most appropriate statistics to the analysis, and the accuracy of conclusions. This is the basis of the peer review process. Peer review adds a level of scrutiny for the quality of the science in a study before it is published. It is meant to objectively evaluate all the parameters of what makes science good.

What are the limitations of scrutiny in science?

Scrutiny by other scientists is critical to weed out the bad science, as well as encourage and welcome innovative thinking and ground-breaking experiments. The problem is that peer reviewers are people and their quality as reviewers varies widely. As "peers," they are knowledgeable volunteers, not professional reviewers who are taught the art of reviewing. Many of them don't know more than the researcher about their subject of inquiry. Most reviewers do not understand statistics at the level needed for complex studies and professional statisticians are not usually part of the peer review process. And, further, many reviewers are resistant to innovation within their field of science.

And that's not all. It's well known that many investigators publish their *positive* studies, those that support their hypotheses, and not the negative studies, which are equally important to scientific discovery.[9] Positive studies are also more often cited in the works of others so the authors can conclude to have found support for their hypotheses as they ignore studies that don't

---

[9] See Selena Ryan-Vig. Publication bias: a problem that leaves us without the full picture on the benefits and harms of treatments. Evidently Cochrane. 2023.

support them.[10] This inherently shapes the body of knowledge and the story we tell about the subject of study.

It's also well known that studies depend on their funding sources.[11] Science is expensive and the need for funding often results in asking very specific questions that serve the funding sources' interests while not asking other questions. This can leave gaping holes in knowledge that could better serve the interests of the scientific community as well as the public at large.

The National Institute for Health (NIH), a major funding source for science in medicine, is beholden to congressional approval for the research it funds, so it's directed by special interests, leading to bias in the questions asked. The U.S. federal government has not legalized cannabis, for instance, and continues to restrict access to NIH research dollars to study it, though cannabis is legal in many states and has been shown preliminarily to be a highly effective treatment for several health problems, including pain, nausea, anxiety, insomnia, and seizure disorder in children. The lack of substantive science to support these observed health benefits is directly linked to the lack of available funding. At the same time, massive numbers of NIH dollars go toward research on subjects represented by powerful lobbyists who wield large amounts of political capital, especially drugs and vaccines. This is not an indictment of what subjects are emphasized by NIH support per se, but just to show how politics leaves its imprint on scientific knowledge.

Another important funding source for studies in medicine are pharmaceutical companies whose bottom lines benefit from study outcomes that support the use of their drugs, vaccines, and devices. Their funding is directed to research that benefits them most, while not asking other questions that are highly relevant to solving human problems. There are no large well-designed clinical studies that compare drugs to lifestyle therapies for preventing or treating illness. There are no such trials comparing cholesterol-lowering drugs head-to-head with healthy diets for the prevention or treatment of heart disease, for instance. While studies looking at the health effects of multi-variable diet and lifestyle factors are inherently more

---

[10] See Bram Duyx et al. Scientific citations favor positive results: a systematic review and meta-analysis. J Clin Epidemiol. 2017. PMID: 28603008.

[11] See Alice Fabbri, MD, PhD, et al. The Influence of Industry Sponsorship on the Research Agenda: A Scoping Review. Am J Public Health. 2018. PMID: 30252531.

Karyn Shanks MD

complicated than looking at the effects of a single variable, such as a drug, the importance of such studies for understanding what we need to become and stay healthy is irrefutable. Of course, answering questions about the benefits of lifestyle factors versus drug effects would potentially take massive profits away from drug companies.

The problem isn't with the special interests of pharmaceutical companies seeking profits. The problem is with the medical community and society at large accepting the findings of drug company trials as knowledge that best serves all our interests to the greatest extent possible. The medical community ignores that key questions have not yet been asked, questions that may yield much more important knowledge. We adopt the new drug with some positive effects without asking what else there is to know.

It is also widely known how pharmaceutical companies actively suppress the publication of study outcomes that don't lead to increased revenue.[12] In addition, many medical journals are supported by advertisers and special interests who are allowed to have a say in which studies are published or not. It's all bad science.

In medicine, it's critical that the questions posed are relevant to human need. And, also, that the studies are well designed, the statistical analyses are appropriate for the study design, and the conclusions drawn by the investigators are as accurate and unbiased as possible.

SO, WHAT IS SCIENCE, REALLY?

What ultimately becomes scientific knowledge is determined by the questions that are asked and *not asked*, the completed studies that are published and *not published*, the relevance of the studies to the real world and how well they answer peoples' real needs, the accuracy of the statistical analyses, and the thoughtfulness by which study outcomes are translated to solve real world problems.

Furthermore, there's the issue of what constitutes acceptable knowledge *within a society.*

---

[12] Joseph S Ross MD MHS, et al. Promoting Transparency in Pharmaceutical Industry-Sponsored Research. Am J of Public Health. 2012. One of many articles addressing drug company distortion of the medical literature.

Even if new knowledge has jumped through all the right hoops for scientific discovery, that new knowledge may not fit the accepted norms of what we already believe is true. We have countless examples of this bias against knowledge society and culture are not ready to accept. It has been estimated that an average of seventeen years elapse between discovery of paradigm-shifting new knowledge and the acceptance and application of that new knowledge to real-life contexts.[13] And there are many examples in medicine of up to thirty years between ground-breaking research and wide acceptance in the clinical setting. The gene hypothesis, which we'll be looking at more closely in the next section of this book, is an important example of an idea that has held on far too long, despite research that should have supplanted it long ago. I would argue that its acceptance as a dominant paradigm in medicine has gone well past the thirty-year mark. Science has shown that our genetic code is not set in stone, as it was believed for decades after the discovery of DNA. Rather, the expression of that code changes constantly, *adapting* to our circumstances, a process known as epigenetics. While epigenetics has been an important research area for over fifty years, the gene hypothesis still dominates how medicine is practiced, and it's still stuck in our heads that we're sitting ducks to our genetics.[14]

It is very clear that the process of scientific inquiry must fit acceptable norms (including applying a reductionistic scientific method to complex humans). Who decides what those norms are? Who gets to scrutinize that body of knowledge and expel any assumptions or interpretations that don't fit their parameters for acceptability? For centuries, and persisting today, those authorities have been men, adhering to the logical, rational, linear thinking style, helping lock in the accepted norms, assumptions, interpretations, and agendas (we'll circle back to the male thinking style shortly).

Therefore, what we hold as the most objective process for generating the "facts" of science, and the "truth" we define ourselves by, is not actually objective at all. It is a methodology inspired by ideology and opinion like everything else. It's chock full of vulnerabilities and potential inaccuracies.

---

[13] Z0ë Slote Morris, et al. The answer is 17 years, what is the question: understanding time lags in translational research. J R Soc Med. 2011. Doi: 10.1258/jrsm.2011.110180.

[14] Gary Felsenfeld. A Brief History of Epigenetics. Cold Spring Harb Perspect Biol. 2014. PMID: 24384572.

Karyn Shanks MD

Understand that I'm not saying science is bad. Science is stunning. Where would we be without it? How immeasurably better are our lives because of it? What I'm saying is science is a human construct and all scientific knowledge is influenced by the stories, politics, strengths, and frailties of people. *Science is a story.*

CHAPTER FIVE
The biomedical model of disease: how scientific "facts" are applied to humans.

The biomedical model of disease arose from the explosive growth in the physical sciences during the seventeenth century. Key assumptions of this model were derived from everything we've talked about so far—the human body as a machine, the scientific method, reductionism, and the "experts" in medicine.

WHAT IS "DISEASE?"

What IS a disease? Diseases are intellectual constructs designed to help describe and categorize the things that can go wrong with the human body. These constructs are created to make questions about illness and treatment effectiveness more amenable to investigation using the scientific method. They're also a language tool to make it easier for medical professionals to communicate about what's wrong with the patient. As such, disease categories are simple, easy to define, rigidly classified, with strict rules about identifying who "has" the disease or not, typically consisting of lists of symptoms, physical findings, and abnormal biomarkers.

Based on our discussion so far, do you see a problem with that?

It's reductionist. It's simplifying a complex problem to make it easier to research and streamline communication about it. We're defining human beings and their health—yours and mine—based on the presence or absence of disease constructs developed for investigational purposes. We're asking all our questions for further research based on that simplified construct, and we're seeing people through that highly simplified lens. The problem is, what may work for scientific investigation and understanding general ideas about the health of populations of people, falls apart when we work with individuals. We forget to circle back to the complex, unique, dynamic, and sophisticated human who can't possibly fit into the confines of a disease category.

In the context of a real person, a disease is a hypothesis, isn't it? It says, "based on these signs and symptoms, here's what we think is going on and what we've learned about possible treatments."

A disease is a story about what has been observed in the research lab and how we talk about patients who have signs and symptoms about what was studied.

The disease construct has value in how we *begin* to understand what happens with people when they're sick, what might help them, and how we can start the process of communicating with them and about them. But how is it limited?

People aren't machines. We can begin our work with the disease idea, the hypothesis, the simplified story about what's going wrong. But then we must shift our perspective and expand our lens. We must always remember we're applying our disease story to a real complex human.

This is what's most dangerous about the disease model based on humans as machines. Once we start talking about diseases in the context of a real person, they stop making sense. What begins as a fixed abstract idea to help us study and understand and facilitate communication about the health problems of real people, takes on a life of its own, a story we misconstrue as "the truth." Something very important gets lost when we apply fixed abstract ideas to humans. We forget the individual. We forget that disease is a story, a classification language, *applied* to an individual, but is not the real experience of a real person living their unique dynamic equilibrium of illness.

My body was viewed as a machine when I presented to my doctors time after time with recurrent injuries to joints and muscle attachments that wouldn't heal. Each injury was considered separate from all the rest. Each injury was given a diagnosis, like biceps tendonosis, knee strain, hamstring tear, and so on. Through the reductionistic lens that understood my body as a machine with problematic parts, those diagnoses were precisely correct. But because no one viewed me through a wider lens that could see me as a unique complex human, there was no effort to explain why I kept showing up with injuries that seemed to come from nowhere. Therefore, I remained injured and vulnerable. But as soon as I saw myself through a wider lens, that explained the repeated injuries as well as the intermittent fatigue no one was even interested in, I better understood. And in that understanding, as a person with EDS hypermobility syndrome with low blood pressure that goes with having unique stretchy connective tissue, I quickly learned what I had to do to address my problems more deeply and sustainably. While EDS hypermobility is still a diagnosis, it sees me through a wider lens. It gets me enough that I've been able to manage my problems much more successfully.

And it's not just me, is it? I've worked with countless clients who've lived this same journey of frustration with a medicine based on over-simplified diagnoses of populations. That just don't get them.

HEART "DISEASE" IS DOWNSTREAM TO THE REAL PROBLEM.

Let me give you an example of a common disease story that leaves people sorely misunderstood.

Heart disease, also known as cardiovascular disease or coronary artery disease, is the number one chronic disease worldwide in both men and women, responsible for over nineteen million deaths globally in 2020.[15]

The story of heart disease in western medicine focuses on three things:

- Risk factors are associated with damage and dysfunction of the heart, such as uncontrolled high blood pressure, high cholesterol, diabetes, and smoking.
- Defining the extent of reduced blood flow to the heart and the degree of heart dysfunction.
- The application of medications and procedures to restore blood flow to the heart and improve or preserve heart function.

Where is the lens focused?

---

[15] American Heart Association (AHA). 2022 Heart Disease and Stroke Statistical Update Fact Sheet Global Burden of Disease. 2022.

Karyn Shanks MD

On the heart. Seems reasonable, since the heart is in trouble and needs immediate attention.

But what's missing?

The larger *context* of the heart problem. This story doesn't consider the larger equilibrium and all its components that leads to vascular damage and heart dysfunction. That's the wider lens we keep talking about. Nor does this story consider the larger context of the high blood pressure, high cholesterol, diabetes, and other metabolic consequences that hurt the heart.

"Heart disease" is a diagnostic classification, simplified for research, and narrowly focused on a single organ. However, when we widen our lens to look at that equilibrium, the broader context of people with this problem, what do we see?

Yes, we see decreased blood flow to the heart, heart dysfunction, and for many folks, the pain and exhaustion due to a heart with reduced ability to provide oxygen and nutrients to all the cells of the body. When considering a person with heart disease's most urgent needs, this is exactly right. People might die. People are suffering. But when we look upstream to what's *causing* the heart dysfunction, we realize we're dealing with a much *larger* problem— the heart is *downstream* to the larger problem.

Now, we all know the common "risk factors" often associated with heart disease, right? Most of us know how untreated high blood pressure, high levels of cholesterol in the blood, smoking, and diabetes can all be associated with heart disease. It might be slightly less common knowledge, but many of us are also aware how untreated obstructive sleep apnea, autoimmune disorders, sedentary lifestyles, persistent high stress, and nutrient poor diets are associated with heart disease.

How do we know this?

From the science on heart disease.

But have we gone as far upstream as we can go to really understand the *causes* of heart disease? Are these risk factors the causes?

No.

So, what do I mean by *cause*? What's the difference between a cause and a risk factor? And what do I mean by downstream versus upstream?

This is important, so bear with me for just a moment.

Let's think about downstream versus upstream. The problem right in front of us is downstream. The symptoms, sensations, and changes in our bodies we can feel and see and that create our suffering—our pain and fatigue. My frequent injuries. The heart attack. These are all downstream.

We all know there must be a cause for what we experience, something that happened before we started to suffer. The cause is upstream. What happened before we were aware we had a problem? What were those events? And how far upstream should we go?

Like many of life's problems, it's ideal to solve them as upstream as possible, to get all the way to the cause. For example, if a river near your home is polluted, that's a problem, isn't it? You can purify the water as you need to drink it. That addresses the problem immediately in front of you. But if a powerplant upstream continues to dump pollution into the water, you're not actually addressing the cause of your problem. And there's more at stake than your need to drink it. If the contaminated water continues to pollute your neighborhood, affecting your neighbors, saturating the soil in your garden where you grow your food, and your pets are drinking it, you've still got a whole lot to be concerned about. You still have an array of problems, even though you fixed the problem in front of you by purifying your drinking water.

To really solve your problem, you have to address the powerplant upstream dumping pollution into the river. That's the cause. It's the most upstream issue leading to your problem. You get the picture.

So, let's go back to heart disease.

For someone experiencing heart disease, the immediate problem is the chest pain, shortness of breath while going for their usual walk, or the heart attack that suddenly came out of "nowhere." These problems are downstream from the cause.

If we read the medical literature, heart disease is described as a condition in which there's not enough blood and oxygen going to the heart muscle, which is "caused by" blockages within the coronary arteries consisting of lipid-rich plaques.[16] But they're not causes, are they?

If you keep reading, the literature will go on to explain how high levels of LDL (low density lipoprotein) cholesterol is the usual "cause" of the blockages that lead to reduced blood flow. According to the literature, LDL would be the cause of the cause (blockages, plaque, reduced blood flow). But we still haven't gone far enough upstream to understand the problem.

_____

[16] Rai Dilawar Shahjehan and Beenish S Bhutta. Coronary Artery Disease. StatPearls. 2023.

Karyn Shanks MD

What happened upstream that led to the blockages? Could it be as simple as high cholesterol, untreated hypertension or diabetes, or smoking? These are upstream to the problem, but are they causes? Are they upstream enough to have the most positive effect on peoples' lives to make them less vulnerable if we made corrections at that level? Do we get all the way back to the powerplant dumping pollution into the river?

What is the most upstream cause of heart disease as we know it?

In my opinion, we haven't gotten there yet. We still need to go farther upstream to keep people safe. Keep in mind, in the fullest disclosure, mine is a story too. It's all story. But I'm telling my story in the most accurate way possible given the facts as I've found them in the scientific literature, knowing full well that this literature and, thus, my story will continue to evolve.

The true upstream cause of heart disease is a systemic inflammatory syndrome.[17] It comes about because the immune system is persistently activated in ways that result in lasting widespread damage throughout the body. Immune activation is a highly complex process with many causes. Short-term immune activation is a normal process of a healthy body, leading to protection and healing as it was intended. *Persistent* immune activation is problematic, as it creates constant destructive inflammation without the opportunity for repair. Heart disease has been shown to be associated with many, if not all, persistent inflammation-producing diseases, such as autoimmune disorders, diabetes, obesity, hypertension, chronic infections, gum disease, persistent stress disorders, and chronic depression. Heart disease is also highly associated with socioeconomic factors that increase inflammatory stress, such as poverty and living in dangerous neighborhoods.

The intense inflammation present in heart disease leads to damage not just to the heart but to all the vasculature and every organ of the body. We see this in the wide array of other "diseases" that share inflammatory causality with heart disease, such as peripheral vascular disease, kidney disease, obesity, stroke, and dementia. What else belongs in this list? All the reported "risk

---

[17] See Elena Barbu et al. Inflammation as a precursor to atherothrombosis, diabetes, and early vascular aging. Atherosclerosis: From Molecular Biology to Therapeutic Perspective. 2022.

Ejii Matsuura, et al. Is atherosclerosis an autoimmune disease? BMC Medicine. 2014.

factors" for heart disease—high blood pressure, high cholesterol, diabetes, and obstructive sleep apnea.

Does fixing the heart address the larger upstream inflammatory syndrome? Does placing a stent in a coronary artery or surgically bypassing an arterial blockage fix the larger problem? Does a beta-blocker, statin, and aspirin—the mainstays of pharmaceutical management of heart disease—address the larger upstream problem?

No.

When heart disease is treated with the state-of-the-art drugs, surgeries, and procedures of western medicine, focus is on the *downstream* manifestations of a systemic problem. The fix may very well improve blood flow to the heart and the rest of the body, but it's temporary. These fixes don't ask *why*. They don't expand to see and understand and address the whole. They don't help people address the underlying inflammation and its true upstream causes. They don't help people change their pro-inflammatory diets, pro-inflammatory sedentary lifestyles, chronic infections, disordered microbiomes, or unresolved trauma and persistently high stress—all the issues that get closer to the most upstream causes of heart disease as a systemic inflammatory disorder.

So, peoples' hearts are fixed but *they remain vulnerable.*

Of course, I've simplified this story to keep it from running on too long. There are myriad other factors that play into heart disease that we don't fully understand. There are genetic factors. There are people who show up with heart attacks who lead healthy lives and have normal cholesterol levels and no obvious risk factors. And there are people who live past the age of one hundred who feel great, have no signs of heart disease, but they smoke, eat high cholesterol diets, and enjoy life! See, we're complicated.

Back to that lens that moves in and out. We need that here. Rather than defining "heart disease" as a condition that looks the same from one person to the next, totally focused on the heart, with predictable trajectories, requiring the same treatments, we tell a different story—a more complete and accurate story. By telling the story of upstream system-wide immune activation and inflammation with downstream effects to the heart, with discernable causes capable of being understood and addressed in sustainable root-cause ways, *we'd be able to help countless people suffer less*. We'd treat the person, not the disease. In fact, we'd be able to *prevent* these problems altogether. Once heart disease is obvious, the train has run off the tracks.

See? It's complicated. But meeting a complicated problem with a more sophisticated approach could save nineteen million lives a year and help countless more.

One more thing. When we look at heart disease as the downstream effect of a larger problem, what is it *really*?

It's a symptom. Heart disease is a symptom.

And what is a symptom?

Right. It's the language of the body telling us what it needs. A language designed to lead us on a path of inquiry to understand the deepest, core-level, upstream problem calling for our attention.

We can say the same thing about most other common "diseases": Type 2 diabetes, hypertension, hypothyroidism, obesity, depression, insomnia, and so forth. Like heart disease, they're all symptoms, downstream of the root cause problems. And like heart disease, if all we do is fix the downstream symptom without addressing the upstream origin, we remain vulnerable.

OUTLIERS LOSE OUT.

In addition to favoring downstream effects over root causes, research constructs, by virtue of their reductionistic design and over-simplification of the subject matter, are inherently strict about what constitutes a disease. This strictness leaves out people with the illness who are a bit different, outliers if you will. That may be fine for research, but in the real world, there are all kinds of outlier patients who fall through the cracks because their doctors are using a diagnostic yardstick that doesn't fit them. I see these people in my practice all the time, who are sick but are told "there's nothing wrong" because they don't fit into a disease box.

A classic example is Lyme disease. Many folks with Lyme disease, a tick-born illness associated with borrelia bacteria, look nothing like the classification system used by the Centers for Disease Control (CDC). That system, meant to be a reporting and research tool, is used widely in the U.S. as a diagnosis and treatment guideline. As a result, many people very sick with Lyme disease haven't been diagnosed and treated at an early stage. Or, they haven't been diagnosed at all and succumb to downstream devastation that could have been prevented by addressing their illness early and upstream.

It's important to remember that experimental conditions are artificial because they're purposefully simplified for the experimental process itself. Therefore, while many experimental outcomes of medical science give us important clues about human illness and treatments, they are inherently incomplete. They were never meant to become diagnostic or treatment guidelines, but that's what's happened. For the practice of medicine to be the most relevant to people's lives, it must hold both the research findings (reductionism) and the contexts of real human experience (complexity) *at the same time.*

CORRELATION IS NOT CAUSATION.

One more thing about medical research and the biomedical model of disease before we move on.

It's important to resist the powerful temptation to assume causality when two factors are observed together. Just because two events occur together doesn't mean we understand whether one caused the other. It can be dangerous to make that mistake. Scientists are supposed to sort this out for us, but they often don't.

For example, there is a statistical correlation between eating ice cream and accidental drownings. Does one cause the other? No. Eating ice cream does not cause people to drown, but people eat ice cream and swim at a higher frequency during warmer weather. There's no causation here.

How about less obvious examples?

Smoking is correlated with a higher risk of many kinds of cancer. But not everyone who smokes gets cancer. In fact, many heavy smokers don't get cancer. They're correlated because smoking increases the *tendency* toward the very complex equilibrium of cancer. The relationship between smoking and cancer is real, and gets close to causation, but it's not direct or absolute. So, when we say smoking *causes* cancer, it's not precisely true. It would be truer to say, "smoking *in addition* to many other factors that must be present at the same time, causes cancer." You may think I'm splitting hairs here, but I've seen and experienced how locking down a story can get us in trouble. A locked down story represents a locked down mind that isn't available to learn something new.

Karyn Shanks MD

Here's one more less obvious example of correlation not being the same as causation. While the discovery that microorganisms contribute to a wide spectrum of human diseases led to huge leaps in our understanding of contagion and the need for public health hygienic practices to reduce outbreaks of illness, did we really learn that microorganisms *cause* disease? Or is the relationship more complicated than that?

For viruses, bacteria, and fungi to cause disease there must be a susceptible host (the person who gets sick) whose immune defenses are not up to the task of warding off an infection. For many diseases related to microorganisms, the susceptibility of the host is the *most* important risk for the disease.

No matter how you slice it, that's not *pure* causation. There's a much more complex equation involved in the person-microorganism relationship leading to disease. And we all know this, right? How we're more likely to catch a cold when we're stressed? Or, God forbid, shingles (reactivation of chicken pox virus) when we're *really* stressed? And what did we just learn from the SARS-CoV-2 pandemic about human susceptibility? From the onset of the pandemic, it became clear that those most likely to die or require hospitalization were the most vulnerable because of *pre-existing* problems leading to immune dysfunction: diabetes, vascular disease, hypertension, obesity, cancer, and so on. What *caused* the severe disease that led to the deaths and hospitalizations? The virus? Or the human vulnerabilities?

It's easy to blame the microorganism for our getting sick. It keeps the story simple. It's also profitable to blame the microorganism, since billions of healthcare dollars go to combatting infectious diseases every year. But, like heart disease, combatting the infectious disease is a downstream battle. The upstream solution is to make humans less vulnerable. See, it's a relationship. It's complicated. But if we addressed the human vulnerability to disease—to heart disease or viruses—might we be way further ahead than we are? Might we suffer less?

Causality is tricky. And if everything I just said doesn't convince you that viruses alone don't make us sick, fair enough. But consider this: how upstream do we need to go to make ourselves less vulnerable to getting sick? Is it enough to try to shield ourselves from viruses? Is that even possible? Wouldn't it make more sense to go as far upstream as possible to strengthen our immunity by creating robust human resilience?

PAUSE AND BREATHE.

Invite a better story.

How do we disentangle ourselves from what we believe *for sure*? From what the experts have told us is true? From what the entire body of frontline medical literature tells us is true because it operates within a very particular paradigm of thought? Because it tells stories all day long while calling them "the facts, the truth, and how it is?"

First, breathe. So deeply. And again.

I want you to know something very important. Your inner healer is there, the one who gets you and knows what to do. Sometimes it's just a little twist in the gut when you know you're misunderstood, not listened to fully, or when parts of your story are dismissed as irrelevant. It's the small subtle voice that whispers so quietly sometimes it's hard to hear, and even when we hear it, it's hard to trust. How can we possibly know more than our doctors about what we need?

How do we tap into that inner healer who knows what to do? How do we learn to trust it? To feel safe with it?

Now we know. We're *all* storytellers. Even our doctors and scientists.

Stories are both our problem and solution.

So, invite a new story, a better one, a story that gets you, that serves *you*, that heals *you*.

We're going to invite and practice your new story. To do that, you recruit the powerful energy of neuroplasticity (the brain that evolves) and all your brain circuitry to support and strengthen it.

Consider the parable of the grandfather who told his granddaughter a story about two wolves fighting. One wolf was full of negativity, self-doubt, and darkness. The other wolf was full of positivity, lightness, and hope. The granddaughter asked which wolf wins, to which her grandfather answered, "whichever one you feed."

In that spirit, let's feed our new story.

Maybe it looks like: *I need to do some research next. I need a new doctor. I need more sleep and to eat more vegetables.*

Or, how about this? *I need more time to contemplate this. I need to see this current strategy through longer, it's too soon to walk away. I'm on the right track but there's more I need to do.*

You get the picture.

With your new story in mind, or clear intentions to *receive* your new story, I invite you to stand or sit comfortably. Close your eyes. Hands over heart.

I am brave to notice the stories that no longer serve me—I may have called them "the truth," "the way things are," "the diagnosis that shows what's wrong with me." I can now see how they failed to understand me. They've disempowered and disconnected me, and not taken me as far as I need them to.

My stories are so pervasive they've been in the structure of my reality. I now hold them with compassion, knowing they helped me belong and feel safe in some way at some time.

With great gentleness for myself, I consider how there may be a new story. One that is completely new to me and may go against everything

I've always held as true. I take my time. I breathe into the possibilities that are there even if I don't yet believe in them or know what they are.

This new story may simply be … I trust myself. I trust my healer within. I feel her hand on my shoulder. I hear her small quiet voice. I let her guide me. Even in my darkness and uncertainty and feeling lost, I dare to trust I'm guided toward healing.

WHAT KEEPS MEDICINE STUCK IN REDUCTIONISM?

Why do we still operate by seeing people as a simple sum of parts? Why do we keep our gaze laser-focused on what's right in front of us, what's most downstream, ignoring the whole? Why do we do this when we know in our deepest core it's not enough?

As we've seen, reductionism is deeply problematic for understanding complex humans. So, what keeps it alive in western biomedicine in an era when our medicine should be more nuanced and sophisticated?

Four things:

- Reductionism facilitates the scientific method, the primary source of knowledge in science and medicine.
- Reductionism is an innate adaptive strategy of the human mind.
- Reductionism supports acute, urgent, and catastrophic medical care.
- Reductionism is highly profitable.

We've already considered the first of those points. Reductionism makes the experimental process more controllable and the conclusions (when they're made responsibly) more reliable, even though this design will inherently bias *in favor of* simple and *miss* the complex. This is okay when we're all clear that experimental outcomes are one small part of the story about understanding and helping people. Knowledge straight from the research lab by itself isn't enough to help complex humans or complex populations of humans to thrive.

Reductionism is an innate adaptive strategy of the human mind.

The second reason we lean toward reductionism is the way the human brain operates. How *people* operate. Humans have enjoyed an evolutionary advantage by keeping things simple, certain, and predictable. Or at least we tend to view our lives in ways that make things *appear* simple, certain, and predictable, even when they're not. It's helped us survive complex environments and overwhelming circumstances.

Psychologists call adaptive brain strategies "cognitive biases."[18] They give us a sense of control over our lives by reducing our perception of complexity, uncertainty, and ambiguity. We feel safer when things seem simpler and within our control, even if that means remaining ignorant to the whole truth. The certainty of reductionist principles and the certain simple stories they generate help us feel safe.

Beyond a sense of control, reductionism is *rewarding*, a powerful biological strategy that can be hard to resist. In medicine, reductionism rewards *everyone* for a quickly executed job well done. Physicians are rewarded for solving the simplest problems directly in front of them. Not problems upstream—those take time. We may *never* see the results of preventing a downstream problem with an upstream preventive strategy, because prevention means no one suffers. There's nothing to fix. But we get huge rewards for discernable action toward a tangible problem. Instant payoff makes us feel accomplished.

And for the patient? Feeling better now rewards us with a tangible fix. We don't have to wait for it. We don't have to have faith. *That's* what we keep asking for. When we're asked to shift our gaze upstream, away from our most immediate and distressing problems, we're expected to invest in outcomes we can't yet see and perhaps won't see for a while. We're challenged to have faith that healthy food, an exercise plan, and a diligent sleep schedule will pay dividends much later, but not today, not right now. Our need for the fast return on investment is part of what keeps reductionistic healthcare alive even while we ask for something better.

---

[18] A thorough review of human cognitive biases: The Decision Lab. Cognitive Biases.

Reductionism in medicine saves lives in the short term.

Reductionism and the disease model are a perfect fit for relieving suffering quickly and for saving lives in acute, urgent, and catastrophic situations.

There are times when we need urgent relief of our most distressing symptoms—pain, for example. Or we need to stop complex problems that are about to kill us in their tracks, even if they aren't addressed at their most upstream causal level. We need the cancerous tumor surgically removed and the chemotherapy that will address remaining cancer cells, so our own immune systems can take over to do the rest of the healing. We need stents placed in our coronary arteries to prevent the heart attack and recover our energy. We need the broken bone fixed, the life-threatening infection treated, and the accidental drug overdose reversed.

These are the times when we need help from a team of experts trained in the art of fast analysis using state-of-the-art diagnostic technology, who can rapidly mobilize well-established emergency treatment protocols. Reductionism and a rapidly deployed disease-focused protocol in this context is lifesaving. No question. It's genius.

And we all have some level of experience with this, don't we?

Several years ago, I had a spontaneous retina tear in my right eye—it wasn't due to an injury, it just happened. I depended on the expertise of my retina specialist who repaired my retina with great care and precision. Her approach was based on state-of-the art reductionistic biomedical science. It saved my eyesight, even if it did nothing whatsoever to explain the underlying cause or what I could do to prevent a recurrence.

These are the problems our modern system of biomedicine is brilliant at: precise, fast, effective diagnosis and management of urgent and life-saving problems.

So, why don't we have two parallel systems of medicine? One for urgent and catastrophic problems based on the reductionistic disease-focused biomedical model and another one for chronic problems based on a more complex, systems-based, whole-person model?

This question brings us to the fourth reason reductionism and the biomedical model of disease remains so dominant in medicine and why the obvious question about two systems of medicine is yet to be a question at all. Because it serves the most powerful masters of all: money and power.

Karyn Shanks MD

Capitalism is a lousy healer.

As we've discussed, western biomedicine thrives on framing human suffering as "diseases," "dysfunctions," or "something is wrong." Because as long as we're "broken" when we're sick or suffering, the directive is clear: we need to be fixed. And that fix, with all the services and commodities that come with it, generates tremendous profits. Some people get very rich on the disease model of medicine. The aggregate cost of diagnosing and treating heart disease is projected to grow from $555 billion in 2015 to $1.1 trillion in 2035 in the U.S. alone.[19] Atorvastatin, widely considered to be the gold standard statin drug to reduce cholesterol and treat heart disease, continues to generate over $2 billion in annual sales for Pfizer, even after a generic became available.

Profits like that lock in all the assumptions and practices that propagate them. By teaching us this is "the way" to end our suffering, it ensures that we keep asking for the commodities it has to offer. Because we want our fix. Whatever it takes. With all the bells and whistles that make us feel we're getting the best medicine can offer—high-tech imaging, lab tests, drugs, specialists, and endless follow up care.

As our medicine has evolved, technologies have advanced. Super specialization of doctors came along to align with those advances. In some ways, the growth of high-tech medicine over recent decades has resulted in better patient outcomes for certain problems (those urgent and catastrophic problems). But the enormous profits enjoyed by hospitals, clinics, and drug companies have helped drive a more technological and specialist-oriented response to peoples' needs, with less of a focus on health, more focus on fixing catastrophes *after they've already happened*, and with less consideration of what makes real people well. There's vastly less profit in that.

To be fair, we can't limit our concern for profits driving commodities solely to conventional western medicine. The profit motive is very much alive in the worlds of natural, alternative, and integrative medicine as well. It's just as insidious how the profit motive takes advantage of suffering vulnerable people seeking solutions. There are scams, unfettered promises, and conflicts of interest everywhere.

---

[19] Centers for Disease Control and Prevention (CDC). Health Care Expenditures in the United States, 2020-2021.

Who pays for the high-tech catastrophic care everyone expects to receive? Most people don't have a clue how it all shakes out in backroom deals between insurance companies, government agencies, and medical corporations. With insurance companies brokering deals directly with employers, the patients have become non-participants in how their own healthcare is funded, while insurance companies enjoy enormous profits with seemingly no oversight of their practices. The average cost per individual of coronary artery bypass surgery, the most common type of heart surgery performed on adults in the U.S., was $123,000 in 2018, not including insurance premiums. This is more than twice the annual salary of most U.S. citizens, who clearly could not afford this procedure without insurance. The considerable cost of technologically advanced medicine has led to a burgeoning insurance-industrial complex, which enjoyed revenues of $1.25 trillion and profits of $69.3 billion in 2022.[20] Where do those revenues come from? That's right—out of our employers' pockets, and out of *our* pockets, effectively slashing what we have left to spend on staying healthy.

It used to be the commodities of medicine were the physicians bringing their knowledge and compassion to bear on peoples' suffering—listening, consoling, and doling out simple medicines and advice to mend the sick and relieve their suffering. Or midwives tending to women during pregnancy, childbirth, and the early days with new child, as well as other essential medical tasks. The price for those commodities were real exchanges between people, in village barters or small amounts of cash. We knew what we were getting and paying for. Those decisions were made within our relationships with our doctors, uniquely positioned to most know what we need, not by insurance companies directing our care to lock in their profits.

What do we know about the low-tech, low-cost art of listening in medicine? By listening to the person's story—without interruption—a savvy physician can solve the puzzle of the illness most of the time.[21] No fancy tests. No bells or whistles. All while activating the healing power of connection, empathy, and

---

[20] Wendell Potter. Big Insurance 2022: Revenues reached $1.25 trillion thanks to sucking billions out of the pharmacy supply chain—and taxpayers' pockets. 2023.

[21] JR Hampton et al. Relative Contributions of History-Taking, Physical Exam, and Laboratory Investigation to Diagnosis and Management of Medical Outpatients. British Medical Journal. 31 May 1975.

Karyn Shanks MD

safety. When people are heard, they know they matter. When they know they matter, they heal better.[22]

But listening, the single most successful diagnostic *and healing* tool available to physicians, is time-intensive and profit-poor, and it has been lost within the chaos of the medical-industrial-insurance complex.

We've talked a lot about upstream versus downstream and causality. Let's apply those ideas here. What *is* profit for the corporations and experts so deeply embedded in the profit motive of the medical-industrial-insurance complex? What do they get from it, *really*? Beyond the American dream of capitalism and support for innovation, why is it so irresistible? What's upstream of the profit that disconnects all of us from what matters most?

It's what we've been talking about—how the core trauma of disconnection has landed in all of us. Profit is success. Success is worthiness. Worthiness, like belonging, is essential to our survival. We need it to feel safe. Profit bolstering a sense of worthiness in a human individual or collective is a classic signature of trauma. *Why would anyone look to profit so robustly at the considerable expense and suffering of others if they felt worthy? Why would anyone participate in such a system, allowing their helplessness to supersede their impulses to change it, if they felt worthy?*

What might happen if society and the powers-that-be gave up the tremendous profits of medicine, particularly those in tech, pharmaceuticals, and insurance, to better serve individual and collective needs and advance medicine to a higher level of sophistication and relevance to peoples' real needs?

Well, the whole system would fall apart. But beyond that?

The yardstick of success and worthiness measured by enormous profits for the rich, the classic signature of the American dream, would be lost. *Our* yardstick of success and worthiness measured by what we believe will fix us would be lost. Without huge profits, the drugs, tech, and advanced-medicine-at-our-fingertips could no longer sustain itself. It would have to change. We'd lose the safety in what we've always known. But while there'd be growing pains, I believe we'd discover and come to appreciate how enormous profits

---

22 Justin Jagosh et al. The importance of physician listening from the patients' perspective: Enhancing diagnosis, healing, and the doctor-patient relationship. Patient Education and Counseling. 2011.

have no place in the care of human beings. We'd see how we've been barking up the wrong tree all along.

It feels overwhelming, doesn't it? How do we even begin to change such an entrenched social-cultural construct that keeps us sick, suffering, and stuck?

Like everything else. First, we breathe. We create space for something new to emerge. Then, we soften our stories, soften our minds. And into that space, that softness, we ask: what's my next step?

PAUSE AND BREATHE.

Just breathe.

Sigh it out. Shake it off. Allow yourself to soften.

WHAT ELSE LOCKS IN THE STORY: PATRIARCHY AND THE TRAUMATIZED BRAIN.

Aside from power politics, profit motives, and our own cognitive biases, what else locks in the mind-body divide story, and lots of stories, keeping them so entrenched in our culture-bodies-minds?

- A male-dominated culture and the logical, rational, linear thinking style.
- Our traumatized brains.

How patriarchy locks in the mind-body divide cultural narrative.

The scientific revolution came about during a time of intense patriarchy. Men dominated all branches of the sciences and mathematics, as well as government, religion, and all the most powerful social institutions. Women were scarcely allowed a voice inside their homes, much less in the greater world.

While men and women are heterogenous groups that can defy generalizations, gender-specific differences in thinking style have been observed. As we increasingly understand the influence of epigenetics, neuroplasticity, gender roles, and social-cultural factors on thinking style, these differences are less certain today, and it is likely that thinking styles are more complex, fluid, and gender-neutral than it was once assumed. That said, men, the dominant force of the scientific revolution up until recently, were associated with a preponderance of logical, rational, linear, and analytical thinking styles. Women, as a group, tended more toward holistic, creative, intuitive, and integrative thinking styles.

This is important because male dominance of influential societal institutions allowed the male thinking style to determine how discovery and analysis of discovery were approached. Crucially, the male thinking style determined what constituted *valid knowledge.*

Therefore, the male thinking style engendered the mind-body divide, the scientific method, reductionism, and the biomedical model of disease. Further, it wields its powerful influence to actively dismiss new ways of thinking that challenge its status quo. Again, this has led to many important advancements in how we understand ourselves.

But it also keeps the narratives locked in.

As such, the story of medicine doesn't evolve or lead to new questions the way it was meant to. It's become a victim of its own logic, rationality, and linearity. While these are important attributes of focused observation, this way of thinking is inherently limited. Without creative imagination about what's not seen, intuitive inspiration for new ideas, and a holistic view of how parts fit a much more complex whole, the story stays stuck. It can't grow. It no longer serves our increasingly complex needs. This failure to evolve from the logical, rational, linear, locked in thinking style in our culture keeps us disconnected from ourselves, as well as sick and stuck within a pandemic of human suffering and chronic illness. We need the creative imagination and intuitive wisdom of the female thinking style to help us find our way back to wholeness and healing.

How the traumatized brain locks in an unsustainable narrative.

How is it possible not to feel traumatized when we've been sick, suffering, and failed by a healthcare system we've trusted our entire lives?

We're traumatized as hell, but we tend to say, "I'm a failure," "I don't fit in," "there's nothing they can do for me," "I'm broken."

When we "slip through the cracks," our brains understand that as we're not safe.

What does a traumatized brain do to restore safety?

Think of what we do when we're scared.

We try to keep things quiet, simple, and small as possible. We want things to stay the same. We hide from anything too complex, new, or uncertain. Often, we bluster, become dogmatic, and judge the hell out of anyone who doesn't agree with us or support us exactly the way we need them to.

What happens when we have an entire society of scared people with traumatized brains?

You got it.

We polarize. Because we're right and they're wrong. And we either give all our power away to the "experts" who we ask to fix us, or we seize power for ourselves to bully and disempower others.

Sound familiar?

It should.

We've all been witnesses—and participants to some extent if we're honest—to a traumatized society on a grand scale this past decade, in our response to the SARS-CoV-2 pandemic.

The traumatized brain *loves* the male thinking style of logic, rationality, linearity, and analysis. During the SARS-CoV-2 pandemic, many of our traumatized brains loved how our medical experts called out the crisis, sounded the alarm, locked us all down, and feverishly worked on strategies, drugs, and vaccines to save us from our common "enemy."

Alternatively, some of us glommed onto voices calling out our healthcare system with cries about "conspiracies," "big Pharma," "snake oil."

Many of us felt well protected even as we handed our power away to the "experts" we believed understood us, understood the problem in its totality. We trusted that their specialized knowledge and wisdom would help them figure out how to keep us safe.

Only they didn't.

They failed us long before SARS-CoV-2 emerged when they didn't make it clear how vulnerable we all were because of the global pandemic of *preventable* chronic illness that came long before SARS-CoV-2. But we didn't know it. We were sitting ducks. We were shocked when catastrophe hit.

They failed to grasp the larger picture of what the SARS-CoV-2 pandemic was all about—a collision between a savvy virus and a *highly vulnerable population of people*—and therefore failed *us* with overly simplistic and largely ineffective strategies that focused solely on the virus while ignoring how the problem is about our relationship *to* the virus.[23]

This is not to say the initial crisis response was all wrong. Given that we didn't know the full scope of the problem, much of it was right. The emergency strategies saved a lot of lives and reduced a lot of suffering. But the crisis phase of COVID-19 kicked our butts, didn't it? The global economic burden alone was estimated to be between $77 billion and $2.7 trillion in 2019.[24] Most of us lost something huge—people, businesses, opportunities. So depleted and so laser-focused on the downstream catastrophe, we never circled back to use a wider lens, to see the bird's eye view of the problem as far upstream as possible. To this day, we've not evolved from crisis management to creating upstream sustainable solutions to the core-level problems that made us, as a global population and individuals, so vulnerable to the SARS-CoV-2 virus.

From the very beginning of the pandemic, we were shown our vulnerability. We saw how many of us were more susceptible hosts to a savvy virus by virtue of that vulnerability. That the multitude of common chronic problems that affect so many of us worldwide—heart disease, diabetes, hypertension, obesity, smoking, lung disease, cancers, and others—also made us sicker and more likely to die from the effects of SARS-CoV-2 infection due to how these illnesses weaken our immunity. But did knowing that help us shift our perspective upstream to how those vulnerability factors placed us more at risk? Could we *hear* a message that would ask our traumatized, risk averse brains, needing to keep things certain and the same to focus upstream? To imagine personal, community, and worldwide strategies that could address

---

[23] RE Jordan. COVID-19: risk factors for severe disease and death. BMJ. 2020.

[24] Ahmad Faramarzi et al. The global economic burden of COVID-19 disease: a comprehensive systematic review and meta-analysis. Syst Rev. 2024.

the immunologic vulnerability of chronic illness and create more meaningful safety than strategies that focus solely downstream?

Why isn't it obvious to all of us that the most sustainable solution to our biggest problems revealed by the pandemic was to focus upstream and help the world solve the root problems?

It's not just the experts we ask to fix us that are culpable, though, is it? We're all part of the problem. We're all trying to stay safe. It all goes back to what we said before. We're disconnected from ourselves and planet Earth. This disconnection has left us with an unprecedented global crisis of chronic illness and planetary destruction. It's left us scared and disempowered and clinging to old stories that no longer serve.

But the good news is here as well. We're here together right this moment looking upstream. We can breathe into that.

PAUSE AND BREATHE.

Calling back our power.

How do these words make you feel?

"You can direct your own healing."

If you're like me, it feels exciting, but daunting. *Who the hell am I to heal myself?*

Right question. But the wrong connotation.

Who the hell am I is the cry of a traumatized person, isn't it?

It says, "I'm giving myself way more credit for knowledge, wisdom, and power than I have the right to, than I've been taught to, or perhaps have given away to experts I now ask to fix me."

But it *is* mine. Yours. Ours. We *can* direct our healing. And we *must.*

Karyn Shanks MD

This is another part of accepting our assignment to heal that needs to be addressed.

To heal, we must call our power back.

The power we were born with, our legacy from the Earth, but that we're taught not to recognize or trust. It's there all the same. We're now called to name it, claim it, and place it into action.

We'll remember to be gentle, won't we? We're scared. We were taught to fear our own gorgeous power. We're restoring safety here too.

Let's take a comfy seat, hold our beautiful hearts, and use our powerful words.

My Dear Precious One,

Yes, YOU.

I see you. I see how magnificent you are. Your beauty. Your purpose. Your power.

Even though you may suffer. Even though you may feel forgotten, lost, and hopeless. Even though they may not be able to fix you.

I see you.

And even though you may not believe me right now, I see you nonetheless. I know you. I believe in you. I hold you, as I hold myself, with the most tenderness and compassion I have.

As we learn to hold ourselves with tenderness and compassion, we begin to trust ourselves.

As we begin to trust ourselves, we trust our power. It's there. It's our true essence. It's our legacy from the beautiful Mother Earth we became disconnected from, that they turned us away from.

In trusting our power, we call back all our essential connections—to ourselves, to one another, to the Earth, herself. In all this, as we see ourselves, we belong.

Karyn Shanks MD

CHAPTER SIX
What's the difference between fixing and healing?

What are our bodies, our feelings, *our planet* asking for in our pain, suffering, and feeling stuck?

To remember who we are.

To blast through the false narratives, frustration, and exhaustion to remember who the heck we are. Gorgeous beings of wisdom, wholeness, and self-healing, even if we are hovering around an unsustainable equilibrium of suffering.

Where do we begin?

First things first, right?

We accept our assignment to heal.

Then, we tell our new story of healing as we upend the old one that's been holding us back.

How do we do that?

Stop asking to be fixed.

Instead, ask to be *healed.*

Broken things need to be fixed. Broken is part of an illness story that simplifies what's going on, so we fit into the disease box that western biomedicine has created to explain and help us. The aim of western biomedicine is noble. The goal is to heal. Only we can't heal that way because it looks at us all wrong.

It may keep us alive so we can *go on* to heal. By heading off the heart attack, repairing the retina, or putting the cancer into remission, we buy time. But fixing is not the same as healing.

So, what *is* healing?

Healing begins with understanding the deeper, wider context of the story of human suffering and illness.

Healing sees us within the dynamic context of our lives. It means understanding the terrain of all that makes us who we are. That's what we'll be exploring in the next section of this book, *We flow*. This terrain consists of our gene expression, life experiences, environments, lifestyle habits, mindsets and beliefs, communities and culture, ancestral legacies, and purpose.

"Heal," derived from Old English *Haelan* and Proto-Germanic *Hailjan*, both mean "to make whole."

So, *healing is wholeness*. Not fixing. Not a diagnosis. Not a disease-specific treatment protocol. But reconnecting to who we really are. The laws and exquisite beauty of the Earth we carry inside these miraculous bodies. Our intrinsic wisdom. Healing is wholeness. Wholeness is our flow. Flow, as you'll soon see, is ours to direct.

What happens when we reconnect to all this miraculousness inside us?

We belong. We feel safe.

You know this in your bones.

LAST WORDS.

What happens to us when we take these bodies—wired to belong, wired to feel safe in that belonging—into the spaces of western biomedicine? The clinics, offices, emergency rooms, and hospitals we turn to for help when we're in need, when we feel the most vulnerable? Spaces that may be filled with the most caring people on the planet but who tell us in countless implicit ways: *your body is not your mind, your mind is not your body, your body is a machine composed of parts that need to be fixed, you are this disease.*

What happens when we're *rushed* through these spaces? We don't have time to tell our own story. Our doctors don't look at us and can't listen in their hurry to document our visit in their electronic medical records systems *and* get to the lineup of other patients on their busy schedules. They no longer touch us, instead lean on the ease and medical-legal protection of diagnostic imaging. Even though we know the diagnostic and healing power of the unrushed story. Even though we know the connection and safety we experience through deep listening, eye contact, touch, and empathy. When we're shown we matter.

This is what happens: we learn we don't belong. Not to ourselves, not to our bodies, not to our stories. Not to our own truth.

What happens when we don't feel like we belong?

We don't feel safe.

When we don't feel safe in our own bodies, what happens inside us?

All that gorgeous biological wisdom designed to get us back to safety is activated. That makes us feel scared, anxious, and vigilant to restore safety.

Because safety is belonging. As one of my mentors puts it, "safety isn't the absence of danger, safety is connection."[25]

We're *traumatized* by western biomedicine. Even when it pulls us back from catastrophe so we can go on living, it traumatizes us. It traumatizes us from the moment we are born. It traumatizes us as we land in the culture of our families and communities who believe in its healing. It traumatizes us with its teachings that when we're hurt or suffering or sick, we're broken and need to be fixed. And the one to do the job is the expert outside of us. We're traumatized in how we turn away from our own wisdom and agency from the very beginning. No fault of our own. No fault of anyone. We're *all* traumatized. We're all doing our best within that trauma.

So, what do we do now?

We accept our trauma and hold our suffering with compassion. Compassion moves us toward restoring safety. We turn our attention with reverence and curiosity toward the story of who we are and who we're meant to be.

In the next section of this book, *We flow*, we see how our sacredness meets the new 21st century science of human potential and the Life School wisdom we've always had but didn't know to trust. Emboldened by this knowledge and fortified by the belonging and safety we're reestablishing within us, we take our next powerful steps to change our brains, change our stories, change our futures, and step into our incredible potential, that we may not have known we had.

With all that, we step out of the pain, suffering, and chronic illness that brought us here in the first place. We reclaim who we truly are—whole, innately wise embodiments of the Earth. Her laws, her genius, her beauty. Yes, we can finally breathe. *This* is who we are.

---

[25] See Stephen Porges. Our Polyvagal world: How safety and trauma change us. 2023.

SECTION TWO
We flow.

Remember how we flow?
Rhythms and waves carrying the life force energy of our sacred Earth within
us. Rendering us sacred.
This flow is her law. We carry this wisdom in us whether we acknowledge it or
not. We are sacred whether we acknowledge it or not.

CHAPTER SEVEN
Flow is in us.

What would it feel like to see ourselves—no matter how sick, suffering, or stuck we feel—as intelligent, sacred, gorgeous beings of wisdom always guiding us toward our wholeness?

Not "broken" when we feel sick.

Not "defective" when we are suffering.

Not "unworthy" when we are stuck.

We'd recognize how broken, defective, and unworthy the stories we were taught are. They are not *our* stories. Not about us at all.

Because now we know. "Broken," "defective," and "unworthy" aren't true. They're *never* true. These words are not who we are. They're someone else's stories that disconnect and disempower us.

Without these stories getting in our way, we'd flow, wouldn't we?

WHY "FLOW?"

Flow is how it feels when we ...well, *flow*.

Flow is a visceral experience of the energy currents that run through us, our *lifeforce*. Flow is at the core of what we want, regardless of how we ask for it. We want to be in our groove, to be ourselves, to feel like the person we were meant to be. We want to flow like a river. We want spontaneous vitality that moves us forward fluidly, without having to swim through mud all the time. Like the many kinds of rivers, we want many kinds of flow—sometimes we'd like to slowly meander under the great blue sky, while other times we'd like to surge foreword with unstoppable power. But always flowing, always forward progress with robustness and ease, always trusting ourselves, trusting our flow.

Flow is an attribute of all nature. It describes the continuous and harmonious movement of a natural system through space and over time. We can see this flow in the movement of water, the wind in the trees, and the change of seasons.

Humans flow exactly like the rest of nature. We *feel* our flow. We experience it. In this sense, it's subjective. We can perceive our flow however we want. We can acknowledge what makes us feel like we're flowing (*I really feel like myself when I'm playing music.*). We can inhabit our flow (*I'm totally in my groove.*). And we can direct it in our own way (*I know exactly what I need to do to feel my best.*).

I flow when I'm feeling well, my energy is high, and my head is clear. When I'm getting enough sleep, eating healthy foods, moving my body a lot, spending time in nature, sitting regularly in meditation, speaking my truth, asking for what I need, and doing work aligned with my purpose. Those are my needs for flow.

I've had difficult times in my life—chronic pain, severe fatigue, a lack of direction. During these times, it's felt like there was no flow.

The same is true for my clients. Their greatest anguish when they don't feel well is losing their sense of flow. They may call it other things, like "I'm stuck," "I don't feel like myself," "I don't have energy or motivation," or "I can't do what I need and love to do." But those are their way of saying they've lost their flow.

WE'RE ALWAYS FLOWING.

Truth is, we're flowing even when it doesn't feel like we are.

We might feel like we're swimming in mud. Burdened by pain, overwhelm, lack of energy, or chronic illness, it feels like we can't access our flow.

But even glaciers flow. Mountains and continental land masses flow. We just can't see their movement through how our human lenses perceive time and space. We see mountains and land masses as permanent, when, in fact, they are constantly moving and changing in geological time.

The same is true for us. We flow even when we don't know it. Our lifeforce is still there, it's just not flowing with robustness, trust, and ease.

Karyn Shanks MD

How do we get to *optimal* flow? The flow we can feel, that we want, that moves us like a river?

Optimal flow is what athletes, artists, and musicians call "the zone." The zone must be consciously tended, we can't just rely on it to happen automatically.[26] When we carefully craft the best conditions for flow, like athletes, artists, and musicians, we can get to the zone, flowing like a river, reveling in our *lifeforce with robustness, trust, and ease.*

Achieving the zone is not accidental. But it is accessible to all of us through directed intention and practice that includes:

- An energized focus on our intentions—where our minds go, our energy flows
- Purposeful preparation—we take care of our needs.
- Daily practice for a well-developed skill set—our practice makes progress
- A deep commitment to the process—courage and compassion.

Here's what I most want you to know.

Flow is Earth's law.

We can flow without conscious awareness of the potential within us, not knowing we're at the helm of our bodies, the helm of our stories, and the helm of our healing. There's still healing. We're still whole. It's all still dynamic and miraculous, our very best equilibrium at that time, with those circumstances. But that equilibrium may still be pain, suffering, and illness. Our flow without conscious awareness and direction will not be all we're capable of.

But knowing we're at the helm of our bodies, our stories, and our healing, and crafting the conditions for optimal flow—getting in the zone—is a whole other level of transformation, healing, and stepping into our potential.

By consciously activating the potential within us, we step into the zone, optimal flow, our lifeforce with robustness, trust, and ease.

This section of the book is all about how to achieve optimal flow.

---

[26] Stephen Kotler. The Rise of Superman: Decoding the Science of Ultimate Human Performance. 2014.

REDISCOVERING YOUR FLOW.

How do we craft our lives for optimal flow so we can settle into our exquisite wholeness? To activate our lifeforce with robustness, trust, and ease? To heal our pain, suffering, and illness once and for all?

What are the elements that lead to flow and how do we access and activate them in our everyday lives?

How do we transform the swimming-in-mud flow we're in now to flow that is totally kick-ass? That blasts open our potential to heal, to be all we can be?

First things first. Let's look to twenty-first century science—the science of possibilities—to help us reclaim our flow.

CHAPTER EIGHT
The 21ˢᵗ century science of Directable Human Potential.

T he scientific basis of this book's premise—that there is a wise healer within us who embodies Earth's laws, who can reimagine their stories to change their life circumstances, direct their outcomes, and embody their full human potential—is rooted in what I call the *21ˢᵗ century science of Directable Human Potential.*

This science consists of a large, well-established, extensively vetted body of work that includes:

- Epigenetics.
- Neuroplasticity.
- Core functional systems biology.
- Transformational psychology.

Taken together, this body of science has ushered us into an era in which we are no longer stuck in simplistic, unchanging notions of who and what we are as humans. Everything we ever thought was true about what we could expect of our life's outcomes has been called into question. We are not fixed. Not our bodies, not our minds, not our spirits, not the vast potential within us. We are marvelously complex, continuously adapting to life's circumstances, completely available to reinvent ourselves as we wish. Our equilibrium of healing, flow, and where we want to be is largely in our hands.

Now, is this science better than the old science on which we built our entire system of medicine? Is it better than the science that shaped our understanding of who we are, and what happens to us when we're sick, and how we heal?

Yes. But it's not either-or. The new science is *evolved* science. To borrow Sir Isaac Newton's famous phrase, it 'stands on the shoulders of giants' of the old science, but it has uncovered more. It has discovered, measured, and accounted for human dynamic complexity and deep intelligence down to the genetic level that allows us to redefine what healing really means.

This science supports what our bodies have known all along and that urges us to reclaim the Earth's transformative laws operating inside us. These are the engines of our *innate ability* to achieve resilience and shift from an equilibrium of suffering and illness to an equilibrium of healing. Nothing is permanent. Anything is possible.

And the best news of all? This science is not complete. It continues to evolve. Our new paradigm of human potential and possibilities can only expand and become more relevant to us as it grows.

EPIGENETICS.

Epigenetics is the science that says our genetic expression is not set in stone. We are not our parents or grandparents. We are not sitting ducks just waiting for our genetic legacy to kick us down. Our destiny is fluid and responsive to what we do to *curate it* rather than simply accept it.[27]

This is key: we can actively shift our genetic expression to change our outcomes. All of them. To move us to a better dynamic equilibrium. To achieve the potential and possibilities we may never have dared to dream of. We were *born* to heal. Epigenetics links our terrain of healing (coming up shortly!) to all our life's outcomes—our equilibrium, our flow, our gorgeous potential.

NEUROPLASTICITY.

Neuroplasticity is how epigenetic processes are expressed in our brains. This transformative energy allows our brains and all their connections to

---

[27] Deepak Chopra MD and Rudolph Tanzi PhD. Super Genes: Unlock the Astonishing Power of Your DNA for Optimal Health and Well-Being. 2015.

learn, grow, and heal. To change in form and function. To continuously regenerate, expand in complexity, and evolve in sophistication. This process can easily be seen as our children develop, but it is also unfolding in all of us as adults.

The brain can heal itself.[28] And as we learn to direct this neuroplastic potential, we learn and grow, accessing our potential and possibilities.

The keys to accessing our neuroplastic potential are practices we'll be exploring deeply. First, through meeting challenge with curiosity—the challenges life brings us and the challenges we choose. Second, through support of our brains' needs by tending our terrain of healing. Without challenge and nourishment, our brains are just as likely to shift us backwards, to atrophy, devolve, and degenerate.

The ability to respond to challenge is another way to describe learning. The key to deep learning in adults is not just challenge. It's knowing *what* to learn (What part of my life needs my attention right now?), *when* we need to learn it (Is this the right time to take this new challenge on, do I have the time, patience, and support to do it?), and exercising the commitment to put that new knowledge into immediate practice. Consistent practice deepens learning by activating neuroplasticity and laying down new neuropathways in the brain.

CORE FUNCTIONAL SYSTEMS BIOLOGY.

We are integrated, multidirectional, complex, dynamic biological systems that constantly seek their best equilibrium. This is Earth's law and the biological imperative of being human. These biological systems are the engines of our health, resilience, and transformational energy.[29]

This is us. Not machines, not fixed, not simple, not identical to everyone else, not stuck. Unbroken.

---

[28] Norman Doidge MD. The Brain's Way of Healing: Remarkable Discoveries and Recoveries from the Frontiers of Neuroplasticity. 2015.

[29] Leonard A Wisneski. The Scientific Basis of Integrative Medicine, 2nd edition. 2009.

Institute for Functional Medicine. What is Functional Medicine? IFM.org.

One of our core biological systems is how we make the energy to drive everything about us. This includes the *Brain-Thyroid-Adrenal-Mitochondrial energy operating system (BTAM)*—the biology of energy; and *the Autonomic Nervous System (ANS)*—the biology of safety. We'll be exploring both systems.

Beyond energy, our systems biology includes the chemistry and infrastructure to run all the business of the human body:

- Detoxification and biotransformation.
- Digestion, absorption, and assimilation of nutrients.
- Immunity, defense, repair, and inflammation.
- Communication, transportation, circulation.
- Movement: skeleton, muscles, joints, and connective tissue.
- Our microbiome.
- Our brain and nervous system.

TRANSFORMATIONAL PSYCHOLOGY.

Transformational psychology is the practical science of how we use our powerful minds to harness the energy of neuroplasticity, shifting our closely held stories and beliefs into greater alignment with who we are and who we want to be. It includes how we personally direct our terrain of healing to harness the energy of epigenetics, to support our bodies and minds, to shift them into more robust equilibria. It understands our bodies and minds are not separate. Transformational psychology views human experience through the embodied lens. We must support both to support the whole.

Transformational psychology understands trauma as an embodied process. It explores the wisdom of trauma to reestablish safety and create resilience.

Karyn Shanks MD

CHAPTER NINE
The dynamic healing principles of the human body.

The twenty-first century science of directable human potential satisfies our savvy, show-me intellects that need to feel justified. It closes the circle of wisdom with science. Now, we'll explore how this science of possibilities shows up as the dynamic healing principles within us, that we'll use to shift out of suffering, into the vast potential within us, living our flow.

So, how do we create our most kick-ass flow? Our lifeforce with robustness, trust, and ease?

We must look way, way upstream for this. We have to reach where three primary laws of planet Earth flow into our own veins, creating the dynamic healing principles of the human body. They are:

- The primary urge of your body is to heal.
- Your body is innately wise.
- Resilience (energy + strength + adaptability) is your birthright.

These laws are *our* laws. And as you'll see, they upend the powerful cultural stories that have kept us sick, suffering, and stuck.

FIRST LAW: THE PRIMARY URGE OF YOUR BODY IS TO HEAL.

Your body will always reach its best possible equilibrium given present circumstances. Chronic illness and suffering are equilibria; robust health and wellness are equilibria. The healing potential is always there. Your outcomes depend on the available resources to support that healing.

You absolutely know this law of the Earth. You see it and experience it every day, you just didn't know it applied to you.

We introduced this law in the first section of this book, describing how we see it in nature and how she recovers from the worst possible catastrophes without any intervention whatsoever. How she miraculously emerges into new landscapes in ways we never expected. How was that healing even possible?

Though it seems like one, that kind of transformation is not a miracle. It's what the Earth is designed to do. Nature heals no matter what. She always rises to her very best equilibrium. What equilibrium she can achieve depends on the available resources—nutrients, sunlight, biodiversity.

What's an "equilibrium?"

In nature, an equilibrium is the point of balance that stabilizes a system (an ecosystem, an organism) at its optimal state given all the forces acting upon it. These "forces" are the available energy and resources balanced with the needs of the system. When the needs of the system are greater than the energy and resources available to meet those needs, the system must downshift its equilibrium. The available energy and resources will be shunted to the highest priority areas needed for survival. Not all the needs of the system will be met. It will be less resilient. And the ecosystem or organism will not thrive in all the ways it could. An ecosystem may lose biodiversity. An individual may fail to grow or reproduce. It may not survive.

When the needs of the ecosystem or organism are fully met by the available energy and resources, it will thrive, reaching or exceeding its expected potential. The ecosystem will be able to expand biodiversity, creating additional resources for all. Individuals will grow and reproduce and thrive.

Accordingly, human healing is an equilibrium. It's the very best version of ourselves we get given present circumstances, the energy and resources available to support our needs. That's why we say healing is a "primary urge" of nature. We always reach the best possible position we're capable of. It's never just halfway. It may not be the cure we're looking for—our best equilibrium may still be suffering, pain, and chronic illness—but it's the best we can possibly be given our present circumstances. Nature never shortchanges us.

Karyn Shanks MD

The lesson of this law is this: to shift into a better equilibrium, change your circumstances. To rise out of pain, suffering, and chronic illness, change your circumstances. Give yourself the experiences you need. Nourish your body with healing resources. The circumstances, experiences, and resources we can control, that make us who we are, are what I call "the terrain of healing." We'll unpack the terrain shortly, then use it as our roadmap as we practice our *Unbroken* core resilience steppingstones.[30]

SECOND LAW: YOUR BODY IS INNATELY WISE.

Pain, suffering, fatigue, all the symptoms of illness, and all your sensations, feelings, and energy states are the language of your body telling you what it needs to shift into a better equilibrium. Your body isn't the problem, the conditions that favor an equilibrium of suffering are the problem. Your body is *never* wrong.

This law links to the first. In our suffering, pain, and chronic illness, our bodies are responding to their circumstances with the highest wisdom. That wisdom is expressed through the body's nuanced and highly sophisticated language: the language of sensations, feelings, and energy states. This law is how your body *expresses* the equilibrium it's in and the needs it has. All the symptoms and sensations of illness and loss of function, rather than being "what's wrong with us," are the wisdom of our bodies, the nuanced language guiding us toward discovery of our needs for healing, for upshifting our equilibrium.

This is a mind-bending concept because we're so used to blaming our bodies. How do we shift our understanding of our suffering, to know it as language and wisdom, rather than an account of the ways in which we're broken? We keep touching on how we're storytelling creatures. As such, our words are important. They're miniature stories that invoke a whole lot of meaning based on what we've been taught before. So, we must use our words so carefully.

What words do you use to describe how you suffer? See if you can name a few right now.

---

[30] See page with graphic.

Do any of those words or phrases blame you or blame your body?

These are words *I've* used in the past: "Oh, shit, there's that terrible pain coming to get me again!" Or "Ugh, my headache is back again!" Or "Oh, God, what's wrong with me?"

What happens if you choose different words to describe your suffering that also link you to your possibilities?

Like "Hmm, there's that pain again, let me look at it with curiosity." Or "It feels a bit sharp, warm, achy, and tingly; I wonder what that means?" Or "I feel tightness and constriction here, let me hold it." Or "I feel stuck but I'm curious what might happen if I tell someone and ask for help."

The old stories that blame us or our bodies for our suffering or that tell a bleak story help perpetuate our vulnerability and helplessness. They make us feel less safe. They ignore the inherent wisdom in our bodies' sensations, feelings, and energy states to guide us toward what we need to heal.

Honoring our bodies' wisdom means changing our stories about them. We can begin to shift our stories by changing the words we use. By changing our words, we shift our relationship to our inner experiences. We can use our words to create safety and to show us what's possible. Using words with conscious awareness keeps our old stories out of the picture. We focus on our bodies' language of sensations, energy, and feelings directly, without distortion through blame or catastrophizing. We're guided toward what we truly need.

Of course, choosing words with conscious intention is a challenge when we're suffering, isn't it?

Let's practice briefly right now.

Name your problem or pain. Breathe without trying to change or fix it. Tune into how it feels in your body—how does it show up as sensations, feelings, or energy? Acknowledge what you experience as the wisdom of your body.

Can you hold it without judgement? Without catastrophizing? Without telling a story about it? Continuing to breathe, can you welcome it with curiosity?

See if you can take it one step further. Ask: what do you need? Breathe and let your question go.

See what you just did?

You treated your body with respect, *yourself* with respect. Not wrong, but wise.

Karyn Shanks MD

THIRD LAW: RESILIENCE IS YOUR BIRTHRIGHT.

Resilience is the equilibrium that supports us through life's changes and challenges without losing robustness. Resilience, in fact, *requires* change and challenge. It's our circle of life: we create it, and it creates us.

Resilience is the energy of healing. It's not about fixes or doing the "right" things. Resilience leads to healing and healing is wholeness, but the disease paradigm confuses us. We've been taught to polarize our experiences—broken versus fixed, sick versus well, diseased versus not diseased, stressed versus relaxed, and so on.

But none of these represent who we truly are, dynamic beings of experience, not either/or states of existence. We're constantly flowing along a vast continuum—an equilibrium—of experience, thought, emotion, energy, and biology.

We never land. We flow.

How do we flow optimally? How do we reach our zone, our best equilibrium? Our lifeforce with robustness, trust, and ease?

Through resilience.

The third law of our humanness is about our potential for resilience. In nature, resilience is the adaptability in any system to adjust to the forces acting upon it without losing function, without injury. Organisms that are resilient have achieved an equilibrium of robustness. There is enough physiological, emotional, and psychological reserve that challenging circumstances are not diminishing. A resilient species can survive drought or a loss of habitat. A resilient individual can pivot when their home is destroyed, or their food supply is interrupted. They rebuild or migrate. In the face of such challenges, resilient organisms do more than survive, they thrive.

The same is true for humans.

As we discussed in the first section of this book, all biological systems prioritize survival and safety over all else, including us. When we adapt to a persistent survival equilibrium, we may sacrifice higher levels of function to remain in safety. Resilience is a level of adaptation that allows for robustness *and safety*. There's ample energy and resources to manage the challenge, remain in safety, *and* maintain an equilibrium of robustness. Just like the tree that grows strong roots *and* a wide trunk, big branches, copious leaves, and seeds to create the next generation.

As humans, we can expand on this definition of resilience. Resilience is our adaptive potential to successfully manage all life's changes and challenges, the "forces" acting upon us, without sacrificing robustness. This adaptability requires the availability of all resources to meet our structure-function-energy needs. But human resilience requires something more: *courage and curiosity*.

Courage helps us step up to our challenges, despite the risks. While some of us are risk adverse, tending to avoid challenge and view it as something that's bad, others are less afraid and more likely to view life stress as positive. Studies show how those who understand life stress as necessary and meaningful enjoy healthier, happier, and longer lives than those who view stress as negative.[31] A positive mindset about challenge leads to positive behaviors that shift stresses from lonely, diminishing experiences to those that are supported and lead to learning, practice, and confidence.

Curiosity allows us to actively explore, helping us learn and grow. Curiosity is an attribute of the courageous. It's also one we can learn and will be practicing a lot through the remainder of this book.

Beyond adaptability, resources, energy, courage, and curiosity, there's something else we must have to create a deep well of resilience: *challenge, itself.*

In the human body, adaptative growth and healing in response to challenge is called "hormesis."[32] This physiological adaptation occurs at the level of genetic expression, leading to greater robustness as our bodies grapple with difficult circumstances.

Hormesis is thought to have helped organisms adapt to harsh environments in earlier times of life on Earth. Our remote ancestors faced great uncertainty and navigated complex environments to stay alive. They worked hard and endured many threats to their survival. The same challenges that lead to improved function in our ancestors, are health-promoting for us. Such as:

- Varied movement under heavy loads.
- A wide variety of postures.
- Near-constant movement throughout the day.

---

[31] Alia J Crum, et al. Improving Stress without Reducing Stress: The Benefits of Stress is Enhancing Mindset in Both Challenging and Threatening Contexts. 2014.

[32] Mark P Mattson. Hormesis Defined. Ageing Res Rev. 2008.

- Curious and actively investigative minds.
- A highly varied diet of real food.
- An untamed, continuously changing, often harsh, living environment.
- Living according to the solar cycles of light and dark.

Many of these challenges can be encouraged through choices made in our daily lives. Some more advanced challenges that lead to positive genetic and physiological adaptations in humans are periods of fasting, small doses of environmental toxins and radiation, extremes of temperature, and oxygen deprivation.[33]

But how do we start to make ourselves more resilient in ways that are accessible to us in our daily lives?

You're creating resilience right now, though you may not realize it. If any of what you're reading is new to you, challenges you, or excites you, you're shifting your genetic expression toward robustness.

What's the hardest thing in your life right now?

Name it. Notice what happens to your body. What are the sensations, feelings, or shifts in your energy? Breathe without trying to change or fix anything.

Ask: what do you need? Breathe. Let the question go.

You may feel anything but resilient right now. But let's revisit the "ingredients" for resilience once more:

- Energy.
- Strength.
- Adaptability.
- Resources.
- Courage.
- Curiosity.
- Challenge.

In the early pages of this book, I recommended exploring our practices with a beginner's mind. *That's* curiosity. That's the positive mindset in the face of

---

[33] Suresh IS Rattan and Marios Kyriazi, editors. The Science of Hormesis in Health and Longevity. 2018.

life stress that challenges you, that leads to resilience. And courage? You're here, aren't you?

What else do you need?

Name one thing from that list. Just one. One you can manage right now. What is it? What's your next step? Breathe into the question for now without expecting an answer. Sometimes the questions are the bravest thing.

Let me leave you with this: the key to resilience is knowing you're built for it and are fully capable of it. Whatever you lack, you can learn. And the harder your life, the more potential for resilience you have. You were created to adapt to your hard, varied life on this planet. So, this is what we're going to do— reconnect to the creative wisdom within us and reclaim our place at the helm of our bodies, the helm of our emotions, the helm of our minds.

Together, we'll accept our life's challenges, *inviting* them into our lives, knowing they're not just inevitable but necessary to become robust beings of incredible potential.

How we grapple with challenge is the crucible from which resilience emerges—a personal healing terrain dialed in to support our needs for energy, strength, and adaptability.

CHAPTER TEN
Our personal healing terrain.

O ur personal healing terrain is all that makes us *us*. It is composed of all the internal and external influences and experiences that create and shift our biology, our bodies, and our selves. By getting to know our terrain and how to work it to our advantage, we shift ourselves into an equilibrium of resilience to rise out of pain, suffering, and illness, and to expand into our potential and possibilities.

Let's see if we can make this easy. We've established that mind, body, spirit, and planet are not separate. They're intimately interconnected. They are all one, really, we just don't have the language for it, so it's hard to say and hard to conceptualize. So, let's make up a new word to represent the whole of us—body, mind, thoughts, stories, emotions, gut feelings, spirit, soul, energy, and all our interconnectedness within ourselves and with others, our communities, our planet, and our Universe. One big fat all-inclusive word.

How about TotalGloriousOneness? TGO for short. Or go ahead and create your own word. I want us to become stakeholders in claiming the totality of who we are in our lives and in this world. To really carry the truth of it in our bodies, that everything is connected and everything we do affects everything.

So then, what's the terrain of our healing?

Can you guess?

Yes. *Everything.*

It's everything that has an influence, positive or negative, on our state of being. Our health. Our happiness. Our growth. Our energy. Our flow. Our potential as humans. Our ability to change the trajectory of our lives. Our TGO.

But we don't have to discuss *everything* in this book. And you don't have to consider *everything* to heal. We can break this down into the simplest elements of our everyday experience and draw everything we need to know from that to jumpstart, sustain, or upshift our healing.

Here's how I've come to think about the terrain of our healing from the science of human potential and the wisdom and experience of countless keen observers of our human lives (including myself, my many savvy clients, and so many of you!). Our personal terrain of healing is the dynamic relationship between our:

- Gene expression.
- Environments.
- Life experiences.
- Lifestyle habits.
- Mindsets and beliefs.
- Communities and culture.
- Ancestral legacies.
- Purpose.

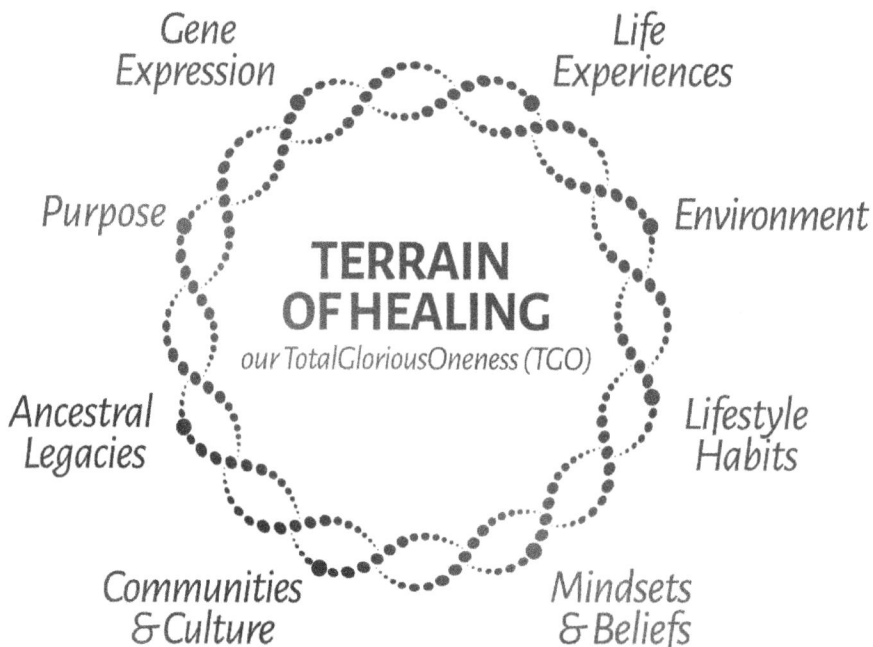

Gene Expression   Life Experiences

Purpose   Environment

TERRAIN OF HEALING

our TotalGloriousOneness (TGO)

Ancestral Legacies   Lifestyle Habits

Communities & Culture   Mindsets & Beliefs

Karyn Shanks MD

Each aspect of this terrain shapes us. And each aspect is identifiable and under our control. We have the capacity to heal, to shift our equilibrium, and move more deeply into our potential as humans by working with each of the components of our terrain.

Notice how the terrain elements are interconnected. They overlap and are multi-directional, interweaving biology with perception and personal meaning. The terrain is messy, but so are we. Considering the terrain elements this way will make sense as we head into our *Unbroken* core resilience steppingstones—the practices that activate our terrain—in the next section.

Notice how some of these terrain components support and elevate us, while others hold us back.

How will we know which aspects of the terrain to work on?

Our bodies will always make it clear to us in their exquisite, nuanced language through sensations, energy states, and feelings, where to direct our attention.

Let's take a closer look.

GENE EXPRESSION.

Oh my gosh, this sounds scary. How science-y do we need to get about genes and gene expression to heal ourselves?

Truthfully? Not very. We can leave most of the details for the science geeks. But we do need to understand a few basic concepts to take more meaningful control over how we make our genes work for us. We're not sitting ducks to "bad genes" after all.

First, we must unlearn a big idea that arose over half a century ago when genes were first discovered: the gene hypothesis. Despite being a hypothesis, which is supposed to grow rather than get stuck, it rapidly became a narrative so powerful it still has a stranglehold on how we think about ourselves, even as it has been thoroughly upended by current science. It's such a sticky and powerful narrative, it continues to be a cornerstone of mainstream western biomedicine and how it is practiced. (Remember when we talked about the medical-industrial-insurance complex? That's why. The gene hypothesis is highly profitable.)

Genes are the functional units of our heredity composed of strands of DNA and support proteins called histones. Some genes serve as sets of instructions used by our cells to manufacture proteins involved in all aspects of our bodies' structure and function, while other genes are involved in controlling the protein-coding genes. Genes are packaged into twenty-three paired structures called chromosomes mostly found in the nuclei of our cells, though some are found within mitochondria, the energy-producing parts of our cells.

With the discovery of chromosomes in the mid-twentieth century, the gene hypothesis was born. It said we *are* our genes. The narrative rapidly took medicine by storm: our book of life—all structure and function and risk for disease—was thought to be predetermined and fixed at birth, contained within these genes. Since we inherit our genes from both our parents, their genes establish the probability of what will happen to us. The only thing to do was to sit back and wait for our book of life, our genetic destiny, to come true—and when things go wrong, ask the "experts" to fix us.

Then came the human genome project, launched in 1990, with the goal to map all the genes of the human genome. Some believed that this information would establish the ultimate cure for all diseases, which were still thought to be immutable manifestations of the genetic familial legacy contained within our genes.

The genome project found over twenty-two thousand protein-coding sequences in humans. Our genome is largely the same as those of all other mammals and ninety-three percent the same as all living organisms on the planet, including the tiniest invertebrate microorganisms! More importantly, ninety-nine percent of the DNA discovered in humans were sequences that did not code for proteins the way scientists believed they would. They initially referred to this as "junk" DNA, implying that it had no value or purpose because it didn't fit what scientists were expecting.

Since these discoveries, however, more curious scientists have established that non-protein coding DNA function as *regulatory elements* for DNA expression, switching genes on and off to either activate or repress the process by which genetic information is turned into proteins. It turns out, these regulatory molecules touch every aspect of our lives. Because everything we experience—what we eat, how we sleep, all our feelings, *everything*—talks to our genes. Our terrain.

These findings helped upend the gene hypothesis and gave rise to the new science of epigenetics. Epigenetics tells us that our genetic expression is not fixed, it's fluid. Our genes shift their expression in response to everything that happens to us. The physical structure of our DNA stays the same, but the regulatory elements within the genome are continuously monitoring our terrain and shifting genetic expression responsively.

So, what does this mean for us and our healing potential?

Instead of genes determining the potential of who we are and who we can be, we are created by our environments and life experiences. Our genes don't cause most disease, dysfunction, and suffering, *our environments and life experiences do.* Our genes may contribute risk or predisposition or a certain measure of probability that we will develop certain health outcomes. But our environments and life experiences shift those inherent qualities in profound ways.

The strength of determining your outcomes varies among genes. Based on your parents' genetics, we can predict things like hair and eye color. There are also a handful of diseases that are strongly predicted by genetics, such as chromosomal abnormalities (Down's syndrome, for example) and single gene disorders (cystic fibrosis and Huntington's disease, for example). But *the vast majority of gene-related problems* are the result of interaction *between* genes and the environment.

We may not have control over the chromosomes we inherit from our parents, but we do have control over most environmental influences and life experiences that modify gene expression and, thus, open new possibilities for healing.

Here's our challenge, though. The gene hypothesis is stuck in our heads, isn't it?

I'm just like my mother. My mom and grandma both had hysterectomies, I will too. My dad had diabetes, guess I will too. Depression runs in my family. I am my disease. This is who I am.

I know this so well—it lingers in my head too. Both my father and grandfather had Parkinson's disease. They both died from its terrible effects. My dad developed an aggressive form of Lewy body dementia as part of his disease and died within a few years of the diagnosis. His final days were mostly alone in a care center during the lock-down phase of COVID-19 in 2020. It was a tragedy. I catch myself worrying about my own future and considering carefully what to do to avoid what appears to be a powerful family legacy. Fortunately, I know about epigenetics and neuroplasticity and core Functional Medicine systems biology. I know I can shift my genes and my biology into a more favorable equilibrium than my dad and grandpa.

Sound familiar? We always assume we're set up for what happened to previous generations of our families. Or, that whatever disease we've been diagnosed with is "who we are" and was always meant to be. That we have no recourse.

Now, it could go down that way, right? Our outcomes depend on what we do with our environments and life experiences—with our personal terrain of healing.

ENVIRONMENT.

Your environment, as experienced by your genes, is everything that influences them as they are tucked away in the nuclei and mitochondria of your cells. This means the genetic environment is, well, *everything*. We now know that everything is connected. Therefore, everything that happens *to* you and *around* you—everything you feel, think, sense, ingest, get close to, and do—will in some way touch your genes. Your TGO.

For our purposes as we explore the healing terrain, we'll limit "environment" to what's in our *external* environment—the external factors outside our bodies that are taken into us in some way to affect our genetic expression.

What's in your environment that your genes will be exposed to or affected by?

- Pollutants, toxins, and irritants.
- Natural phenomena like sunlight, the phases of the moon, weather patterns, and temperature.
- All the elements of Earth's biome—the microorganisms, plants, insects, and animals.
- Everything that engages with your senses—people and their energy, sounds, smells, visual stimuli, what you taste and touch.
- Everything you take into your body—food, drink, air, what touches your skin.
- Anything from your environment that invokes stress and survival responses within you.

Why do such a wide range of environmental exposures and experiences affect our genes?

They all have a biological effect on us as they interface with our bodies. This biology communicates with our genes, which shifts their expression in adaptive ways, changing your life outcomes. Now, such adaptations may not be desirable. They might lead to equilibria that will sustain you. That's why it's important for you to understand what aspects of the environment support you and what doesn't.

We'll get back to these environmental factors to explore how you can optimize yours as we dive into the nine *Unbroken* core resilience steppingstones a bit later. You'll learn what you can do right now to shift your genetic expression in a direction that supports your healing.

LIFE EXPERIENCES.

Life experiences are, of course, everything that happens to you in your life.

Just as important as how these experiences directly affect your gene expression and biology is how you *feel* about them, how they shape your understanding of yourself and the world, and how they influence your future behavior.

What we're most interested in is how these experiences change you on the inside. Rather than focus on the events themselves, we want to consider how you responded to those events. How did they make you feel? How did they influence your perceptions, beliefs, and the stories you tell about yourself, others, and the world? Did your experiences make you feel safe? Were your survival impulses activated? Did they provoke lots of stress? Or did they empower you, enliven you, and elevate you? How did they change your behavior?

Your life experiences and reactions to them have a biology. That biology consists of all kinds of molecules that bathe your genes and shift gene expression. Your interpretations about what happens inside you—your beliefs and stories—and your responses to them continue to shape your gene expression, biology, and your life outcomes. In this way, your biography becomes your biology becomes your biography and so on. It's a cascade of life experience, gene expression, biology, and life outcomes that feedback on themselves.

Let me give you an all-too-common example of the kinds of life experiences that can hold us back.

You may have heard of the Adverse Childhood Experience, or "ACE," test.[34] This is a list of ten questions designed to ascertain harmful events, such as abuse, neglect, or household dysfunction, that may have happened to you as a child. Higher scores correlate well with what most of us would expect— problematic behaviors later in life, such as addiction and relationship problems, as well as mental health challenges such as depression, anxiety, and suicide attempts. But what may come as more of a surprise to you, is that higher ACE scores also predict chronic health conditions such as diabetes, heart disease, cancer, and autoimmune conditions.

While the ACE test is far from perfect as a measure of childhood stress and trauma—it does not assess for stress outside of the household, protective factors, or differences among individuals—it provides insight into the genetic and biological effects of life experiences and how they can lead to a host of common chronic and deadly illnesses later in life.

This research on childhood stress and trauma used to scare me. When I took the ACE test many years ago, my score was worrisomely high. Shit, was I doomed to suffering, chronic illness, and an early death because of my childhood experiences? Then I learned about other research looking at the positive effects of *repairing* childhood trauma. How the repair process in childhood (*Sorry honey, mommy yelling isn't about you, it's about me*, and so on) leads to well-adjusted children. It is probably best if that repair happens in childhood before the trauma can cascade into years of dysfunctional adaptations and problematic behavior. But, in my book, repair is repair. I've done tons of therapy. I've learned to work with my body and feel my feelings. I practice self-compassion every day and hold my feelings in safety as they arise. I have worked hard to create relationships based on trust and authenticity. And I raised two incredible boys, now incredible men. Through loving them and learning from them, I have been able to give them what I did not get as a child. That, in and of itself, has been healing. And seeing how I didn't ruin them after all, I realized the cycle of trauma stopped with me.

---

[34] NPR. Take the ACE test—and learn what it does and doesn't mean. 2015.

Karyn Shanks MD

What did we just say about challenge? Even terrifying and completely disempowering challenges can become life-enriching and resilience-building when there's repair. At any stage in life.

Based on epigenetic principles, the biology and gene expression of childhood trauma is modifiable. We now know we can purposefully shift the direction of gene expression and biology. By understanding the biological and genetic harm of traumatic life experiences, we have clues about how to unwind what happened inside us because of those experiences. We have a clear direction for creating conditions for healing that we will continue to unpack.

LIFESTYLE HABITS.

You knew we'd get to these, didn't you? How we choose to live each day absolutely determines our genetic and biological life potential. One hundred percent of the time. No free passes, loves.[35]

We know more about the genetic-biological-disease risk aspects of lifestyle than any other parts of the terrain, but our lifestyle choices can be the hardest to change when we want to improve our life outcomes.

Why?

We'll explore this more as we dive into the *Unbroken* core resilience steppingstones in the next section of this book. But briefly, our lifestyle choices aren't really choices at first—not until we're looking for answers to our problems and claiming agency over our lives. If they were simple choices, without any emotional baggage tied to them, we'd make them easily, wouldn't we?

Some of lifestyle is pure habit. It's how we learned to do things. The habits suit us just fine until there's friction. We don't feel as well. We've been reading about how to prevent problems and live longer—we want that! Something inspires us to look at how we do things, and plan changes we want or need. While it may take planning and patience, when it's *simple* habit change and

---

[35] Karyn Shanks MD. Heal: A Nine-Stage Roadmap to Recover Energy, Reverse Chronic Illness, and Claim the Potential of a Vibrant New You. 2019.

there's nothing big standing in our way, we can do it. But sometimes changing lifestyle habits isn't so easy.

Lifestyle habits can represent deep traditions that tie us to our people. They are what our families and communities do. They are how we belong. These well-worn, thoroughly practiced habits help us feel connected and safe.

Lifestyle habits can bring us comfort and solace. We use many of our lifestyle choices to soothe and settle our frazzled nervous systems, to make us feel more alive, to ease our anxiety and lift our spirits.

Changing lifestyle habits can be hard. Change challenges us to learn and practice and reckon with what the old habits do for us. What they *really* do for us. We bump into our unmet needs and unhealed wounds.

As we move into our *Unbroken* core resilience steppingstones in the next section, we'll practice many lifestyle changes. We'll be doing it with tenderness and compassion, creating safety, showing reverence for what our habits, even those that no longer serve, have done for us.

For now, consider the following lifestyle habits that we know powerfully influence genetic expression, biology, disease risk, vitality, longevity, energy, and resilience:

- Diet.
- Sleep.
- Rest.
- Movement.
- Sitting.
- Stress balance.
- Play, fun, and laughter.
- Connection with others, community.
- Meditative and mindful activities.
- Time in nature.

MINDSETS AND BELIEFS.

Mindsets and beliefs are stories we tell ourselves over and over. They're what we know for sure—our minds are "set." They're how things have always been.

Mindsets and beliefs have powerful biology that can heal us in a heartbeat or shut us down.

We'll spend a lot of time looking carefully at the mindsets and beliefs that limit us, as we have with the mind-body divide and the disease paradigm.

I'm reminded of an experiment I once heard about. When fruit flies are placed in a jar without a lid, they all fly out to freedom. But when they're placed in a jar *with* a lid, after first trying to escape, banging themselves against the walls, they settle for flying within the confines of the jar with contented little looks on their faces (I'm sure). After a few days, when the lid to the jar is removed, most of the fruit flies don't even try to get out, though a few adventurous outliers hightail it right out of there.

You could argue that fruit flies don't have minds or mindsets. But somehow, they learned and adapted to the limitations of the closed jar. *They* became limited. Most of them couldn't unlearn their limitations, though a few did. Like the fruit flies, people can get stuck in their limiting beliefs about what is possible. Who do the outliers in the fruit fly story represent? Yes! You and me.

We've also all heard anecdotes of people who were told how long they had to live. Sure enough, those who believed the doctor's prophecy died in precisely that timeframe. Then there are the ornery ones, who reject their doctor's dictates, who go on to live long and vibrant lives despite a grave diagnosis.

Studies show our beliefs about how we'll fair in the face of challenging circumstances—catastrophes, high stress, trauma—determine our outcomes, rather than the circumstances themselves.[36] In other words, if we believe we'll fall apart when our lover leaves us, we'll fall apart. If we believe we'll die when our doctor tells us we're going to die, we'll likely die. But if we believe that what doesn't kill us makes us stronger, guess what? That's exactly what happens. The bad thing that happened that we trust will make us stronger leads to all kinds of good things in our biology that help make us more resilient. We're strong and adaptable. And it makes sense, doesn't it? We live like we're *living* rather than dying.

This is what we talked about before. We're built for change and challenge. The clincher is that we must believe it.

---

[36] Alia J Crum et al. Improving Stress without Reducing Stress: The Benefits of Stress is Enhancing Mindset in Both Challenging and Threatening Contexts. 2014.

COMMUNITIES AND CULTURE.

As communal-cultural beings, we're intrinsically wired for connection. Survival is not possible without it. When connection is robust and nurturing, we thrive.

Beyond belonging, the traditions of our communities and cultures shape who we are. They can keep us safe and nourish us in countless ways. But they can also hold us back.

Our families, neighborhoods, schools, churches, governments, community organizations, and cultural traditions can shelter and protect us. They can hold us in our sacred truth. They can empower us to grow and evolve into who we're meant to be. But many of the ways we're held by our people are not empowering. They don't show us the truth. They don't encourage us to become who we are.

Disparities in community resources, support, and opportunities among groups of people lead to profound and measurable differences in health and life outcomes via their effects on genetic expression. Poverty, systemic racism, exposure to violence and insecure environments, and reduced access to quality healthcare, food, education, and countless other cornerstone social resources are all linked to greater risk for chronic illness, mental health problems, addiction, homelessness, joblessness, and early mortality. The common thread for these classic signatures of cultural trauma is lack of safety, a tragic social equilibrium of disconnection that maintains a world of hurt.

Culture has a collective biology that leads to population shifts in genetic expression.[37] This leads to problematic outcomes for whole communities of people through generations. The core problem isn't with the bodies, experiences, and lives of these people, though, is it? The core problem, the problem most upstream, is with the unsustainable equilibrium of social injustice.

Communities and culture are critical aspects of our personal terrain that can be the most difficult for us to see and change. A lot of trauma lands within all of us here. Deep inside. Poisoning us with stories that keep us down or keep others' down. Not one of us is safe if someone else is not. Remember? We all belong to this sacred Earth, the great web of life. We're all one.

---

[37] Rachel Yehuda et al. Holocaust Exposure Induced Intergenerational Effects on FKBP5 Methylation. Biol Psychiatry. 2016.

Karyn Shanks MD

ANCESTRAL LEGACIES.

The ancestral part of our terrain is really a subset of communities and culture, but it deserves special recognition for the ways in which it shapes us profoundly from before we were even born.

We now know how the epigenetic expression of our ancestors' experiences becomes a part of our legacy. The deep safety and connection of a thriving village can land in our own genes through parents who welcome us and love us beyond measure. Likewise, the chaos and turmoil of a disenfranchised community of a society's outcasts can challenge us from the moment we're born.

Our earliest caretakers are given the sacred responsibility for meeting our needs as infants, children, and evolving humans. Research on early childhood development reveals how there are two primary non-negotiable childhood needs: attachment (connection) and authenticity (being who we are).

In ideal circumstances, both needs are met. When the parental figures in our lives nourish us from the moment of conception, hold us in absolute safety, assuage our hunger and thirst, touch us, look us in the eye, and reflect to us through their facial expressions our beauty, lovability, and innate magnificence for precisely who we are, we thrive.

In less-than-ideal circumstances, the need for authenticity must give way to preserve attachment. The safety of connection is sacrosanct. As small children, we can't survive without it. Connection keeps us fed and protected in our vulnerability. Many of us have had to trade aspects of who we are for the belonging that keeps us safe. We stay quiet. We withhold our true feelings. We accept blame for the deficiencies of others. We bargain away our worthiness and lovability. We strive endlessly for unattainable perfection. We keep our light from shining. This is the price for survival and having our most urgent needs met that must be reckoned with when we awaken to it later in life.

How does healing ancestral trauma relate to our terrain?

Trauma has a biology. The biology of trauma and persistent stress drives physiological processes that lead to chronic illness, mental health problems, and addictions.[38] This includes all our adaptations to stay safe and preserve our connections. All kinds of pain and suffering that keeps us stuck. The

---

[38] Nagy A Youssef. The Effects of Trauma, with or without PTSD, on the Transgenerational DNA Methylation Alterations in Human Offspring. Brain Sci. 2018.

terrain of ancestral trauma will keep us tethered to life experiences, lifestyle habits, and tenacious mindsets and beliefs until we see it, hold it, and heal it.

PAUSE AND BREATHE.

I see you. I hear you. I feel you. I know you. I am you.

We keep talking about trauma.

You might ask, how does that relate to *me*?

I assure you, not one of us has been spared. We may call it "stress" or "old wounds" or "the way it was back then" or "the way the world works," but trauma has landed in us all. The trauma of our childhoods, ancestors, communities, the planet Earth. All of it. What lands in some of us, lands in us all. We're all connected.

This is important. Trauma keeps us stuck. In pain, suffering, mindsets, and persistent behaviors that keep us from moving ahead, from achieving our dreams.

Is there any place in your life where you feel stuck? Call it whatever you like, but *that's* trauma.

So, what do we do about it?

You know where we must start, don't you?

Hands on heart. Let your beautiful heart know you're there. Drop in. Breathe. Hold whatever is there with reverence and compassion. Without trying to change or fix it, just hold.

If you don't feel beautiful at this moment, if you question whether you deserve reverence and compassion, I have a few words for you.

I know this about you just as I know it about myself. You are a person doing her best. You've always done your best, though you may not have given yourself credit for doing so.

I know this. I know who you are. I see you. I hear you. I feel you. And I welcome all of you and your feelings. Right here in this present moment. I welcome you as my sacred ally of this planet Earth. Sharing this earthly experience of humanness. Of healing. Of the necessary suffering that has kept us alive.

Trauma is not permanent. It flows. It's what happened inside us that led to an equilibrium of pain and suffering. But we know we're epigenetic, neuroplastic beings of miraculous potential. We are all these things regardless of what we believe, of what we've been told, of the stories that have shaped our thinking. But to know, accept, and activate this potential inside us? We're unstoppable.

So, let's use our powerful words together right now.

Standing here, hands over our hearts, our hearts beating as one, we simply hold. We breathe. We rest. Without fixing or changing or judging, we hold, hold, hold.

With compassion for precisely who we are and where we are at in this difficult life. With reverence for where we've been, what we've survived, how well we've survived, for how resourceful we are. We're so bad ass. And the farther we've fallen, the harder we've fallen, the more bad ass we've had to be.

I see you. I hear you. I feel you. I know you. I am you. Because we're all one. No matter our experiences. I'm no better than you. I'm no different at the deepest levels of our needs as humans. Of our sacredness.

Let's breathe that in right now. We're all connected. We're all sacred. Holding that, holding ourselves as all that, is how we compassionately direct our healing.

PURPOSE.

Purpose is the aspect of our terrain that inspires us to get up in the morning. It can light our fire or exhaust us, but either way it infuses our lives with meaning.

Purpose is often misunderstood as the thing we're looking for that will make us feel good about who we are. It's often defined *for us* by strong family and cultural narratives about who we "should" be, how to be "good," and what makes us "successful" as people. Purpose is what so many of us yearn for and spend our lives searching for. If we could just find that passion, amazing job, or perfect partner to make us feel our lives have the most meaning. In this way, purpose becomes a story of our dissatisfaction and unworthiness.

While purpose may well make us feel good about ourselves and what we choose to do in our lives, it's become disconnected from who we truly are *intrinsically*. Rather than flowing through our bodies, it's floating around *out there* somewhere, in the expectations and dictums we've taken into us. It's unattainable.

I propose we work with purpose as the life path of our most authentic selves. Whether we believe this purpose is gifted to us from a wisdom source greater than ourselves, fully self-created, or some combination of both, it's what gives our lives the most meaning. And, just like us, is always in evolution. So, as we're discovering ourselves, our purpose is always unfolding before us.

We might understand our purpose through these questions: What do we hold most dear just because? What compels us to action without regard to reward? What feels necessary to fully expressing who we are?

Our purpose may be related to our families, other people, a job, or aspirations of some kind, but it's not those things, themselves. Purpose is more the thread of meaning in what we do that provides our reason for living and that expresses who we most authentically are.

So, *purpose = authenticity*.

By making authenticity our purpose, we can become more aligned with what we love, what we believe in, and what we're curious about. We can connect more readily to our own authentic creative impulses.

Looked at from another angle, everything we do to become more who we authentically are, to express who we authentically are, to walk through the world as our whole true self, well, *that's* purpose. What else do we need?

Karyn Shanks MD

Purpose is in our bodies. It has a biology. And like the rest of our biology, it has a lot of influence over how our genes are expressed and how our life outcomes unfold. It's a key part of our personal healing terrain. Studies show how the strength of purpose guiding and galvanizing our actions has a direct link to mental and physical health, cognitive function, and longevity. It's a powerful resilience factor, promoting a more positive approach to life's challenges while mitigating the effects of stress on the body.[39] We'll be working with purpose a lot as we turn to our *Unbroken* core resilience practices.

THE TERRAIN OF HEALING IS OUR ROADMAP.

That was our roadmap, friends, the terrain of all our healing, all that makes us *us*. The terrain is all the places we live our lives, even the places we're unfamiliar with, that are hidden from view or are uncomfortable to look at. But it's us regardless, our TotalGloriousOneness, our TGO.

Where can our roadmap lead us?

At its best, dialed in to meet our unique needs, the roadmap leads to resilience—the strength, energy, and adaptability we need to successfully flow through the changes and challenges of life without losing robustness.

What do we need to dial in our terrain?

Resources. Knowhow. Energy.

We've been working on the resources and knowhow. Let's look at energy next.

---

[39] Victor J Strecher. Life on Purpose: How Living for What Matters Most Changes Everything. 2016,

CHAPTER ELEVEN
Energy: the heart of our flow.

Energy is the heart of our flow. But it's not just what we feel. Energy runs the business of our bodies. It keeps us alive. It helps us do all our chores.

WHAT IS ENERGY?

We contain many kinds of energy. There's lifeforce energy. Chemical-biological energy. Creative energy. Mental energy. Spiritual energy. Big bold gym energy. Sexual energy. Chi, prana, and Kundalini energy. All kinds. You name it.

In physics, energy is the capacity for doing work. In our bodies too. As such, energy fuels all function, everything our bodies do from gene expression, to making energy, itself, to running across the street.

Recall how the highest biological priority for human organisms is survival. Therefore, energy is the foundation of everything it takes to survive, like:

- Movement.
- Seeking shelter.
- Reproduction and parenting.
- Finding nourishment.
- Finding and maintaining connection.

Beyond survival, energy is also the basis for human creative expression, for wonder, awe, authenticity, intellectual growth, and spiritual evolution.

Energy is the foundation of our TotalGloriousOneness , our TGO.

Energy doesn't appear magically, though. We have to make it. By working through our terrain of healing, we'll optimize the availability of essential resources for energy production while healing and protecting the structures where energy is made in the body.

Because survival is the priority of our energy systems, only when survival needs are met is energy available for everything else. So, in survival mode, when there's high demand for the energy of safety, or when essential resources for energy production are insufficient to meet all our needs, survival comes first, and robustness and creative expression are last.

There are two key biological energy systems I'd like you to know about. These are the two energy-functional pathways within our bodies that make our existence possible. They're at the heart of our ability to live, stay safe, heal, and thrive.

Do you need to know about these two systems in detail to thrive? No. But it helps you see how incredible you are, intrinsically wired for great potential.

These two energy-functional pathways are the genius inside you:

- The Brain-Thyroid-Adrenal-Mitochondrial energy operating system (BTAM): the biology of maintenance energy within the human body.
- The Autonomic Nervous System (ANS): the biology of safety.

First, please know this lesson will be grossly over-simplified. In fact, calling anything about our biology by a simple name, like "Autonomic Nervous System," makes it seem like we're talking about a simple thing. It's not a simple thing. It's not a thing at all. It's a highly sophisticated complex system that is so completely interconnected with all our other systems that it is impossible to put into words all the exquisite details. In addition, there's much we don't know about energy in the human body. It's an intricate, tangled, and uniquely individualized equilibrium. That said, we'll learn a few foundational concepts to understand ourselves better.

WHAT IS ENERGY DEPLETION?

This is the part of energy most of us can relate to. It's often the reason we think about energy at all: we don't have it. Especially how it *feels* when we don't have it. We might call it "fatigued," "no get up and go," "low motivation," "no mojo," or "swimming in mud," but it's all the same. Energy depletion is the common denominator for all the ways we experience fatigue and is also a key player in all persistent suffering and illness. Energy *always* needs to be addressed as part of our healing. Healing and recovery from illness is an energy expensive process.

I'm exhausted. I'm depressed and unmotivated. I don't have the energy to play with my children. I don't feel like my usual vibrant self. I don't feel safe. I want my life back.

All the ways we experience energy loss has a biology. And this biology is a very useful framework for helping solve the puzzle of suffering and illness.

At the most foundational level, energy depletion is the result of an equilibrium that involves compromised mitochondrial function. Mitochondria are your body's energy powerhouses. They're tiny organelles found inside most of your body cells where chemical energy, known as ATP, is produced. Chemical energy forms the basis for all other energies experienced throughout the body: motivation, mojo, flow, lifeforce.

Loss of energy occurs when the mitochondria can't produce enough energy to meet your needs. What causes that?

Any hindrance within the environment of our cells (which is largely influenced by the environment outside our cells) that affect mitochondrial function will result in energy depletion. General causes of mitochondrial dysfunction and energy depletion due to decreased supply include:

- Damage to mitochondrial structures (due to toxins, inflammation, infections, and so on).
- Damage to cells (due to toxins, inflammation, infections, and so on).
- Decreased resources (nutrients, oxygen, and so on) necessary for energy production.
- Decreased signaling regarding energy need (hypothalamic, pituitary, thyroid, or adrenal dysfunction, for example).
- Hypoxia (insufficient oxygen getting to the mitochondria).
- Blood circulation problems (to transport oxygen and nutrients to the mitochondria).
- Problems with enzymes and other aspects of energy chemistry.
- The cell danger response (see below).

These problems are exacerbated when there is an increase in demand for energy (in addition to decreased supply) in the body due to:

- Illness.
- High stress.
- Exercise and exertion.
- Healing.
- Pregnancy.

The cell danger response.

Energy depletion can also occur in the presence of signals the body perceives as dangerous.[40] This may be the result of a grave or persistent illness, lasting or particularly high levels of stress, and severe or unresolved trauma. In these situations, the body will biologically downshift into a survival state known as the "cell danger response" to preserve energy and resources. The constellation of symptoms that often accompany the cell danger response (fatigue, weakness, orthostatic intolerance, postural orthostatic tachycardia or POTS , and pain) conserves crucial survival resources and keep the person unmoving and quiet to preserve energy as they heal. Though it is often misunderstood as the illness itself, the cell danger response is a *healing cycle*. We commonly see the cell danger response in chronic infections, the aftermath of severe infections (post-COVID), environmental illnesses, and other severe illness or traumatic events.

THE BRAIN-THYROID-ADRENAL-MITOCHONDRIAL (BTAM) ENERGY OPERATING SYSTEM.

Polly, an Iowa farmer and mother to a special needs child, developed drop-dead fatigue at the age of 40. She also experienced vertigo, severe insomnia, brain fog, and extreme intolerance to all forms of exertion. She spent five years going to doctors and specialists who couldn't find anything to explain her symptoms. As we began our work together, I threw out a "wide net" in terms

---

[40] Robert K Naviaux. Perspective: Cell danger response biology—the new science that connects environmental health with mitochondria and the rising tide of chronic illness. Mitochondrion. 2020.

of collecting her history and ordering diagnostic tests that would help us thoroughly assess her BTAM for causes of the energy deficit/mitochondrial dysfunction to help explain her symptoms. What we discovered was Lyme disease and several tick-born co-infections. Treatment of the infections in addition to a comprehensive whole-person support strategy (nutrition, sleep, movement, addressing trauma) lead to full recovery of her energy. As she recovered, she told me how incredible it felt to feel energy moving through her body again, especially her heart.

With Polly, as with many of my chronically fatigued clients, we had to address the cell danger response, the healing cycle that decreased mitochondrial function to keep her safe. First, we had to remove the biological danger signals (Lyme disease, co-infections, nutrient deficiencies, lack of sleep, unresolved childhood and adult trauma) and address her unmet needs. Once biological safety was in place and she felt better, we could address the trauma of being persistently ill and not knowing what to do. Of having slipped through the cracks of many doctors who told her "Nothing is wrong." In some ways, this was the defining factor of her stories: *My body is wrong. I'm wrong. I'll never recover.*

By now you know, the stories we tell affect everything. They shift our gene expression, our biology, our brains. They determine our outcomes in powerful ways. Powerful stories, like fear of lost faith in recovery is one of the energy nodes we must heal. Fear, itself, is a survival strategy. Just like the cell danger response, it's a healing cycle. But once the danger has passed, it no longer serves. Polly learned to recognize this. She thanked her fear, focused on her newly opened heart (energy!) to guide her, and lived her new flow.

The brain, thyroid gland, adrenal glands, and mitochondria make up a vital energy operating system that is responsible for managing all the maintenance energy needs for the body. It provides energy for waking up in the morning, doing the daily chores, and working through your favorite exercise routine. Most of the work of the BTAM is going on in the background so we don't even have to think about it. It's providing fuel for our breathing, heart rhythm, detoxification pathways, muscle function, and all the maintenance functions of the human body. And quite a task that is. But when everything's dialed in just right? Yes, we flow!

I've taken the liberty of reorganizing this energy operating system framework from the conventional "HPA axis" (hypothalamic-pituitary-adrenal axis) because this way makes so much more sense.

The "old" way says the HPA axis is responsible for "the stress response." But I find that designation misleading. First, the operating system is bigger than only the hypothalamus, pituitary gland, and adrenals. Second, stress is only part of it. It's *really* an energy system. Referring to the "HPA axis stress response" implies the system only works when we're stressed. Not at all true. It also implies that "stress" is something unusual and bad, so bad we must have an entire system in our bodies to address it. Wrong again.

First, what's stress? Well, we all know the popular, everyday definition: stress is what *feels* bad, overwhelming, and so on. No one likes to feel stressed out.

What we *should* be talking about when we say "stress" is challenge. And we need challenge. Challenge is the crucible for resilience, remember? But challenge requires energy. Lots of energy.

So, we have this whole gorgeous BTAM energy operating system to create that energy.

And we need a big brain to help us sort that all out, don't we?

Let's look at each of the players in the BTAM more closely.

The brain.

The brain is a ginormous sensory organ. It takes in all kinds of information from the environment, both outside and inside our bodies. The brain perceives, creates meaning, and coordinates responses, usually in an instant without our conscious awareness. In this way, the brain helps us adapt and thrive through shifts in biology, movement and behavior, learning, and the meaning we assign to our lives.

The hypothalamus and pituitary glands, both located in the brain, are key players in the BTAM. They make communication molecules called hormones and neuropeptides that travel throughout the body to signal what resources are needed. A priority of the brain-hypothalamus-pituitary apparatus is to make energy to support all vital maintenance functions of the body.

The brain is also taking in information about sunlight and seasons to help manage sleep, another key part of supporting energy production. Sleep promotes energy through energy conservation (we use less energy while we're sleeping), energy production (energy hormones and mitochondrial function ramp up while we sleep), detoxification (protects the structures involved in energy production from damaging effects of toxins and irritants), and production of the hormone melatonin (induces sleep).

Outside the brain are the key receivers of whole brain communication about our energy needs—the thyroid, adrenals, and mitochondria, the other BTAM nodes. Let's look at their roles in producing energy.

The thyroid and adrenal glands.

The thyroid and adrenal glands work in concert to help create and mobilize energy by responding to communications from the brain.

The thyroid gland sits at the base of the neck just above the sternal notch. It acts as a thermostat, much like the one in your home. By adjusting your thermostat settings, you're regulating the amount of fuel delivered to your home's HVAC system, which then heats or cools your house.

In response to TSH (thyroid stimulating hormone) from the pituitary gland in the brain, the thyroid will produce the hormones thyroxine (T4) and triiodothyronine (T3). They control the amount of work done by the cells through regulation of oxygen consumption (oxygen is used to make chemical energy, ATP, within the mitochondria) via changes in genetic expression. Thyroid stimulation increases the need for oxygen and all the other resources (carbon atoms, nutrients, enzymes, for instance) required for energy production.

The adrenal glands direct how much fuel becomes available for your body, responding to ACTH (adrenal cortical tropic hormone) sent from the pituitary gland. They are also keeping track of the demands that thyroid hormones are placing on cells to do work. The adrenals make carbon atoms available (derived from glucose, fatty acids, and amino acids) to produce the energy needed for cellular work.

The adrenal glands sit on top of the kidneys and consist of two parts: the inner adrenal medulla and the outer adrenal cortex. The adrenal medulla is part of the Autonomic Nervous System, or ANS, which we'll talk about shortly, producing epinephrine (adrenaline) and norepinephrine (noradrenaline) in response to signals from the brain during acutely challenging situations. The adrenal cortex makes the energy hormones cortisol, aldosterone, and DHEA in response to ACTH from the pituitary.

The role of cortisol is to make carbon atoms available for conversion into energy. Cortisol also helps suppress non-vital biological functions to conserve energy, such as reproduction, digestion, and growth, during times of high challenge. This helps us focus our biological energy on survival when challenge is high.

Aldosterone helps maintain blood volume and blood pressure through its effects on the kidneys. This action helps maintain circulation of the carbon atoms made available by cortisol and transports them to all the cells of the body where they will be converted to energy. Circulation is also supported by the pituitary neuropeptide, anti-diuretic hormone (ADH), fluid and electrolyte intake, and movement.

DHEA's primary action is related to the brain, priming it for growth and learning, key parts of responding successfully to life's challenges. It ameliorates the potentially harmful effects of persistently high cortisol levels, which can lead to immune suppression, delayed wound healing, bone loss, insulin resistance, and depression.

What is "adrenal fatigue?"

There is a popular concept in recent years called "adrenal fatigue ," in which the adrenals become the focus of explanations for why fatigue occurs in those who are persistently overwhelmed or chronically ill. The adrenal fatigue diagnosis is a misnomer, as it's rare that the adrenals alone would be responsible for fatigue. While isolated adrenal gland failure can occur, adrenal dysfunction associated with fatigue is almost always the result of depleted resources needed to support *the entire* BTAM energy operating system, rather than the adrenals alone. We also see BTAM-wide dysfunction with systemic inflammation from infections, allergens, autoimmunity, and toxin exposure, often part of the cell danger response to keep us safe by shutting us down.

So, "adrenal fatigue" is an oversimplification of more complex BTAM dysfunction or the cell danger response. We may support adrenal gland function in the settings of persistent overwhelm or chronic illness, but it should always be part of a more comprehensive support strategy.

Mitochondria.

These tiny subcellular organelles are the powerhouses of the body, producing the energy that fuels all biological processes. As such, they play an integral role in all health and illness. As you can imagine, it's vitally important we consider what resources mitochondria need to function at their most optimal level (nutrients, oxygen, and so on). It's also important that their delicate structures are protected from external and internal challenges to their integrity (by toxins, infections, and allergens, for instance).

What's happening with our BTAM when we're tired?

When you're tired, sick, or feel you've lost your flow, understanding the BTAM provides a logical framework for sorting out the language of your body, what it's trying to tell you about what it needs through its sensations, energy states, and feelings.

When you've lost your flow, you're experiencing an energy deficit.

What does the language of a struggling BTAM look like?

- Fatigue, exhaustion, sleepiness during the day.
- Exertion intolerance.
- Muscle weakness.
- Muscle soreness and stiffness.
- Brain fog and cognitive dysfunction.
- Depression.
- Intolerance of upright position.
- Headaches.
- Sleep disturbance.
- Gut problems such as IBS and poor digestion.
- Irritability, frustration, and anxiety.
- Hormone imbalances and infertility.

Ultimately, these are all signals of mitochondrial dysfunction. Since mitochondria manufacture the energy you need throughout your body, any problem in the BTAM will manifest as an energy deficit because the mitochondria can't do their job to make energy.

Karyn Shanks MD

What are common causes of mitochondrial dysfunction?

- Insufficient sleep.
- Sleep disorders (sleep apnea, snoring, nocturnal movement).
- Nutrient poor diets (nutrients run the chemistry of energy production).
- Sedentary lifestyle (causes loss of mitochondria and slowed transportation of resources through the body).
- Depressed mood.
- Acute and chronic infections.
- Allergies.
- Environmental toxins (through excess exposure or impaired detoxification).
- Persistent stress.
- High levels of acute stress.
- Persistent inflammation from any cause.
- The cell danger response.

These are only the most common causes—there are many more!

Chronic fatigue syndrome (CFS), also known as encephalomyelitis (ME), is a debilitating, persistent form of BTAM/mitochondrial dysfunction. The Institute of Medicine estimates as many as 2.5 million Americans suffer from CSF/ME and many more people with this syndrome have not been identified.[41]

In my experience, many of these folks have slipped through the cracks of a medical system that places people with persistent severe fatigue and exertion intolerance (key diagnostic requirements for the CFS/ME diagnosis) into a disease box. While they may be accurately diagnosed, the problem is that CFS/ME are descriptive diagnoses only. They don't identify the specific cause. While there can be comfort in fitting an accepted diagnosis (it feels better than being told "nothing's wrong"), they're often no better off because while the diagnosis suggests there's a cause and treatment for "the thing" that's wrong, there are as many causes of CFS/ME as there are people suffering from it. The only common denominator among CFS/ME sufferers is the energy deficit somewhere within the BTAM that explains all their symptoms. And the true

---

[41] CDC: Myalgic Encephalomyelitis/Chronic Fatigue Syndrome. www.cdc.gov.

cause is usually multifactorial—there is a confluence of things contributing to the energy deficit (nutrient deficiencies, a chronic infection, and a sleep disorder, for instance). A careful person-specific analysis of all symptoms, a meticulous timeline of all life events, and scrutiny of key aspects of their systems biology will reveal the BTAM needs to restore energy.

How to decode the language of BTAM energy deficit.

Often the causes of fatigue are obvious—not enough sleep, too much stress, overwork, no exercise. These are usually easy to identify.

When fatigue is more persistent, such as in Polly's case, it's important to carefully follow the energy nodes within the BTAM—the brain, thyroid, adrenals, and mitochondria—and how nutrients, oxygen, and energy can circulate throughout the body. We begin by asking two essential questions:

- What are the unmet needs (nutrients, water, oxygen, sleep, movement, self-compassion, safety, and so on)?
- What's in the way (toxins, irritants, infections, allergens, negative energy, damaging habits, disempowering stories, and so on)?

By relentlessly asking these two essential questions about each energy node in the BTAM energy operating system—is it the brain, the hypothalamus or pituitary glands, the thyroid gland, the adrenal glands, the mitochondria, or is it transport of the energy throughout the body?—we discover the causes of our energy deficit equilibrium. This leads to strategies for shifting into an equilibrium of energy repletion and healing.

Though the questions are simple, the process can get complicated. Most of the time persistent fatigue is caused by *many* unmet needs and obstacles to healing that are present at the same time. You may need to work with a professional who can look at you in a comprehensive, systematic way. It will be challenging to get this from a practitioner of conventional western biomedicine with their disease-focus and time constraints. You need someone trained in all the details and idiosyncrasies of human systems biology, preferably with a whole-person and trauma-informed approach.[42]

---

[42] See the database for certified Functional Medicine practitioners in your community. Many of them work by telemedicine as well. www.ifm.org.

Karyn Shanks MD

THE AUTONOMIC NERVOUS SYSTEM (ANS): THE ENERGY OF SAFETY.

If the *Brain-Thyroid-Adrenal-Mitochondrial (BTAM)* energy operating system meets our energy needs for daily maintenance operations of the body, the *Autonomic Nervous System (ANS)* modulates that energy production and directs it toward survival. These two energy systems are highly integrated, with overlapping roles in vital maintenance function and safety.

Beyond maintenance, we must have a reservoir of energy at the ready for urgencies and emergencies. As such, the ANS—while always active at baseline levels to support automatic functions like breathing, heart function, blood flow, digestion, and immunity—also directs energy and action impulses to quickly help move us out of harm's way, then return to a stable, supportive equilibrium of safety. Though we often associate the ANS with how it can make us squirm (more on this in a bit), it's a healing system at its core.

How does the ANS help us achieve an equilibrium of safety?

Neuroception: how we 'read the room.'

It all begins in the gorgeous sensory organ in our heads—the brain. We need to be able to read danger instantly and accurately. Our brain does this for us, mostly without our conscious awareness. We read the room, so to speak, through an internal surveillance process called "neuroception."[43] We react before we realize there's anything to react to. We may feel scared and look for a way out. Or we feel comfortable and decide to stay. Neuroception and ANS responses happen automatically. We don't have to think about them.

The ANS circuits.

The ANS mobilizes powerful energy in both the face of and retreat from danger. In danger, we have to act quickly to get ourselves or others out of harm's way. Once the immediate danger has passed, we may need to shiver or shake to release the energy of urgency and fear and call in our reinforcements to support us. Through the ANS experience, we're both staying alive and

---

[43] Stephen W Porges. Polyvagal Theory: A Science of Safety. 2022.

learning to support our future safety. Our ANS also helps us shift from danger toward restoration, calm, and relaxation.

The ANS consists of three primary circuits to keep us safe and on a healing trajectory.[44] These circuits originate in the brain or spinal cord and connect to billions of nerves. They deliver information about safety to every organ and cell in the body.

The Sympathetic Nervous System (SNS).

The SNS is responsible for "fight or flight" responses to perceived danger, post-emergency tremble and shake responses, and anxiety. Its energy supports active learning, alertness, trust, and social engagement.

The Parasympathetic Nervous System (PSNS), ventral branch of the vagus nerve ("ventral vagal").

The ventral branch of the vagus nerve is the most evolutionarily evolved ANS circuit. It restores and calms, adapting us to relaxed social engagement, trust, wellness, and growth.

The Parasympathetic Nervous System (PSNS), dorsal branch of the vagus nerve ("dorsal vagal").

We share this more evolutionarily primitive ANS circuit—part of what we often call our "reptilian brain"—with many of Earth's creatures who utilize this circuit to play "dead" when attacked. Similarly, humans use this circuit to help us survive danger through immobilization, freeze responses, and disassociation. It's also involved in passive social engagement and intimacy, supporting relaxation when one feels safe.

Each circuit of the ANS automatically mobilizes different energy strategies for safety, but not to the exclusion of the others. The SNS and both vagal

---

[44] Deborah A dana. Anchored: How to Befriend Your Nervous System Using Polyvagal Theory. 2021.

branches of the PSNS are always active to varying extents, blending according to perceived and programmed needs. The goal is to have all the ANS circuits activate and blend harmoniously to hold us in the best possible equilibrium for our safety and wellness needs.

How the ANS circuits blend.

In the presence of environmental cues of threat, the brain reads the level of risk through neuroception, then automatically shifts into the ANS circuits that best address our perceived needs.[45] The higher the risk, the more SNS and dorsal vagal circuits take priority. Cues of safety downshift SNS and upshift ventral vagal circuits.

The blending of ANS circuits scale based on the present cues of safety, including neuroceptive inputs, past experiences, and how we interpret cues. While there are infinite combinations possible, these are the six primary ANS functional energy strategies:

- **High Emergency (mobilization with fear):** *high SNS, low PSNS "fight or flight"* states in response to real or perceived danger. Movement to confront or get away from danger is instantaneous. Associated feelings are fear and anger. The perception is "I'm not safe."
- **Overwhelmed**: *high SNS, low ventral vagal PSNS,* though danger has passed or there are persistently high levels of challenge without adequate restoration. This strategy can feel a lot like high emergency SNS states, though the perceived "emergency" only exists in stories, beliefs, ruminations, and unresolved trauma.
- **Active engaged readiness (mobilization without fear):** *balanced SNS and ventral vagal PSNS* that support learning, creative activities, play, and friendly competition.
- **Relaxed:** *high ventral vagal PSNS* in restful, calm, and meditative states.
- **Shut down (immobilization with fear):** *high dorsal vagal PSNS "freeze" states* in response to unsurvivable danger (prey plays dead

---

45 Stephen W Porges. Polyvagal Theory: A Science of Safety. 2022.

when in the grips of a predator) or dissociative, depersonalized, and emotionally numbed states that occur due to severe unresolved trauma.

- **Trust and intimacy (passive without fear):** *balanced SNS with ventral and dorsal vagal PSNS* in relaxed social engagement and intimate relationships.

Which energy strategy are we in right now? If we're relaxed or in trust and intimacy, our SNS and ventral and dorsal vagal PSNS are supporting us in relaxed social engagement. We're in a good place. We're more apt to be in our flow and ready to manage the changes, challenges, and uncertainties that come our way. We're resilient.

What if the energy strategy we're in is overwhelmed or we're shut down and checked out? How do you think we'll fare when challenges come our way? That's right. It's hard to thrive through challenge when we're scared or disconnected. You can see how which ANS circuits are activated says a lot about our capacity for resilience.

Remember, however our ANS reacts, this is the language of our bodies offering us its wisdom about what we need. It's not wrong, it just might not be serving our current needs. Our off-kilter ANS is not there to kill us, it's our healing circuit. It's kept us safe in some way and can teach us what we need right now. The ANS is part of the genius of our bodies even when it feels wildly uncomfortable, destabilizing, or immobilizing. It's easy to understand why we sometimes experience ANS activation as "something's terribly wrong with me." We often reject what's uncomfortable, passive, or requires our trust. But sometimes we need discomfort to get us out of harm's way. And sometimes we need to stay quiet and small (passive) to survive what seems unsurvivable. Discomfort and passivity are important survival strategies, our bodies' genius.

How do we learn to trust ourselves and our bodies? How do we return to our home base with ventral vagal connected energy?

Here's the lesson about the ANS. As much as it operates automatically to help you survive, you also have enormous conscious control over it. You can direct it to your own advantage. You can turn down the intensity and ramp up the support.

ANS discomfort is hard, not bad.

My hope is we can break through our trepidation about the ANS to see and appreciate its sheer gorgeous brilliance. To use it as a tool to reclaim our flow.

One of the most destructive aspects of the mind-body divide that disconnected us from our bodies' truth and genius is how we interpret any level of discomfort as meaning something is wrong. This is especially true for how many of us experience the energy of our internal biology of safety, the ANS, especially when SNS anxiety or dorsal vagal disassociation are high.

Persistent mental health struggles so many of us are familiar with are associated with ANS discomfort. They have names like depression, social anxiety disorder, and so on. I love how labeling them as such has helped destigmatize these experiences so people can seek help with less fear. However, it concerns me how putting experiences associated with persistent ANS discomfort into a disease box. For many people suffering common mental health disorders, their symptoms are addressed, and that can be incredibly helpful, but many remain vulnerable because the treatments don't address the upstream causes of their suffering. They may shift out of the extreme discomfort of high SNS (anxiety) or dorsal vagal activation (disassociation, depression) through strategies like drugs and cognitive behavioral therapy, but they may still feel unsafe. The proof is in the pudding: conventional treatments for mental health disorders have a high relapse rate.

Many of us experience the prickly anxiety of the SNS and shame-ridden avoidance of the dorsal vagal PSNS as bad and unpleasant. And something to be gotten rid of as soon as possible. Because it's *uncomfortable*, so something's *wrong*. It hurts. Something's wrong with *us*.

Here's where holding our bodies' wisdom with reverence and curiosity is the hardest. The ANS can be the loudest, harshest, most urgent, and scariest of our bodies' energy processes because its job is to keep us safe, sometimes to *hurl* us to safety. Isn't that amazing? And yet no part of us is as misunderstood or feared.

We'll be exploring and working directly with our ANS throughout our work with the *Unbroken* core resilience steppingstones in the next section. We'll be asking our hard sensations and feelings: "What do you have to teach me?" "What do you need?"

PAUSE AND BREATHE.

I'm safe. I'm right here.

If a speeding car is about to hit your kid, you have no choice. The neuroceptive genius of your brain will see it before you do. You and your fully activated Sympathetic Nervous System (SNS) will be racing into the street to grab your kid before you consciously know what's happening. This is beautiful wisdom in the body. We don't want to change this, do we?

How about the new lover who's *sure* to abandon you? What do you think happens then? Same as the car speeding toward your kid. Your SNS kicks in, with all that adrenaline trying to catapult you the hell out of there before they dump you. Only this time, there's nothing to run after. There's no clear danger, just the expectation that it might be around the corner. So, you can't use the adrenaline energy for what it was designed to do (to move you quickly out of harm's way). It's just you and the anxious stories of hurt and loss. This is *also* the beautiful wisdom of your body, doing your bidding.

We all do this. We tell stories that bring our greatest fears to life. There's value to this if we're paying close attention. We can look carefully at our scary stories and learn what we're afraid of. We can evaluate them for their present moment accuracy. Maybe they're fears of a very young part of us who is yearning to be healed.

How can the stories that torment us also help us heal?

We can hold those stories with compassion, gaze upon them with curiosity, and ask them for their wisdom. We let them lead us to healing by asking them what they need from us.

But these stories are hard. Therefore, it helps considerably to have strategies to directly shift our ANS circuits from danger to safety.

Let's take a moment to practice shifting into ventral vagal safety.

You've already been practicing one—activating your safety circuit: mind-hands-heart-feet-breath. Let's add to that.

Take a comfortable seat. Close your eyes. Breathe.

Place one hand behind your head, palm pressing against your occiput (the bony prominence just above your neck). This part of the head is immediately adjacent to where the vagus nerve exits your brainstem, carrying the impulses of your PSNS. Touching this area sends sensory information back to your vagus nerve. It says, "I'm safe, I'm right here."

Place your other hand firmly over your heart. You're telling your heart, "I'm safe, I'm right here."

Breathe and rest while holding your head and heart. As you breathe, repeat "I'm safe, I'm right here," as many times as you'd like.

Now, keeping your hands where they are, open your eyes and without turning your head look all the way to the right, as far as possible without discomfort. What do you notice there? Hold your gaze for 30-60 seconds as you continue to breathe. Bring your vision back to center and rest a moment here. When you're ready, without turning your head, shift your gaze as far to the left as you can comfortably and hold. Again, notice what's there and hold for 30-60 seconds. Return your gaze to center.

Rest here for as long as you need. *I am safe. I'm right here.*

You've just sent tactile and visual safety signals directly to your vagus nerve and heart while activating your safety circuit (mind-hands-heart-feet-breath). This helps shift your ANS into a ventral vagal dominant state, one of relaxation and active engaged readiness.

You can stop anytime during your day, take a few easy conscious breaths, place a palm against your occiput and one on your heart, and use your powerful words: *I am safe. I'm right here.*

LOOKING AT FATIGUE AND THE CELL DANGER RESPONSE THROUGH THE LENS OF POSSIBILITIES.

We've looked at fatigue all wrong, haven't we?

Something's very wrong. Something that's stopped us in our tracks, stopped our lives. We've looked desperately for our fix yet nothing's worked. We've tried everything. Medications. Supplements. Devices. Food plans. Every. Magic. Bullet.

We're either told there's nothing wrong or given a diagnosis that's just a description or looks too far downstream to help us in the way we need. CFS/ME. Adrenal fatigue. Thyroid fatigue. POTs. Long COVID.

We remain exhausted. We feel stuck. Devastated.

What happens when we feel we've slipped through the cracks of the system of medicine and experts we've asked to help us? When none of their fixes fit us? When none of their strategies help us? When we feel alone and unheard and unseen? When our true needs don't matter? Even when we're in the most loving of hands yet the way they see our problems are all wrong?

We feel unsafe.

What happens inside us when we feel unsafe?

Without knowing, without even trying, we activate our SNS and dorsal vagal-mediated survival biology. Our nervous system sees us and comes to our rescue—or at least that's its intention. That biology activates and *adds to* the cell danger response. But it adds to our fatigue, our despair, our trauma.

What do we do now?

We must bring ourselves back to safety.

Let's keep this simple.

First step. Stop. Breathe. Breathe space all around that fatigue, despair, and trauma. Breathe space around how your life has been upended. Without trying to change or fix anything. Breathe. Let go of the diagnoses. Let go of the fix.

Second step. Hold everything inside you, every sensation, feeling, and energy state, hold it. Just hold. Let it be true. This is where you are right now. This is the language of your body, the language of you and your wisdom. Hold that. Breathe.

Third step. As you hold, consider this. This wisdom of you is not wrong. It's your guide. It will become your portal to healing. True healing. Healing that occurs upstream. That meets your true needs. Welcome it as it is. Say it out loud. *I welcome you, all of you, I hold you with compassion and reverence as the wisdom inside me. You are safe with me.*

Fourth step. Activate your safety circuit. Breath-hands-heart-feet-mind. Repeat.

Fifth step. Ask your body: what do you need? Then let your question go.

Repeat this sequence as many times as you'd like, but at least once daily. You're calling in safety. You're shifting out of survival biology, out of high SNS overwhelm and dorsal vagal disassociation and shut down. You're shifting into high ventral vagal PSNS safety and calm presence. You're honoring how you feel as the portal to your healing. You're honoring yourself.

LAST WORDS.

We're incredible beings, aren't we? So complex. With all that intelligence laser-focused on keeping us safe and supporting our TotalGloriousOneness (TGO).

The 21st century science of *Directable Human* makes it clear to our gorgeous scrutinizing intellects that we're putting our trust in the right place—in ourselves and our unlimited potential to heal. Even when it's complicated. Even when it seems impossible. Even when it's messy as hell. Our untapped potential is there regardless just waiting for us to access it.

The Earth's laws inside us and the dynamic principles of our amazing human bodies remind us: we can't *not* heal, we're all wise, and we're born to be resilient.

Resilience is, in fact, an equilibrium we have complete control over.

Our terrain of healing, that is us and provides the energy that sustains us, keeps us safe, and helps us rise. While not always comfortable, this wisdom helps us reclaim our wholeness.

We are energy. We are flow. We are resilience. We are wisdom and healing.

Now, how do we connect what we've learned so far to what to do in our daily lives? How do we *access* our wisdom? How do we *create* the energy and resilience we need to optimize our flow? How do we *manage* the tide of our ANS? And how do we *heal* our pain, suffering, and chronic illness?

In part three of this book, *We rise*, you'll be introduced to the nine *Unbroken* core resilience steppingstones. These steppingstones show you how to shift your equilibrium from pain, suffering, and chronic illness to one of resilience, flow, and amazing TGO through positive changes in genetic expression, biology, and how you learn to see yourself and your life's potential. You'll get to develop the skills you need to unleash the wise healer you already are. Not broken, but temporarily hovering at an equilibrium of suffering. Not stuck, but wise and capable and able to guide yourself to an equilibrium of healing. No longer without hope, already rising.

I see you. I hear you. I feel you. I know you. I am you.
Because we're all one.

SECTION THREE
We rise.

We feel it, don't we?
We can't not flow. We can't not heal.
But consciously tended?
We rise. We remember who we are. Already whole.

CHAPTER TWELVE
The language of rising.

"Rise" is not even in our vocabulary when we're sick, suffering, or stuck, is it? Not until a new story emerges. One that suggests we can flow like a river. That assures we can reach a dynamic equilibrium even when we feel like we're swimming in mud. That promises new possibilities for shifting that equilibrium of swimming in mud to something lighter, freer, that can heal us in ways we've never known before.

You felt it all coming, didn't you? That you're here with me at this moment reading these words tells me you more than feel it, you *know* it. The inspiration, the truth, the deep resonance already inside you. That you are the Earth. Her laws, her brilliance, her genius. They're yours to remember, to reconnect to, to make you shine as brightly as you know you can.

But the story isn't enough, is it? Knowing who we are is huge. But beyond our new story, beyond knowing who we truly are, how can we bring forth our very best equilibrium of healing?

We need a plan.

It's not enough to *see* the lay of the land, our incredible terrain. We need to know how to navigate it to our best advantage. That's what this section of the book is all about. *How* do we rise? How do we expand into the full expression of who we can be? Our flow, our wholeness, our TGO?

We'll get right to work. You're ready. Even if you don't *feel* ready, you are. Take a moment. Take a breath. Embark on this journey of healing with me, holding yourself with courage and kindness through small but fierce steps. A wise person once told me, "You'll know you're on the right track when you feel resistance." Another said, "the obstacle is the path."

Brave your own resistance, brave your path.

TO RISE WE MUST FIRST EXPAND.

We want to go up, don't we? We want energy, joy, optimal flow. We want to rise out of our pain, suffering, and illness.

We can imagine rising, can't we? Despite our suffering, we can feel it. The prize for our earnest intentions and hard work.

How do we land our prize?

How do we create change, achieve our goals, and grow into our new skin?

Let go of the prize.

Let go of energy, joy, and optimal flow. Let go of your goals. Let go of change, growth, and your new skin. Let go of everything you aspire to.

Why?

Aspiration is one hundred percent about the future. While aspiration can guide and energize, it also suggests you *know* where you'll land. *Knowing* anything limits you to where *you think* you're headed—it limits your potential and possibilities.

In this book, we're giving up our old stories based on old ideas about our potential and possibilities. We're giving up what we believe will happen if we do all the "right" things. We're giving up the quick fixes and simple solutions that don't fit us or take us to the deeper levels of transformation we're really asking for.

What are we doing instead? What can we expect as we progress through our lessons and practices in this section of the book?

We're *expanding* into our potential. We're *expanding* into our innate genius.

How?

By creating conditions to shift our terrain, shift our genetic expression, and shift our equilibrium through actionable, practical, small but fierce steps. We're *shifting*.

I'm asking you to trust yourself. To trust the wisdom within you. To trust you'll know what to do and where to go even when you can't see a clear way forward. To trust yourself through uncertainty. To trust the *you* you're becoming.

Why is this important now?

Trust may well be what's held many of us back from what truly deeply heals us. Trust in ourselves and this journey into our wholeness, while unfamiliar, is necessary.

In that spirit, what can you trust in this very moment? And based on that, what is your first actionable, practical, small but fierce step?

Breathe. Hold. Breathe again. Trust one thing. Take one step.

I'm asking you to be so brave.

What one thing do you trust right now?

What one step can you take right now?

Bravo.

INVITE SUFFERING TO BECOME A PORTAL TO THE WISDOM OF YOUR BODY.

Trust one thing. Take one step.

Then what?

Beyond trust and taking small steps with courage, what do we need?

How do we read the language of the body, the language of our emotions and minds to decipher what we need?

We work with the second dynamic principle of our human bodies: *your body is innately wise.*

In this way, suffering is a portal. Pain and chronic illness are portals. Feeling stuck is a portal.

A portal to what?

Your suffering is a portal to the wisdom of your body as it tells you in its unique and highly nuanced language what you most need. Suffering is a portal straight to your genius, your healing, your most sparkly wholeness. Suffering can take us straight to grace.

That's what we want, isn't it? Genius, healing, sparkly wholeness, and grace? Yes!!

But wait.

What happens when I walk straight into suffering? To see, hear, and *feel* my suffering?

We can't escape our suffering if we want to *heal* our suffering. We have to wade right into it. We have to resist the promises that there is a quick and easy fix for it. We have to own it as ours. Because our suffering *is* ours. And our suffering is yearning for our loving care and attention. It's yearning for understanding.

When we can own our suffering, see it, hear it, and feel it, guess what happens? We see and hear and experience its language. It becomes the portal to our deepest and most sustainable healing. Our best equilibrium. Our ability to flow with robustness, trust, and ease.

Our pain, fatigue, and feeling stuck can show us the way. *Our* way. The way that fits us, is designed for us, and is directed by us.

I'm not saying *endure* your suffering. Deciphering the language of your body does not mean don't soothe, comfort, and lessen your pain. By all means, *do* that. We all need that. Reducing pain and suffering can help us *hear* the wisdom.

If you haven't already, I invite you to name the suffering you'd most like to heal. Give it a name: pain, discomfort, tiredness, feeling blah, hopeless, whatever it is to you. That's your portal, the opening to discovering your needs.

Whatever sensation, energy state, or feeling you just named, see if you can hold it for a few moments. Breathe space around it. Allow it to be there without trying to change or fix it. Hold it with compassion and curiosity. Then ask it (literally ask): What do you need right now? How can I help you right now? What do you have to teach me? Then let your questions go.

This is how you invite suffering to become the portal to the wisdom of your body.

The language of suffering.

Suffering says, "I hurt, I'm tired, I'm depressed, I feel stuck, I feel hopeless," and so on. These are the words you use to describe what your body is telling you. But how do we decode the language of symptoms, sensations, and feelings? How do we know what the body is trying to say?

First, we listen. What *are* the sensations and feelings at this moment? We can do that, can't we?

I feel sharp pain in my knees. I feel exhausted and overwhelmed. My head is foggy. I feel despair.

Second, we accept them as they are. We may *want* to change, but welcoming where we are now is the best way to chart our new path. If we move too fast, we risk bypassing our truth for the quick fix.

Third, we decode the body's language. This is more difficult, though, isn't it? When we were taught to disconnect from our bodies, taught our pain was something that needed to be fixed by the experts, we stopped checking in, we stopped feeling, we lost our bodies' language. Just like any body of knowledge, if we don't use it, we lose it, right?

So, we must learn our bodies' language all over again.

We'll learn as we go. We'll be paying attention in present time, holding ourselves and our experiences with compassion, and looking closely at what the body says with curiosity. We'll relearn the language of our bodies, the language of our suffering, and the language of our evolution.

Drop back into your body for a moment and repeat the practice we just did. Revisit the part of you that hurts or is suffering. Call it by its name. Breathe into it. Hold it with compassion and curiosity, resisting the urge to change or fix it. Ask: What do you need right now? How can I help you right now? What do you have to teach me? Like before, let the questions go. Just breathe. Hold your attention there for a moment.

What comes up for you? A big nothing? (That's how I feel sometimes.) A shift in the sensation? (Sometimes a physical sensation can morph into a feeling.) Did anything pop into your mind, a word or sentence or image? Did you experience a rise or loss of energy?

With the body and its language of sensations, energy states, and feelings, anything goes. And we all experience things in different ways. I've learned to not expect answers right away (though sometimes they come that quickly). I'm more apt to receive a flash of insight when I'm not actively looking or listening for it. These insights tend to come when I'm meandering—in the shower, driving, or out on a walk. I wish they'd come at more convenient times so I can write the details down right away, but that's how it often goes for me.

As you practice asking your body questions, you'll get to know how it likes to answer you.

CHAPTER THIRTEEN
Preparing to rise: The *Un*Broken agreements, tools, and muses.

As we begin our more practical work together, let's consider some guidelines for engagement that are perhaps unlike anything you've encountered before. These are the things we need for this journey:

- Agreements with ourselves.
- Essential tools.
- Our muses.

We start with a few simple agreements—promises we make to ourselves. These are not about being told what to do (I don't like that either!) but forging a bond of trust with ourselves. Agreements are how we show up for ourselves, establishing trust and safety through committed practice.

These agreements will smooth your way with the tenderness you deserve (and may not have allowed before) and provide the foundation for a lifelong relationship to deep, sustainable epigenetic and neuroplastic potential. *Your* potential.

Then, we'll be travelling with a few essential tools in our pockets, like a compass or good map (or a smart phone!). These tools will keep our feet steady on the ground beneath us, our gaze focused on our chosen direction, and our hearts and minds open to the changes, challenges, and possibilities before us.

Our muses—our most trusted guides and mentors—travel with us. They're always there for us, but they still love to be personally acknowledged. They reward us with incredible insight and guidance designed especially for us.

FIVE UNBROKEN AGREEMENTS.

Above all else in this chapter, learn these five agreements. If you go no further, you'll be able to apply these to everything you set out to do and do them more successfully, on your terms. What are they?

- Hold yourself with fierce compassion and safety.
- Keep things simple, small, and slow.
- Release what you *think* you know.
- Practice and commit.
- Stay relentlessly curious.

Let's briefly explore these agreements. We'll carry them with us, letting them hold us in their strength and ground us in their wisdom.

Hold yourself with fierce compassion and safety.

A client of mine, Rose, bristles whenever I use words like "compassion" or "tenderness," at least when they're directed toward her. The lack of compassion and tenderness she'd experienced through her challenging life with abusive caregivers and many serious illnesses from an early age made her mistrust those words. One day, speaking of her beloved grandson, her voice softened, tears came to her eyes, and love exuded from her. I asked, "what comes up for you when you think of him?" "Tenderness, compassion, unconditional love," she replied, as a look of shock appeared on her face. "Oh my gosh, I didn't realize I could feel those things." We talked about bringing her grandson to mind, letting herself feel, and remind herself of the tenderness, compassion, and unconditional love she's capable of.

Even if you're not able to conjure self-compassion just now or during any of our practices, no worries, it will come. You're getting your reps in.

Here's the thing. We're all yearning for compassion. *Fierce* compassion. What's more, compassion brings us to safety. Safety is our container for the deepest healing.

The English *compassion* is derived from Latin *compassus*: "to suffer together with."

Compassion places us in immediate non-judging relationship with the objects of our compassion. It says, "I see you, I hear you, I feel you, you matter to me, I feel your suffering."

Karyn Shanks MD

Religious and spiritual traditions worldwide recognize compassion as a bedrock human virtue. Buddhism, Christianity, Islam, Judaism, indigenous North American cultures, and many others recognize how the highest expression of compassion is active—it's *what we do* in the spirit of compassion, to understand and help relieve the suffering of others. Not to fix, but to hold. Fiercely. To suffer together.

Compassion has a biology with vast real estate throughout our bodies.

We have deep brain networks dedicated to compassion.[46] Mirror neurons help us feel empathy for others' experiences. "Prosocial" brain networks support how we respond to the needs of others. The pituitary neuropeptide oxytocin bolsters parental attachment and social bonding by deepening our ability for compassion and responding to others' needs.

Compassion regulates the Autonomic Nervous System (ANS), our biological system of safety. It helps shift us out of fear and into social engagement. This shift into deeper connection improves resilience in many of our biological systems. Heart rate variability increases, helping the heart adapt to cardiovascular challenge. Blood pressure can also adapt more quickly, allowing for variations in blood delivery to vital organs based on need. Blood flow improves, inflammation is decreased, immunity is more robust.

Compassion gives rise to more resilient brains with improvements in cognitive function, intellectual abilities, focus and concentration, and mood.

What's all this gorgeous biology about?

Safety.

Compassion returns us to safety. When our suffering is held in present time, without judgement, we feel seen, heard, felt, and cared about. We *matter.* We reconnect to ourselves.

When an organism experiences safety, its resources can shift into building the resilience that supports its growth, its flow, and expanding into its potential and possibilities.

In this book we're working with *self*-compassion—the same compassion we extend to others we extend to ourselves. That way, we never have to suffer alone. We'll hold ourselves and all our feelings, sensations, and experiences

---

[46] Kelly McGonigal PhD. The Science of Compassion: A Modern Approach for Cultivating Empathy, Love, and Connection. 2016.

reverently, leading ourselves to safety so we can tend to our needs more robustly.

Self-compassion helps us live through challenge and change with growth. The inevitable suffering that is part of being human living a human life can be received with tenderness. It can be asked what it needs. Compassion helps us hold what's hard so we can grow and heal.

One thing though.

Compassion doesn't erase the hard things in life. It doesn't erase suffering. It doesn't erase fear or pain. Compassion helps you hold them. It helps you feel safe in them. Compassion leads you to the truth of who you are, holding you in your wholeness, opening you to *all* your life experiences. A wise teacher put it this way: "When you see the truth, you feel hurt, and when you allow yourself to feel hurt, compassion comes. If you don't allow yourself to feel hurt, you can't feel compassion. That's how our organism functions."[47]

In this spirit, everything we practice will begin and end with compassion. I heard someone liken self-compassion to a muscle. Like any muscle, you have to get your reps in for it to grow. To experience its strength. To feel safe.

Let's pause for a moment to grow and strengthen our compassion a bit more.

What are you struggling with? Today. In this moment. It may be what lead you to this book. It may be what you've identified in our previous practices. Name it, then close your eyes and hold it. Just hold. Breathe. Don't try to change or fix it. Resist judging it. Just give it space to belong to your lived experience in this moment. Without erasing anything you might feel about this struggle, the sensation, emotion, or experience you're holding right now, can you see it with compassion? Can you hold *yourself* with compassion? Just like you would a small child who struggles and needs you. And, who knows, this sensation or feeling may be a younger part of you engaged in the same struggle. Breathe into that part of yourself and hold it so tenderly.

Keep things simple, small, and slow.

We're not on the quick-fix train anymore, are we? We know nothing worthwhile is accomplished overnight. While the fast remedies of

---

[47] A H Almaas. Diamond Heart: Elements of the Real in Man, second edition. 2000.

conventional healthcare may help us feel better in the short-term (and sometimes we need short-term relief), what we're really looking for is healing. Optimal healing requires us to shift our equilibrium at the root cause level. For this, we must address our terrain way upstream in deep sustainable ways.

How do we best accomplish that?

We keep our tasks simple, our goals small, and our pace slow.

I know this flies in the face of how most of us have been taught to operate. We're consummate multi-taskers who bite off way more than we can chew. We walk fast, drive fast, live fast. We're always short on time. Why do you suppose self-help is a multibillion-dollar industry? It thrives on our overwhelm, promising to teach us organization, habit change, and take us on retreats from our crazy lives. Problem is, we can't yoga, meditate, or hyper-organize ourselves out of this mess. We have to change how we operate.

Neuroscience is clear: the simpler our tasks, the smaller our goals, and the less distracted we are, the more successful we can be at just about everything we set out to do. We learn more, perform better, and can make lasting change. And that's key, isn't it? Not a quick fix, but *lasting* change. A different way of living every day.

Our brains are designed to do one thing at a time, not multitask.[48] We can learn to do complex tasks well, but only in a sequential manner. We believe we're multitaskers, but we're not. Even the smallest tasks, done when our attention is elsewhere, will not be done as well as they could be. And the more we try to do at once? The less well we do anything.

We all know this if we really stop to think about it, because relentless multitasking is depleting, isn't it? However, science shows that many of us are not willing to admit to this. We're notoriously poor at self-assessment. For instance, drivers who talk on their phones perceive they are fully attentive to both the conversation they're having and the driving, though studies show attention to both falls off. The competency of distracted driving, even hands-free cell phone use, is comparable to driving drunk.[49]And we all know how it feels to talk to a driver whose attention fades in and out.

---

[48] Edita Poljac et al. New Perspectives on Human Multitasking. Psychological Research. 2018.

[49] David Strayer et al. A comparison of the cell phone driver and th drunk driver. Hum Factors. 2006. PMID 16884056.

Multitasking is stressful.[50] Not only does continuous distraction *feel* stressful, it's biologically challenging as well—cortisol levels stay high to help us cope, and levels of inflammation markers rise because our brains believe we're in trouble. Habitual multitasking makes us feel less safe. When we feel less safe, learning and performance fall way off as our attention and resources are diverted toward survival. It's a vicious cycle when we're trying to learn and create meaningful, lasting changes.

So, how do we optimize our chances for the healing and transformation we're seeking? Not just quick fixes or temporary reprieves?

We give ourselves permission to keep things simple, small, and slow.

Release what you think you know.

The only way to learn something new is to make space for it.

How do we do that?

We approach life's lessons with a beginner's mind. This doesn't mean we don't know anything. We know a lot. We also have knowing within us we didn't realize we had. But I'm not talking about knowing here. I'm talking about what we *think* we know—all the stories we keep telling ourselves.

We've all been 'storied' in a multitude of ways our entire lives, haven't we? We've been parented, schooled, medicalized, churched, coached, and enculturated. You name it. We've been bullied and shamed to stick to the stories we've been taught. And as we've explored, some of our most disempowering and tenacious stories have been about the nature of who we are, our bodies, and how to think about ourselves when we're sick and suffering. It's permeated all of us. We're well-versed in fixes for how we're broken, not understanding we're an equilibrium of genius. We've been taught thoroughly and learned well.

So far, the big new ideas in this book resonate, but when it comes to daily practice of our new knowledge? There'll be lots of competition from "how things have always been" and "what we've always known for sure."

If only the beginner's mind can learn new things, where do we begin? How do we release what we think we know?

---

[50] Deane Alban. The Cognitive Costs of Multitasking. Be Brain Fit.

Karyn Shanks MD

What if we start by identifying ourselves as *having* a beginner's mind? As being capable of learning new things? As being brave to let go of what we think we know, the stories we've always believed for sure?

Release what you *think* you know.

PAUSE AND BREATHE.

This is who I am.

Drop right in. Hands over your heart, let your heart know you're there. Close your eyes, breathe, and rest. Activate your safety circuit. Mind-breath-heart-hands-feet.

Hold yourself and any feelings or sensations that arise in your body with fierce compassion and safety.

Gently notice your thoughts. Without trying to fix or change them, breathe, allow your thoughts to be there. As they flow, see if you can soften. Soften your shoulders, soften your jaw, soften your hips, soften your skin. While allowing your thoughts, see if you can let go of any certainty they have. Let them soften. Without judging or rejecting your thoughts, can you make space for something new, something you don't yet know?

Use your powerful words.

I'm right here. I hold myself and all the feelings and sensations of my body with reverence. I notice my thoughts and stay soft even if they are certain. Even if they are doubtful. Even if they would hold me back.

I can hold my thoughts about the past, present, and future even as I choose something new. I can acknowledge how my thoughts have served

*me in the past even though they no longer do. I can speak and hold my
new truth in my heart. I can hold it all at the very same time.*

*I am a healer. I am already whole. I am filled to the brim with
gorgeous potential. This is who I am. This is who I choose to be.*

Practice and commit.

We're flowing even when it doesn't feel like flow. So, how do we achieve optimal flow, the zone? It's not accidental. It must be intentional. To harness the powerful energy of neuroplasticity, to get our biology activated to realize our goals and dreams, we must practice. Daily practice helps us acquire and deepen the well-developed skill set we must have to experience our zone. And remember, the zone isn't just for the exceptional few, the elite athletes, artists, and dancers. It's for all of us.

A well-ingrained habit requires daily practice for thirty to ninety days, depending on who you ask. Point is, it takes practice to create the new mind grooves of neuroplasticity that allow us to learn and succeed at that learning. Ideally practice occurs when conditions for learning are optimal—when your energy is best, your mind is the most alert, and you are not distracted so the task has your undivided attention. But don't get hung up on waiting for perfection. If we wait for the perfect time, perfect energy, perfect conditions, we won't practice at all.

One of the greatest motivators for me is knowing what's at stake when I avoid practicing what I need. I won't get to feel the way I want to feel. I won't get to unleash my potential. I won't get to heal my suffering. And there's a clock ticking. This is my finite life. If I don't do it now, I might not get to. Interviews with people on their death beds reveals their deepest regrets aren't what they did do, but what they *didn't*.[51]

---

[51] Bronnie Ware. Top Five Regrets of the Dying: A Life Transformed by the Dearly Departing. 2019.

Karyn Shanks MD

How do we manage our excuses, the stories that keep us from getting started with our new habits?

I don't have time. I don't know how. It hurts. It's too hard. I just need one more day.

First, as always, be compassionate toward yourself. Excuses don't make us bad, just vulnerable. We're all vulnerable when we ask to change. *All* of us.

Then, start somewhere. Anywhere. One small, fierce step.

Stay relentlessly curious.

Our final agreement is to stay curious. *Relentlessly* curious.

Why?

Curiosity immediately frees us from preconceived outcomes because it anchors us to the present. It's always asking questions, "what is this, how can I know it better, what does it need, what's possible here?"

Without curiosity, our stories run the show. *This is my pain, it's this thing, it's mine, it's never going to end, there's no hope for me.* Or our excuses. *I don't have time. I don't know how. It hurts. It's too hard. I just need one more day.*

Curiosity transcends all that. It opens us to our unknown possibilities.

Curiosity is such a relief as it releases us from having to know everything. It looks at the same pain and refuses to name it anything at all. When pain becomes a curiosity it's "oh my, that's so interesting, feel how it's kind of pinchy and it comes and goes, I wonder why that is, I wonder what would happen if I ..."

See, with curiosity running the show instead of our stories and preconceived notions, there's an opening for new ways of seeing things.

Curiosity looks at suffering with wonder and openness. It asks, "what are you and what do you need?" Rather than the reductive, "what do we call you, what's your name, what's the diagnosis, how do they fix you?"

Beyond all the possibilities that curiosity opens us to, it also creates space between us and everything we notice, even our thoughts. Curiosity shifts us into being an observer. As the observer, we get to witness things in whole different ways, closer to what they are, and never locked into a preconceived notion. We get to see what we may have never seen before. The curious observer is positioned to learn and imagine possibilities. When we already know for sure, we can't learn, we can't imagine.

Curiosity gives us immediate agency. Because we're controlling the narrative. We're always asking questions. Curiosity keeps us running our own show.

So, let's be curious. We'll shift from identifying with our suffering to observing it. Once we can observe it, we can learn and feel other things, like joy. One of my teachers says, "Joy is not the absence of suffering. Joy is the presence of curiosity. It is the presence of discovery."[52] Discovery is why we're here. It's the only path to healing. Relentless curiosity lets us *live* our healing.

UNBROKEN TOOLS.

Tools are essential for any worthwhile journey.

This book is your tool. Underline what speaks to you and dog ear your favorite pages. Refer to them as often as you need to. If you're listening to an audio or electronic version of this book, take lots of notes and keep them handy. Better yet, gift yourself a hard copy as well. I love holding tools in my hands!

We must also consider our own bodies as tools. The amazing reservoirs of our wisdom and courageous acts of transformation.

We use our breath a lot too, don't we? Breath is an essential tool. Breath connects us to ourselves and all our experiences. It directs us toward the sensations and feelings we need to know—the language of our bodies. Breath tethers us to present time, our only true reality. And we can use our breath to regulate our nervous systems, to soothe and soften what hurts.

Let me introduce you to a few more tools I find essential for the daily practice of healing.

The Life School point of view (POV). If everything we experience is Life School, nothing is ever wasted. Even mistakes and failures. It all has meaning. We learn from it all.

To cultivate a robust Life School POV, we practice two things. First, we stay relentlessly curious. Curiosity keeps us in our flow—learning, growing, and in control of our narratives. Then, the hard but necessary part. We accept full responsibility for how we manage what's happened to us. We call back all the

---

[52] AH Almaas. Diamond Heart: Elements of the Real in Man, second edition. 2000.

energy we've committed to blame and holding onto the past. This energy is precious, finite, and can go to better use. Letting go of blame doesn't mean we weren't harmed. It doesn't mean no one was wrong. But when our energy is tethered to past events, we're *living* in the past. We can't grow in the past.

The Life School POV shifts us into the present. It doesn't bypass the truth about those bad things that happened but holds us in strength. It lets the bad things fertilize our growth.

The Lens of Love. Always love, right? *Always love.* In everything we do. Even as we hold our hardest, darkest feelings, we do it out of love. You know that by now, right? Love isn't all soft and blissful. Love isn't just what makes us feel good. Love can be the hardest damned thing of all.

The Lens of Possibilities. This is the lens we wish guided our science, our medicine, and our futures. It's a lens with a flexible aperture. It opens wide to show us the bird's eye view of what's way upstream, the multiple causes to our problems, and the gorgeous complexity of dynamic human lives woven with the natural world. It shows us our possibilities. This lens can also focus on what's right in front of us so we can get to work on that one small thing that most needs our attention in this moment. It helps us see with laser focus and clarity without getting stuck.

A Journal, gold stars, sticky notes, and permission slips. Finally, writing is indispensable. Writing is a portal too. It helps access wisdom. And it helps us keep a record of the wisdom as it emerges. If I didn't keep a journal of those genius thoughts that pop out of me from time to time, I'd totally forget them!

I think longhand journaling is best. There is a hand-brain-soul connection that is important to activate. Use it to check in with yourself every day and don't forget to give yourself gold stars and A+'s! Sticky notes are great for thoughts and ideas on the fly. They can be attached to the next blank page in your journal.

Not a longhand writer? No worries. Use your laptop or voice memo system.

PAUSE AND BREATHE.

Give yourself permission to heal.

Permission is powerful. And we don't need outside sources — "experts"—to deliver it. We can give *ourselves* permission.

Let's give it a whirl by writing yourself a permission slip.

Grab one of your sticky notes and a pen.

Feel free to use my words or conjure your own.

Dear (your name),

I give you my full permission to heal. Permission to activate all the healing potential within you. Permission to brave the next step, the uncertainty. Permission to slow down, to rest. Permission to open your mind to something new. Permission to believe in yourself, your genius, your potential and possibilities, the Earth, herself.

I give you permission.

Love, Me

Write this longhand, then stick it where you can see it over the course of the day. I also like to fold them up and stick them in my pocket. It feels like a talisman giving me strength.

MANY MUSES.

Every worthwhile journey is inspired by muses—the guides, mentors, and sources of encouragement that soothe, nudge, and energize us on our life's journey.

Outer muses.

Some of our muses are obvious. They're the family, friends, and advisors who know us well. Or they might be our mentors from afar—the favorite authors, teachers, artists, and sages who, through resonant words or sounds captivate us, remind us of some truth we need, and help bring forth our own creative genius.

Generously immerse yourself in what these muses have to say—their words are *meant* for you. I have many well-worn books I keep in key places to help anchor and inspire me. My muses' words can be lifelines. We're never meant to take our journeys alone.

Inner muses.

We're also going to tap into our *inner* muses. These sources of internal guidance have been with us since before we were born. They've tended, lead, supported, and taken charge of us in countless ways. They've kept us alive and shown us our genius.

I like to call these inner muses "wisdom centers," because they converge in complex and mysterious ways to form a wisdom circuit. Learning to tap into and trust this wisdom circuit make us incredibly smart and whole.

What are they?

The head, heart, and gut.

The head is the brain that observes and discerns. It can read the room, tell us if we're safe, and move us out of harm's way. It is the center of our questions—researching, analyzing, and figuring things out. While the head can befuddle us with drama and mistruths, when we stay curious, it graces us with insights and discernment. The head brings its insightful wisdom to bear on our stories: which ones serve? Which ones don't? What's a better story to tell?

The heart is the brain that connects us and knows who we truly are. It holds us and others with compassion and empathy. It is a powerful electromagnetic compass for love. Our intuitive heart wisdom knows who we are. Through its distinctive feelings and sensations in our bodies (*hands over heart, let your heart know you're there*) it tells us: what do we love? What is worthy of our love? What serves love?

The gut is the brain that protects and assimilates. It calmly tells us what's up. Through its enteric nervous system, the gut 'digests' our environment into wisdom. Without a hint of drama, this quiet yet decisive voice delivers up our 'gut feelings.' These subtle intuitive messages about safety, protection, and immunity are never wrong. But can we hear them?

The head, heart, and gut interconnect to create a powerful wisdom circuit. This wisdom circuit is always operating, always in service of you. Our work is to hear this internal wisdom and leverage it to our advantage.

As we continue our work together, do we need to speak the language of head, heart, and gut, learning to distinguish them? No. We'll speak our own language that blends the three. By tuning in and learning to read the wisdom of our bodies, our inner and outer muses will all be there.

CHAPTER FOURTEEN
Rise through trauma.

My client Mary came to see me because of crippling inflammatory arthritis. She was on heavy drugs to relieve the pain. She'd been in a long-standing co-dependent relationship with her daughter, never speaking her truth, always walking on eggshells trying not to make her angry. She started therapy and began exploring what her truth was. She began by writing about it in her private journal. In time, she was speaking her truth to her daughter. It was hard work, but not only did she feel immeasurably freer, she was able to heal their relationship. And not just that, her joint pain completely resolved off all medications. The story behind Mary's story wasn't about a disease, it was about being able to be herself and speak her truth. Suppressed emotions and persistent sadness drive shifts in genetic expression that lead to immune activation and increased inflammation because the body doesn't feel safe. Persistent suffering also drives the panoply of behaviors that do the same. Merging body with mind and emotions allows us to complete the story, to go further upstream to understand more completely what's going on, to heal more deeply.

This is not a book about trauma, per se, but it comes up *a lot*, doesn't it? Trauma, even if we never thought to call it that, is part of our human lives. It shows up in *all* of us in some form at some time. It especially shows up when we try to change. And while the urge to sidestep it is perfectly natural (who wants to hurt, right?), if we don't learn from it, we won't grow. Reckoning with trauma is self-discovery. It's why we're here. When we get to know where we've disconnected from ourselves, though it hurts, it also gives us grace. More than growing into our potential, we're reminded to be more tender with ourselves and others. We're all human. We all hurt.

On this path of healing, a huge part of what we're asking for is change. Change that's good. Change that we want and need. But sometimes a thing we set out to change surprises us. We thought it'd be a snap. So, why did I just crumble into a heap over not eating a cookie, for God's sake? Or trying to move to an earlier bedtime? Or going on a social media fast? Right? See, these old habits aren't just habits. These are the strategies we've used—the cookie, old sleep habits, and social media, all kinds of habits and substances—to help us manage suffering, awkwardness, anxiety, you name it, perhaps for a very long time without realizing that was what we were doing. Sometimes our habits are propping us up. When we try to change them our suffering hits us between the eyes. But many of these strategies, genius as they are to soothe and console and sometimes *save* us, have also led to suffering. Many of them have taken us straight to becoming sick. They *must* be reckoned with.

These trauma experiences embedded in our pain and suffering are often what I call "stories behind the story." They're what we discover to be true behind the story we thought we knew so well. These stories emerge when we try to change.

The story of "I need to stop eating the cookies to lose weight and feel better," becomes "I soothe my pain with these cookies, and when I stop, I feel the pain."

The story of "If I go to bed earlier, get more sleep, I'll feel more rested," becomes "When I go to bed earlier, I feel guilty for all the things I leave undone."

The story of "These social media rabbit holes I go down are wasting all my time," becomes "When I stop looking at social media, I feel left out and alone."

We all know these stories, don't we? They're all signatures of trauma, the ways we've disconnected from ourselves and our true needs to soothe our wounds.

Remember, *trauma is not a character flaw*. Our trauma strategies are not failures. They're not something wrong or damaged about us. They address what happened inside us when the bad thing happened, or when the good thing *didn't* happen when we needed it most. And mostly they're how we managed the pain of not being held in compassion and safety when we were hurt, and when our hurt *wasn't repaired*. Our trauma strategies are how we've survived in the most savvy and magnificent ways. Even when we neglected our needs or our true selves to stay safe. We became quiet, the good girl, the caretaker; or we dimmed our intelligence, our light. To feel better, we turned to habits that weren't good for us. None of that was wrong. Much of it was pure genius. Even if we've suffered from those survival strategies, the old habits served us when we needed them to.[53]

Sometimes the story behind the story of illness is something that happened first before the symptoms arose, like with Mary. The illness becomes what's in the foreground, what we can see right now, what we seek help for. When the illness emerges, it's all we *can* see. It's all we were taught to see.

How about the girl for whom there was a story behind the story *behind the story*? The first story was about recurrent separate injuries and fatigue. The story behind that story was about EDS hypermobility syndrome that tied all those problems together and helped her address them more effectively. But there was another layer—a story behind the second story. That story was about a girl whose body was perpetually in survival mode and used exercise as a strategy to feel good. To feel more relaxed, more alive, and able to focus. But more than that. She used exercise to feel good about *herself*, like a worthwhile human being. The longer her runs and more grueling her workouts, the more accomplished she felt and the less anxiety she experienced about who she was. With so much at stake, it was hard to pull back when subtle signs of injury occurred. Tightness and exhaustion did not slow her down.

That girl was me. While I'm a work in progress and have had lots of good people helping me, I can read the signs of injury now. I can pull back when I need to. I have other strategies, healthier strategies, that address my need to feel worthwhile at a much deeper level.

Obviously, we can't work with the details of your personal trauma here, or mine, or anyone's. It is nonetheless something that's landed in all of us and is bound to show up as we live our healing, so we'll be talking about it and working on strategies to address it as we move through our steppingstones. We'll see how it's part of our genius. How even though it has made us suffer, it has also helped. Because many of us have come to believe our painful feelings and addictions are blemishes or personal weaknesses that we must hide and can't possibly get over (lord knows we've tried!).

From now on we see trauma for what it is. An *equilibrium*. Just like everything else we've been talking about in this book. Trauma is an

---

[53] Zaya Benazzo and Maurizio Benazzo. The Wisdom of Trauma. 2021. A powerful documentary about the work of Gabor Maté MD that looks at trauma as the root of our deepest wounds, an invisible force that shapes all of our lives.

equilibrium of disconnection. The addiction, anxiety, depression, feelings of unworthiness, and all the manifestations of trauma we call "diseases" are equilibria, where we've landed as we've adapted and shaped our lives around unresolved trauma inside us.

You know the good news, though, right? We can shift that equilibrium. We can shift all our equilibria no matter how painful they are, no matter how stuck we feel. That's why we're here. We're *not* stuck. We're *not* damaged. We don't need to be fixed. We need to be held with the fiercest compassion, reverence, and curiosity for what happened to us. We need to be asked, "what do you need?" *That's* what shifts us.

You may choose to work with someone trained in trauma therapy.[54] For our purposes here, we'll always hold ourselves with the fiercest reverence and protect our vulnerabilities. We'll begin and end everything we do with compassion. We'll stay tender, soft, and curious through all our work together. We'll breathe and chant and use our powerful words. We'll tell our new story. About how we're freaking geniuses. How we're expanding into our wholeness. How we rise.

PAUSE AND BREATHE.

What to do with trauma when it arises.

How do you recognize trauma when it shows up in your efforts to change, grow, and heal?

Recall what trauma is.

It's what happened *inside you* when:

---

[54] These psychotherapeutic approaches to trauma go deep and are interactive, giving the client agency and responsibility for their healing, while held in safety, compassion, and relationship: Compassionate Inquiry and Internal Family Systems.

- The bad things that happened weren't repaired.
- The good things that should have happened but didn't weren't repaired.

What happened inside was then carried with you, showing up as uncomfortable sensations, energy states, and feelings. Sometimes as full-blown illnesses. You may know what happened and can tell the story on an intellectual level, but the feelings hang on. They are the relentless painful burdens and the unexpected suffering that hits us between the eyes when we're not expecting it.

How is trauma repaired?

By returning to safety.

Repair of trauma can only occur when we're returned to safety and held there for as long as we need it. Our friend offers their heart-felt apology for hurting our feelings and explains themselves. Our parent apologizes for yelling and explains how it wasn't our fault, it was theirs. Our spouse stays at our bedside every day we're in the hospital and so vulnerable. We learn to hold ourselves. Countless examples in which we're seen, heard, and loved. We're held in connection. We're safe.

When we're very young or vulnerable, our need for repair and safety is met by someone who loves us beyond measure. Our parents or caregivers, our life partners, and friends. When we become adults, many of us can meet this need for ourselves in many circumstances. We can love ourselves beyond measure.

How do we love ourselves beyond measure to repair and return to safety?

First, love is a verb. We often think of it as an emotion, and there is an emotional quality that goes with love. But the love that counts, the love that shows up for us when we're in need, is a verb.

Therefore, we can *learn* to love ourselves beyond measure. We can *practice* loving ourselves beyond measure.

It's important to recognize trauma when it shows up. For our purposes here, I want you to consider anything arising within you that gets in the way of healthy, needed, well-planned change as signatures of trauma. This could be resistance, stubbornness, hopelessness, fear, anxiety, sadness, depression, excuses, or feeling deprived. Even if we're overstating it, let's work with these that way for now.

You've made a commitment to change something about your life so you can feel better. You've chosen one small thing to work on. How about the cookies? Shall we give up cookies? Okay, let's do that.

You set the plan. Then the witching hour comes, the time in the day when you're used to having the cookie. For some of you, it's easy as pie. You breeze through. No cookie. No resistance. No suffering. It's a done deal. Hallelujah.

But some of us have a very different experience. Cookie time comes and just thinking about it brings on a tsunami of suffering. We feel sad. There are tears. We tell all kind of stories. About abandonment, deprivation, and how freaking hard life is. *What?*

What do you do?

Pull yourself up by the bootstraps like you've been taught to do? Get over it? Quit being such a big baby?

Are those ways of showing up as the one who loves you beyond measure?

Of course not.

The cookie was a genius strategy when it was conceived. It soothed the pain of trauma. Not to be taken lightly or dismissed, is it? It was your version of repair and return to safety because they didn't happen when you needed them.

Now, the *source* of your pain and the details of what happened to you can be thoroughly explored within the support and safety of therapy.

But I want you to know what powerful thing you can do right now. And what powerful thing you can do every day even though you have a therapist. (Unbelievable as it is, there are therapists who may not teach you this crucial step.)

This is how love becomes a verb.

How to love yourself beyond measure, a practice:

- Address that part of you who's sad, tearful, and flipping out over her (insert your own pronouns) absent cookie (or whatever it may be) and welcome her like your most beloved. Say, "I'm right here, you're welcome, all your feelings are welcome here with me." And I want you to mean it. This hurting part of you is yearning for you to mean it.
- If you've ever judged or berated her, gotten impatient with her feelings, tried to fix or change her, or rush her before she's ready, tell her you're sorry right now. Literally say it: "I'm so sorry, sweetheart, I'm here right now."
- Taking your time, give this part of yourself all your attention, and send this part of you (whatever sensations or feelings showed up for you, are *you*) compassion, saying your words, letting her know she's safe with you.
- Don't rush this part of you, stay curious. Let her know you see her, hear her, hold her, she *matters*.
- Ask her what she needs from you right now. Literally ask. To be held? To have you listen? To not judge? Whatever comes up is just right.

- Ask her what she needs from you going forward. You can't form a lasting bond of safety in *any* relationship by showing up for a few minutes one time, am I right? Make a commitment to show up every day, as often as she needs.
- Make good on your promises.

That's love as a verb, loving yourself beyond measure.

And what about the judge? What do we do with that part of you?

The judge shows up in all of us. And they're not just you, the evildoer, beating up on a traumatized child. You get that?

We all carry the judge in our psyches. The judge keeps us safe by making sure we follow through on all the prescriptions for behavior we've been given by our families, institutions, and culture. Just a protector whose traumatized too. Hold her with the same love. Love yourself beyond measure.

One more thing.

Self-love is neither an achievement (for doing all the "right" things in life) or a state of grace (for having healed "correctly"). It's a practice. We *learn* it. And even when we slip up (we all most certainly will), we benefit from every bit of the practice. Period.

CHAPTER FIFTEEN
The *Un*Broken Core Resilience Steppingstones.

Wthese (good for you!) and wonder what the heck I mean for others. Either way, you'll land where you feel guided. And *you* will be your guide. Your inner healer will know and without the slightest fanfare you'll see where you need to be. Trust that.

First, what do I mean by *core* resilience?

The core of healing, the core of wholeness, the core of flow, the core of who we are and are meant to be. Resilience is the strength, energy, and adaptability to successfully navigate the challenges and changes of life. And more than that. Resilience is how we *get to* flow with robustness, trust, and ease. What does that say about core resilience? That's right. It's the lifeforce behind our most sparkly wholeness. Core resilience is how we *live* our most sparkly wholeness.

Our *Unbroken* core resilience steppingstones are the practices that help us achieve that most sparkly wholeness. These are the essential transformational practices that activate our terrain, our TotalGloriousOneness, *us*, through profound positive shifts in genetic expression, biology, energy, and our human genius.

With agreements made, tools in hand, and muses at the ready, we're prepared to work our *Unbroken* core resilience steppingstones. If the terrain of healing is effectively our roadmap to our TotalGloriousOneness (TGO), showing us what makes us *us*, suggesting where we need to go and what to do to shift into an equilibrium of resilience and healing, our *Unbroken* core resilience steppingstones are the practices that *activate* this terrain. Our steppingstones literally shift our genetic expression, our biology, our stories, our actions, and all our outcomes—they shift *us*—up out of the mud, lighter, freer. We rise.

Why do I call them "steppingstones" instead of, say, "blueprint," "strategy," or "master plan?"

Imagine steppingstones strategically placed in your garden so you can walk amongst your favorite plantings without slipping in the mud. Or like stones in a stream, where you shrewdly choose to plant your feet so you can cross without soaking your shoes. Steppingstones anchor us as we explore. They help us avoid the muck while gently guiding our way.

Steppingstones allow us to choose.

Moving from where you are now to where you'd like to be, do you want to be told what to do (by an "expert" who may not know you as well as you know yourself)? Or would you rather see the lay of the land for yourself, preferably from a birds-eye view that lets you see the entire vast landscape of choices you can make?

Steppingstones become our life's touchstones. We never truly land, right? We step. Sometimes so lightly we don't stay very long. We step from one to the next, to the next, and back again. We never stay in one place. There are never single options for our healing.

That's how I want the *Unbroken* core resilience steppingstones to be: *yours. For* you and *by* you, from your own perspective, about what you want and need right now, able to move freely among them as you see fit, with no "right" way to step.

This is how I invite you to use this chapter. Allow your inner healer to guide you on a journey that's uniquely yours, defined by you, guided by you. Think of me as your curator of highly discerned tried-and-true options for healing in the deepest possible ways. As mentor with perspectives drawn from vast lived experience—my own as well as my clients'—joined with insights from the 21st century science of directable human potential{ XE "directable human potential, science of" }, the science of possibilities. But here is the most important thing I've learned working with thousands of people over the decades of my career: the strategy that works best is the strategy that's *yours.*

The first three *Unbroken* core resilience steppingstones are what I consider to be foundational to the others:

- Be Present.
- Balance.
- Rest.

While all the steppingstones are crucial, the first three prepare you for the others. In fact, if you work deeply with these first, you may glide through all the rest.

First, let me show you the nine *Unbroken* core resilience steppingstones. When you consciously tend them, these will activate your terrain of healing, your TotalGloriousOneness (TGO), and expand you into your most sparkly wholeness.

The *Un*Broken
Core Resilience Steppingstones

BE PRESENT.
I reconnect to myself through gentle self-awareness, self-compassion, and self-agency, activating my most sparkly wholeness.

I ask: What do I need?

BALANCE.
I trust the wind. I flow with ease. I grow strong roots. Like a sturdy tree.

I ask: How do I anchor my flow, trust the wind?

MOVE.
I move and breathe and have my being.

I ask: How do I move with purpose and joy?

REST.
I restore myself with all the sleep, rest, and play I deserve.

I ask: How do I support my most Divine being?

LIVE YOUR PURPOSE.
I live and love as my most authentic being.

I ask: Who am I at my core? What do I love?

NOURISH.
I am exactly what I eat and drink.

I ask: How do I wisely choose nourishment for my body?

LOVE.
I love myself and all my parts. I hold them in safety with the gentleness they deserve.

I ask: How can I welcome myself—all iterations of me—with tenderness?

LIBERATE.
I let go of the roadblocks to my healing.

I ask: What do I need to get out of my way?

FEEL.
I f trust my feelings, sensations, and energy states as the wisdom of my body.

I ask: What do I notice in my body? Can I welcome it all as my authentic truth?

Each steppingstone will be rolled out with core lessons and foundational practices. At the end, you will be asked to make three promises to help you live the steppingstone authentically, activating the healing potential within you.

As you explore and practice your new steppingstones, be sure to lean heavily on your five agreements:

- Hold yourself with fierce compassion and safety.
- Keep things simple, small, and slow.
- Release what you *think* you know.
- Practice and commit.
- Stay relentlessly curious.

Also, keep your tools close at hand and check in with your muses often.

We'll begin with the most profound healing activator imaginable. The steppingstone which puts you in the driver's seat of all your healing, all your personal outcomes, all your success, and all the magnificence of your human life: *Be present.*

CHAPTER SIXTEEN
First *Un*Broken Core Resilience Steppingstone:

BE PRESENT.

I see through my own eyes. I hear with my own ears. I feel with my own heart. I know with my own gut. This is who I am.

I reconnect to myself through gentle self-awareness, self-compassion, and self-agency. I feel safe and can thrive in this tenderly curated connection. As I do, I get to experience what it means to be the most alive, the most who I am. I get to heal most robustly. This is how I live my most sparkly authentic wholeness.

Some words are *so* misunderstood. Words so beautiful to me seem lost on others, like "presence," "mindfulness," "conscious awareness," and "self-reflection." Even "meditation." They're viewed with suspicion, like they've dropped in from another planet. More than unrelatable, they're scary.

Some might say that being present isn't a choice. *Of course*, we're present, what other way is there to be? I felt that way too, until a time when I realized I truly *wasn't* present.

Twenty years or so ago, I was driving to work along a stretch of country backroad I love so much. As I approached a familiar bend in the road, I was greeted by my favorite barn off to the left. Built in the early 1900's, it's distressed red planks and steep Shaker roof tell old stories of midwestern farm life. On both sides of the road were fields of wild prairie as far as my eyes could see. On that day, the early morning sun struck the wild sunflowers from where it was rising in the east, igniting them in gold, engulfing me in luminous golden light. For those few sweet moments as I rounded the curve, I was one with my prairie, one with the golden light. Stunned, I slowed my car so I wouldn't drive off the road. A thought emerged ever-so-quietly into my awareness, "my life's purpose is about being, not doing, and being right here in this golden light, I am complete, just as I am." The thought was so subtle I might have missed it at any other time. It was a simple, gentle expression of something I'd been chewing on a lot in those days, but as those ordinary words blended with that extraordinary experience, I instantly got it. I knew they were more than just musings of a blissed-out, wandering mind. It was a message for me, a calm but discernable shot of wisdom I'd been asking for my entire life.

When I reflect on that time, I know it was not magic, but a profound moment when being acutely tuned in—*present*—allowed me to receive something incredible, something my soul needed. It was only possible because I'd been practicing being more present through meditation and writing, practices I showed up for every day. To be honest, it could be a slog in those early days of fitting my meditation and writing practices in at the crack of dawn before my boys woke up and we were catapulted into our days. But by showing up every day no matter what, even if for just five minutes (I used to call the short sessions "turbo meditations," and while it felt like a joking oxymoron, I now understand the deep benefits of micro-dosing self-care), it primed me to notice the morning light. It primed me to experience the luminosity of the prairie sunflowers. And on that morning, I believe it primed me to receive the quiet yet clear message I needed to guide the rest of my life.

That message stuck. Since that time, my life has become more about being and less about doing. More about listening and less seeking. More appreciation of what I have and less searching for what I think I need. More connection with what's right here *in* me and *all around* me. I'm more centered, calm, and observant. I'm more intimately connected to myself, my people, nature, and the world around me. I feel so much better. And when I don't? I know the world isn't ending. I'll find my way.

That's what presence is about.

Presence is the awareness, the paying attention, the tuning in that shifts us. It primes us to fully experience our lives. To fully experience *ourselves*—our feelings, sensations, and energy states. To realize we *have* a self to be present to. A self that matters. A self that has needs we can identify. To know our needs

Karyn Shanks MD

matter. To hear the life-shifting insights. To see the sunflowers ablaze with gold, and all the ordinary everyday things in between.

In this way, presence is both a practice and a prize. It's the practice we must learn and show up for that shifts us into an observant existence. It's the prize that gifts us with the incredible things we get to notice, that we wouldn't notice otherwise.

Beyond awareness, presence is the path to all the consciously made choices we make for ourselves as we take this journey of healing. Presence shifts us toward our best choices.

So, what am I saying?

Consider why we're here. Why we're reading this book, working through these practices.

Because we want to heal. We want our lives back, our selves back, our most sparkly wholeness to emerge.

What is all that?

It's self-development, isn't it? Healing is a process of growth.

We talked about healing as wholeness, as the primary urgeof all Nature. That it's an equilibrium inside us, always operating and always doing its best given present circumstances. That's all true. But healing is *also a verb*. It's a process we practice. It's a process we use to shift our present circumstances. In this sense, healing-the-verb is growth and self-development that we consciously direct.

There's just one absolute requirement for the practice of healing.

Presence. Self-awareness. Self-engagement. Whatever you choose to call it. Without our fully engaged selves, there will be no growth, no self-development, no desired change, no healing-the-verb, and no sparkly wholeness.

So.

Presence is our first *Unbroken* core resilience steppingstone. It's the one that is the foundation for all the rest. It makes all the rest *possible*.

When you practice presence like your life depends on it, you get to fall more in love with yourself and the world around you in ways you could never have imagined before. Your life will fall into two overarching eras: "before" and "after." I'm not exaggerating.

WHY IS PRESENCE SO HARD?

So, what's so hard about all that when the payoff is so huge? Why is presence such a 'thing?' Why don't we trust it? Why does it feel so foreign? And why do we have to *practice*? Seems like a process so foundational to human growth and healing should come naturally.

I think it does come naturally. We're born with presence. Look at children, how they laugh and play and imagine and create their way through their days. How fully in their bodies they are, touching their fingers and toes, teaching themselves to walk, then run, ride a bike, playing and creating and experimenting all day. How fully in their feelings they are, freely expressing exuberant joy and soul-crushing sadness without censoring themselves. Children are magical embodied creatures fully attuned to present time and present moment experience of sensations, feelings, and energy states. They practice all day long, calling it "play" or "my favorite things." They respond to their own needs with absolute authenticity.

Then we "grow up." We're taught other ways to be. What's "appropriate" and allowed in our families-communities-culture. We're parented and schooled and coached. We're given templates for successful adulting with lessons to memorize, milestones to achieve, and feelings to keep in check. We learn focus, discipline, and hard work. We learn "how to be nice," "how to get along," and "how to become successful people."

This can leave us traumatized. Our needs as magical exuberant authentically embodied young children weren't met. We traded being who we authentically are for survival. We stayed quiet, small, and obedient. We did what was necessary for safety and connection.

For many of us, this process means we lose connection to our bodies, to present time, to our authentic creative expression, and to our real lived experiences. We disconnect from *ourselves*. We may no longer know how we feel. So used to being told what to do and how to be, we may not know what we want or need.

While presence is our birthright, *we unlearn it.* In many ways, we're bullied out of it.

While unlearning presence may be "normal," because it's what a family-community-culture does, it doesn't help us heal. It leads us away from our authentic sparkly wholeness. It keeps us sick, suffering, and stuck.

Karyn Shanks MD

In this *Unbroken* core resilience steppingstone, we're calling presence back. We're reconnecting to ourselves, all our experiences, our potential and possibilities.

PRESENCE IN TIME AND PLACE.

We'll work with presence in two dimensions: time and place.

First, we'll learn to use tools to help anchor us in present time.

Why is this important?

Because healing can *only* occur in the present. Not the past. Not the future. Right here. Period. Everything worth anything *only* exists in present time. If we're tethered to the past or the future, we miss some fundamental fraction of our real human experience, of who we authentically are. It's too precious to miss.

We'll work with presence as a place. The only place we can truly be in present time. Our bodies. The gorgeous repositories of our wholeness—our biology, structure, function, minds, feelings, experiences, and all our connections to self, family, friends, community, culture, planet. That's right, our TotalGloriousOneness (TGO), the magnificent terrain that is us, the roadmap to our healing.

We'll work with active embodied awareness in present time. Attuning to what's inside us with curiosity and compassion. Shifting into safety and connection. Shifting gently into change.

The simplest hard lessons you'll ever learn.

REESTABLISH EMBODIED SELF-AWARENESS.

To thrive as humans, we need to be seen, heard, known, and welcomed for exactly who we are. Like water and air, we need all this.

But we've established this isn't what always happens. We've talked a great deal about why many of us don't feel seen, heard, known, or welcomed as we are. We've explored the family, community, cultural, intergenerational, and personal trauma we've all been touched by.

We adapted to survive in the best ways we knew how. Along the way, we disconnected from parts of ourselves. We couldn't help it, it's what we had to do, how our organism functions. Many of us disconnected from our own bodies. We don't know what we feel. We may suffer but we are incapable of describing what we're experiencing. Or we don't feel anything. We're numb. Maybe we feel the adrenaline, the high, the exhaustion. But we scarcely hear ourselves think, much less feel. And when we slow down? We don't feel safe.

I've seen clients sob because their pain and suffering are unbearable, but they can't describe any of it. Some can't even point to a location in their bodies where it hurts. Others know they don't feel well, their energy is low, but they're so checked out from their experiences they can't tell the story of their suffering. They don't recall the timeline of events and feel bewildered when I ask for details. Countless more spent years languishing in suffering they believed there was no hope for before they asked for help.

When we're disconnected from ourselves and our experiences, there's only one thing to do: re-establish embodied self-awareness. We have to "get back into the body."

So, for these lessons, we're calling ourselves back.

Back to present time. Back to self-awareness. Back to our bodies. Back to our feelings, sensations, and energy states. Back to ourselves and our wholeness.

The kind of self-awareness that allows us to feel safe is compassionate. It holds us exactly as we are. It welcomes us exactly as we are. It says, "I see you, I hold space for you just as you are, your needs matter, *you* matter, you and your needs are worthy of my full attention."

Self-awareness that gets us is tuned in with curiosity. It witnesses us without trying to change or fix us. More than witness, it tunes in to us with actively engaged interest. It always asks, "what do you need, how can I help you?"

Self-awareness that is tuned in with compassion and curiosity strengthens us. It allows us to act on behalf of ourselves. It helps us move in the world with agency.

So, for our purposes in this steppingstone, we'll work with presence in two foundational ways to reestablish embodied self-awareness.

- Embodied self-awareness with compassion and curiosity: I welcome myself and all my sensations, feelings, and energy states. I create safety for my most authentic self to emerge.

- Embodied self-awareness with agency: *I identify and ask for what I need.*

EMBODIED SELF-AWARENESS FIRST PRACTICES.

Let's start with practices to help us get back into our bodies. Our bodies are foundationally us, though many of us have checked out of our bodies without realizing it. Our bodies connect us to present time and connect us to present moment awareness. These practices will help us both get back into our bodies and feel safe in them.

We'll begin with three simple presence practices:

- Breathe.
- Where are you?
- Breathe, notice your body with compassion and curiosity, create safety.

Breathe.

Here's what I want you to do: place hands over your heart, letting your heart know you're there. Close your eyes, take one deep breath in and out through your nose. Then take another big breath and sigh it out. Take one more, slowing it way down, really noticing how it feels.

There. You did it. That, my friend, was self-awareness. That one simple pause to both breathe and notice yourself breathing.

What did you notice? Was it a piece of cake? Familiar? Awkward? Real?

My point in having you take just a few fully conscious breaths is to show you how presence is not rocket-science. We're not scaling mountain tops here. Presence does not have to be torture. And there are literally no rules other than you must show up for it. Since it may be new for you, it will take practice to get comfortable with it. Practice creates neuroplastic mind grooves that let self-awareness become a piece of cake.

Why start with breath?

There is a whole domain of science on the effects of conscious breathing on our physiology.[55] It slows us down, pulls us into present time, and helps us feel safe through direct effects on the vagus nerve and parasympathetic nervous system. It's all real. Physically, mentally, emotionally real. But to be present we don't have to know how it all works. We just have to be open to its power.

Breath links our awareness to our bodies which can *only* exist in present time. If all we ever do is notice our breath, in whatever we do, we'll be fully engaged with present time, we'll be activating self-awareness. You can't consciously tend to your breath without noticing it.

So, just breathe. This part's simple, isn't it?

Where are you?

No, I'm not being silly. Stop right now, close your eyes, breathe, and tell me. Where are you in your body?

Are you in your head? Your chest or midsection? Or maybe you're somewhere outside your body. Check in right now and identify where you are. Don't over-think this. What's your very first impression?

Place your hands where you sense you are. Now take several deep breaths without trying to change or fix anything, because there is no wrong answer. You are where you are. Allow your breath. Allow yourself.

Now take a slow deep breath and see if you can follow it from beginning to end as it moves through you. Can you feel the cool air enter through your nose? Your chest rise and fall? The warmer air leave through your nose? Can you hear yourself breathe? Take the time to really notice.

Take a few more slow deep breaths. Can you take a deep breath in and then sigh it out? Do it again, this time make the sigh audible. Repeat, slowing down the exhale. Can you feel the vibration your sigh makes in your chest?

Good.

You've just tracked a physical process through your body. You noticed. You were self-aware. And through the practice, you anchored yourself in present time.

Where were you as you noticed your breath, your sigh, the vibration in your chest?

---

[55] James Nester. Breath: The New Science of a Lost Art. 2021.

Exactly! You were in your body. *You are where your attention goes.* Again, not rocket-science.

Which means … you can do this. You can breathe, observe, and practice yourself into your body, into present time, into safety, into directing all your outcomes. It just takes practice.

Breathe, notice your body with curiosity, create safety.

We're going to continue breathing and noticing, this time moving from one end of your body to the other. A body "scan." See if you can pay close attention. Take your time to notice everything.

You can do this practice sitting in a chair or lying down. Make yourself as comfortable as possible, using pillows and blankets if you need them.

Close your eyes. Settle in. Place your hands over your heart, or wherever they feel most comfortable.

Start with the top of your head. Breathe there. Soften. Notice how it feels. Can you visualize the top of your head? Not everyone can "see" what they aren't looking at, so don't worry if you can't. Breathe, soften, and sense what you can. Try gently touching each area as we breathe into it to help you anchor yourself to your body. Touch your crown. Notice how it feels.

Next move to your forehead. Breathe there. Touch your forehead. Soften. Notice.

Move to your jaw. Breathe there. Gently place your hands on each side of your jaw. Soften. Notice.

Keep going. Gradually move to your neck, shoulders, arms, hands, chest, belly, hips, legs, and feet. Take your time. Breathe, soften, and notice.

Finally, breathe into your skin, your brain, and the space around you. Take your time. Soften. Notice.

When you're finished "scanning" your body, allow yourself to relax just as you are. Let go of your breathing and softening. Rest. Without trying to change or fix anything, can you hold yourself, your body, and all the sensations and feelings you experience with compassion? With curiosity?

You just practiced presence using your breath, imagination, touch, and attention to anchor you in present time. By softening you further coaxed your body into relaxation. You activated neurological safety circuits and ventral vagal parasympathetic nervous system pathways for alertness, focus, and calm.

Practice this every day at any time. Hold yourself in compassion. Ask with curiosity: What do I notice in my body? What do I need?

EMBODIED SELF-AWARENESS WITH COMPASSION AND CURIOSITY.

I welcome myself and all my sensations, feelings, and energy states. I create safety for my most authentic self to emerge.

Presence is a major safety signal to our bodies. It says, "I'm right here, I see you, I feel you, I notice you, I care enough about you to be here for you." Compassion and curiosity invite us into this safety, connecting us to ourselves, opening us to our potential and possibilities even when we're scared.

But it feels like a paradox, doesn't it? For some of us, directing compassion toward ourselves is unfamiliar. How do we hold ourselves in compassion and safety if we're not sure they're meant for us? How do we hold ourselves in compassion and safety if we're not experiencing them from the people in our lives? Maybe we've *never* experienced them. It can feel awkward. *Scary.* How do we know it's real? How do we know we *deserve* it?

Compassion and curiosity don't always come easily, but they're *essential* for anchoring us in our bodies. When we disconnect from uncomfortable sensations, feelings, and experiences, we disconnect from our bodies. Likewise, when we hyperfocus on what's 'out there' instead of tuning into what's 'in here,' we disconnect from our bodies. When we disconnect from our bodies, we disconnect from present time. Disconnecting from present time, we disconnect from *ourselves* and our feelings, sensations, and energy states. Disconnection makes it hard to know our needs, to set our course, or steer our ship.

To practice embodied self-awareness with compassion and safety, let's meet ourselves where we are by starting with what we already know. We know a lot already even if we don't realize it.

Consider the following questions.

What do you enjoy doing? What do you love to do? What can you lose yourself in? What makes you feel most like yourself? What sparks joy? What calms and soothes and helps you forget your troubles? What helps you reset?

Name what comes to mind, no matter how ordinary, simple, or mundane they seem. Choose something you already enjoy doing and use it as your presence practice. Set a time for it. See if you can allow yourself to do it without apology, but just because you want to and let that be enough. As you embark on this practice, can you sink into it a touch more deeply than perhaps you're used to? Noticing your breath. Noticing your body in space, your feet against the ground, your skin against the air, your eyes and ears taking in the world around you?

For me, it's walking through the woods. I see the woods every day, but every time I walk through, I find something new. Or I see the same things but hold my gaze there a bit longer, taking it in more deeply, with curiosity, like I'm seeing it for the first time. I walk a bit more slowly. I stop here and there to notice. I take pictures with my phone. I marvel. I delight in how my dog, Jasper, finds the same grassy spots to roll his whole body on. I find my prairie roses or Autumn grasses and notice how the sun touches them. Jasper finds the perfect stick to carry, sometimes for miles. I get into my groove. I pick up feathers—hawk, crow, blue jay. Once I found a bald eagle feather sticking up in the grass, recently shed by an adult nesting nearby. What a gift! Lately Jasper and I have been eating wild black raspberries growing next to our favorite trail, savoring every juicy bite.

That's *my* embodied presence practice.

My husband cooks. I mean, the whole deal. He scours through new recipes, selecting what looks interesting. He's especially excited if there are new spices or different ways to blend flavors than he's experienced before. He plans and shops. He preps, a full "mise en place," (French for "putting in place") with all the little bowls and cups. He weighs everything with a little scale. He's like a man in a trance as he combines, stirs, and tastes, all his senses engaged in the process. The sound of the garlic sizzling in olive oil, the aromas of spices toasting in the pan, the feel of freshly picked lettuces and peppers, the panoply of colors and textures, a feast for his eyes.

That's my husband's embodied presence practice (aren't I lucky?).

You're not limited to just one. All the ordinary everyday things we do for ourselves or others with care are presence practices, which we can strengthen by using our breath, by noticing with curiosity, by holding ourselves through it—all our sensations, feelings, and energy states—with compassion.

Even if you're doing something for someone else, if you're doing it your way, according to your own rhythm, because it brings you pleasure or purpose, and you're doing it with self-awareness, it's yours—your embodied presence practice.

See? Not rocket-science. Not woo-woo. Not exceptional. Just you being you, showing up to whatever you do with conscious self-awareness, compassion, and curiosity.

Having trouble coming up with a presence practice? I know. Sometimes it's hard to think of things for ourselves to do when we spend our days neck-deep in obligations to others. How about these? And remember, your practices can be short, micro-dosing you into profound shifts.

- Walk in nature. If you're short on time, make it a short walk. Use your conscious breathing and keep your senses tuned in (yep, no earbuds!). Feel your feet against the ground, the breeze against your skin, the sounds of leaves crackling or birds singing, the smells of dried leaves and flowers (bend down and put your nose in there— really notice). And look around you. Notice the ground, trees, plants, birds, sky, water, everything. Breathe into all of it.
- Do a seated or lying down meditation. It's not for all of us, but I love it. You might too. Start with just a minute or two, whatever feels doable. Get comfy, close your eyes, or keep a soft gaze somewhere in front of you. Notice your breath—the cool air coming in through your nose, the warm air leaving your nose, the rise and fall of your chest. Rest here for as long as you like. I've included resources for meditation apps you can use for ideas and guided meditations to experiment with. Make this practice yours.
- While doing the dishes, tune into your breath and become as aware as possible to everything you do. Notice your feet on the floor beneath you. Feel the warm water on your hands. How does each dish feel as you touch them and place them carefully in the dishwasher? How does your body feel as you pivot or bend to manage each dish? Return to your breath. Slow your movements down. Be completely present.
- Make art. Putter in your workshop, throw pots, paint, draw, sew, knit, rearrange your furniture, whatever inspires you to create something. See if you can stay connected to your breath while you create. Keep it slow, soft, focused.

- Try something new. Anything you've never done before. Something new in the gym (an awkward balance activity you usually avoid?). Take a class in something you know nothing about. Read something new. Write something. Take a walk on a new path. Extra points if you don't know where it goes. It doesn't matter what you do as long as it's beautifully, awkwardly, anxiously new. But here's the real challenge. Slow it down. Stay consciously connected to your breath. Engage your compassion and curiosity. Be present to it all.

What else can you do? Mow the lawn? Do the laundry? Practice tai chi? Breathe deeply in the shower? Write in your journal? Dance around your house? Sing while you're driving? Listen more deeply to your child or friend?

Yes, all of it! Do something every day. Use your breath. Tune in to your bodies' sensations, feelings, and energy states. Hold it all with compassion and curiosity.

PAUSE AND BREATHE.

Widen your focus, create safety.

Safety is essential to reconnecting to our bodies, to becoming and staying present. Not feeling safe is the reason many of us disconnected from ourselves, our bodies, and present time. Everything we've worked with so far—breath, noticing, activating our senses, softening, compassion, curiosity, holding and allowing who we are and what we know—signal safety. They're all anchors to present time while activating the remarkable neurobiology of safety to soothe and settle our nervous systems. I hope you *feel* safer.

Let's expand our repertoire for creating safety.

Now we'll work with our eyes to activate another important safety circuit. Vision has a long evolutionary history for keeping organisms of all kinds fed, sheltered, mated, safe, and alive. Humans are no exception. The eyes are highly sophisticated visual processors that contain small parts of the brain, the retinas. They sit just behind the eyeballs where they relay information between the environment and the body with a primary goal: safety.

Like all our senses, information between the eyes and brain is bidirectional. So, visual information, such as light, color, and movement, makes it to our brains via the optic nerves. Our brain processes what we see and how we respond to it. That's one direction, from the environment to our eyes to our brains. But we also send information the other direction, from our brains out to our eyes.

Consider a common example of this. When we perceive we're in danger, our pupils constrict, and lenses change shape so we can focus intensely on what's immediately in front of us. When we're relaxed and feel safe, our pupils dilate, our lenses change shape so our vision expands, and we can take in more of our environments. These shifts are mediated by internal experiences via the autonomic nervous system.

This bidirectionality gives us a point of control over our nervous system.[56] We can intentionally shift our vision to modify what the autonomic nervous system is doing. This means we can shift our internal state from high stress to calm, from perceived danger to safety by consciously shifting our focus.

Let's practice.

First, sit or stand comfortably. Take a few easy breaths in and out through your nose. Sigh it out. Soften. Notice. However you feel right now, hold it with compassion. Stay curious.

---

[56] Jessica Wapner. Vision and Breathing May Be the Secrets to Surviving 2020. Scientific America. 2020. Nice interview with Stanford neurobiologist, Andrew Huberman, on using the visual system to regulate stress and the Autonomic Nervous System.

I invite you to look around, wherever you are at this moment, and identify five things. Say them out loud. I see a chair, a tree branch in the window, my dog, and so on. That's all. You're just paying attention to what's there, while allowing your vision to anchor you in present time. This simple practice can be calming when stress or anxiety are high.

Next, take in more of the room. Look at whatever is directly in front of you and notice what's there. Then look way up to the right, all the way to the ceiling. Pause for a moment. Notice. Then look way up to the left, all the way to the ceiling. Pause for a moment. Notice. Finally, turn your head all the way to the left, see what's there. Then, turn your head all the way to the right, see what's there. Then return your head to center, look straight ahead, see what's there. Finally, look straight up to the ceiling above your head. Pause. Notice. Good. You've taken in the room and moved your head around in space, all anchoring you in present time, enhancing safety.

Let's take it up another notch. Look straight ahead. Notice what's there. Focus on one small thing directly in front of you. Be there with it.

Now, *without moving your head or your eyes*, allow your focus to expand out from that one small thing. See how much more of the room you can take in. I just focused on the word "in" at the end of the last sentence. Then, without moving my head or eyes, I expanded my focus, seeing more of what's around me. I saw my hands typing, my laptop sitting off to my right, my other monitors, my desk, and the wall behind my desk.

With that simple practice, you shifted your nervous system. As you expanded your focus from narrow to wide, your pupils dilated, and your lenses changed shape. That visual and structural information proceeded to your brain, communicating expansive engagement of a tuned in, relaxed body. You shifted from sympathetic nervous system activation toward enhanced ventral vagal parasympathetic calm, alert engagement.

Did you notice a shift in your body, in how you felt? If you look closely in a mirror before and after the practice, you'll notice your pupils change in diameter, becoming slightly larger in response to the expanded focus. These are physical signs of safety.

You can use this practice to help you with stress and anxiety. You can also use it as a tool to increase calm alertness. I like to pair it with a few deep breaths and sighs to reset my nervous system while working.

EMBODIED SELF-AWARENESS WITH AGENCY.

I identify and ask for what I need.

This is the hard part of this steppingstone. It's where the rubber meets the road in a very real sense. With our first lesson we practiced embodied self-awareness on our own, doing what we love, and taking it to a new level of tuning in to ourselves. Now, how do we practice our embodied self-awareness with compassion and curiosity *out there*? In the world? With our friends? With our co-workers? With our doctors?

How do we stay in our bodies, in present time, in our *selves*, so we can advocate for what we need? How do we stay safe even when we feel vulnerable or when there's indifference, friction, backlash, or outright challenge to what we ask for?

It's one thing to identify our needs through compassionate and curious self-awareness. But it's a whole other level of courage to *ask* for what we need.

Asking for what we need is hard but necessary. Otherwise, we're alone. Many of our needs don't get met. We're not seen, heard, or known when it really matters. Perhaps when we're the most vulnerable and afraid. Healing-the-verb needs to be seen, heard, and known. We heal most robustly in relationship, in connection.

Self-agency says, "this is what I need, my needs matter, *I ask for what I need*." But this is hard, isn't it? Because many of us were taught our needs don't matter. We learned to subjugate our needs in favor of others'. We disconnected from our needs. We no longer know *what* we need.

So, if we aren't passive heaps of suffering on the floor, we're stoic. We take care of *ourselves*. We pull ourselves up by the bootstraps. We don't whine or complain. We think we're tough and independent. Except we're not. And it's its own kind of passivity to avoid one challenge (asking for what we need) by creating another (going at it alone).

I completely get this. I once thought going it alone was a virtue, until I learned it was a classic trauma response. I learned to take care of myself because no one was paying attention when I needed them to. And I became highly successful at it. I survived quite well and accomplished a lot. I was *rewarded* for it because that's what our fiercely individualist culture thrives on. However, this strategy couldn't address my most important needs. I found that out when I needed help. I needed people to know me, to see my vulnerability, to help me sort things out. It was hard to let my armor down to ask for help. To let people know me, see me, and help me. I took small steps. In response, people surprised me by stepping up *for me*. They taught me I was worthy of care. I learned my needs matter, *I* matter. Gradually, I released the staunch independence I used as self-protection. I realized my power was in my tender vulnerability, my authentic me, not in my ability to go it alone.

How do we achieve embodied self-awareness with agency?

First, we must know in our deepest core our needs matter.

Second, we ask for what we need.

Easy peasy, right?

Nope. Not for me, and I suspect not for many of you.

Therefore, this is something we must practice.

First, we'll engage empathy and turn it back on ourselves. We'll empathize with our own needs, bolstering our emotional conditions for personal agency—knowing our needs matter in our deepest core.

Then, we'll practice setting strong personal boundaries, protecting and energizing us as we ask for what we need and advocate for ourselves in all the arenas of our lives.

Engage empathy: our needs matter.

To exercise agency on our own behalf we must be very clear: *our needs matter.*

Let's work with empathy as a tool to convince us our needs matter.

It takes a lot of self-compassion to ask for what we need, doesn't it?

Many of us find self-compassion to be hard, sometimes impossible. Why is that?

Self-compassion can challenge our closely held beliefs about our worth. Especially out there on the world's stage.

Let's work with an end-around to self-compassion.

Take a deep breath in and out. Land in your body. Rest here for a moment, noticing any sensations or feelings present without trying to change or fix them.

Consider: who do you hold in complete compassion and unconditional love at this moment? Your child or grandchild? A beloved pet? A precious friend?

Bring them to mind. Notice how it feels in your body as you think about them.

Do they deserve the love, compassion—whatever you choose to call it—that you feel toward them?

Of course they do.

Now, drop back into those feelings you have for your loved one. Very gently, see if you can direct those same feelings toward yourself. Don't overthink it, just do it.

Still hard?

How about this. Imagine the part of you who finds this exercise hard. What do they feel? Maybe they're very young. They're afraid. Picture yourself as a precious young one. Direct your empathic feelings toward yourself at that age, just as you would any other young innocent being you love and want to protect.

There you go. You're worthy, just like that.

This is hard. Keep practicing.

ASK FOR WHAT YOU NEED: PRACTICE BOUNDARIES.

Asking for what we need, what we *truly* need, requires fortification, doesn't it?

It's not enough to know our needs matter. Effective agency demands boundaries. Protective boundaries. Strengthening boundaries.

With so many demands on our time, energy, and attention, there would be no possibility of embodied self-awareness without strong boundaries.

Especially 'out there,' where there can be so much friction and backlash for who we authentically are. We must protect ourselves from that. Self-protection is essential to agency. We protect ourselves with strong personal emotional-energetic boundaries.

Like borders on a map? The fence around my house?

Yes. Exactly like that. And more.

Think skin. What purpose does it serve? The largest organ of the body, skin wraps us in a warm waterproof layer that keeps us safe and intact. It protects us from the environmental and potential troublemakers like bacteria and parasites. Our skin "reads the room," communicating information about pain, touch, temperature, and pleasure, all the things we need to know to navigate our lives. It's selectively permeable to let in what we need (sensory information, energy from the sun) and release what we don't (heat, toxins).

Skin is the boundary that keeps us alive and holds us so powerfully in the physical world.

The same is true for our personal emotional-energetic boundaries. Just like skin, they should hold us in strength, keeping us safe, whole, and able to regulate our many relationships, keeping us in those relationships on our own terms—with ourselves, our people, and all the places we inhabit. *That's* agency. Boundaries are all about agency.

Skin is easy. It's just there doing its job. We don't have to think about it. But personal boundaries? We must *create* them.

When we're very young, these boundaries are created for us. Ideally, they are strong, wrapping us in continuous, attentive, fiercely loving protection, while allowing us to explore and freely express our needs. From this place of unconditional love and safety, we learn how our needs for protection, care, and personal expression matter. *We* matter.

As adults, it's our job to create these boundaries for ourselves, even if we didn't learn how, if we didn't have these needs met for us when we were young children. This is the challenge for many of us. So, we must practice.

Boundaries allow us to remain firmly rooted in who we are, calmly centered in our bodies, while participating in our many relationships as we move through our lives. If we become unrooted or afraid, boundaries hold us while we activate our present-moment self-awareness and regulate our nervous systems for safety. We know what to do to guide ourselves back.

When our boundaries are strong, our arenas (home, workplace, social environments, and so on) and relationships (family, partners, friends, co-workers, bosses, and so on) support us and don't deplete us.

Foundational to the language of boundaries is the ability to say "no" without apology. Which raises many questions, doesn't it?

- How do we balance our own needs with those of others?
- Is prioritizing our own needs selfish?
- How do we reckon with a family-workplace-community-culture that depletes all our energy, considers it "normal," and calls it "success?"
- How do we deal with backlash from others for prioritizing our needs?

Let's be clear. For most of us, strong boundaries are not the norm. Exercising strong personal emotional-energetic boundaries is often frowned upon. We're outliers. Some might call us "selfish," "unprofessional," "not a team player," "weak," "bitchy," or "not a good mom, friend, partner."

See? Many of our cultures have normalized the energy depletion and self-neglect that is associated with traditional family, community, and workplace relationships.

This is an important part of what makes us—and keeps us—sick, suffering, and stuck.

Our call, our *obligation* to ourselves is to create strong personal emotional-energetic boundaries. It's the only way to hold us in embodied self-awareness, in present time, in full expression of our whole, true, authentic selves. And beyond what boundaries do for us, which makes them necessary, it's also how we can bring all that strength and authenticity into our relationships, creating connections that are healthier and more meaningful for all.

Karyn Shanks MD

What do strong boundaries look like?

- I choose an early bedtime to protect my sleep even when there are chores to do, or people want me to stay up.
- I eat healthy food even when my family, friends, and co-workers do not.
- I choose to stay sober at the party where everyone else drinks.
- I say no to requests for my time and energy that I do not want.
- I say no to working overtime.
- I say no to common time and energy drains: social media rabbit holes, news consumption, excessive email and text checking, and so on.
- I say no to notifications for social media, email, texts, and news.
- I close the door to my office when I need privacy.
- I say yes to requests for my time and energy only when I've made a clear, conscious decision to do so.
- I express my feelings honestly even though it feels uncomfortable.

You get the message. Would any of these be difficult for you?

How do we know where our boundaries should be to best serve our needs?

First, be clear about what you need. What do you need for energy, restoration, enjoyment, fulfillment, or feeling safe? Are you able to protect those needs? Ask for them? Say "no" to anything that gets in the way of receiving them?

Once you're clear about what your needs are, which ones get met? Which ones don't? Of those that don't get met, why? What gets in the way?

This gets tricky, doesn't it? How do I know if my needs are getting met? Is it when I'm doing what I'm "supposed" to, what I'm "obligated" to, what makes others happy with me? Or is it when I feel fulfilled, rested, energized?

How do we discern our true needs from all of theirs'?

Creating strong personal boundaries helps us identify what we need and decide how best to meet those needs. It doesn't mean we don't negotiate our needs. Sometimes we must. But we always do it from a conscious position so it's a fully embodied choice.

So, let's review what boundaries do for us:

- Declare who we authentically are.

- Help us get our needs met.
- Keep us safely in our bodies.
- Support present-moment conscious awareness.
- Conserve our energy.
- Protect us from toxic or unwanted energy.
- Keep us safe in all our arenas.

PERSONAL BOUNDARY PRACTICES.

Many of us struggle with boundaries for all kinds of reasons we just identified, so we're going to practice.

Let's work on three key areas.

- Boundaries to protect our energy.
- Boundaries to protect who we authentically are.
- Boundaries to ask for help with discernment.

Boundaries to protect our energy.

Sounds easy, doesn't it?

Except for that proverbial elephant in the room, right? If we felt we could create strong energetic boundaries while remaining safe, we'd already have them.

Consider the backlash we often get for how we protect our energy. For pulling back from an overloaded schedule. For going to sleep earlier. For eating healthier food. For taking time away from family, friends, work to take care of ourselves. To exercise, meditate, take quiet time, or pursue a hobby. For not joining the energy-depleting family gathering.

There's a lot at stake here. Our energy is everything. It's our flow. Our lifeforce with robustness, strength, and ease. Our ticket out of suffering.

Protecting our energy tends to require three tasks.

- Identify what we need to protect our energy.
- Declare our need.
- Follow through, no matter the backlash.

And there's probably a fourth here if we're up for it: address the backlash at its source.

Practice creating strong boundaries to protect your energy:

Identify something you need to protect your energy. Keep this simple and small. Examples could be set an earlier bedtime, move more during the day, take a break from social media or news, schedule more rest breaks, or start a breath/meditation practice.

Declare your need. What words would you like to use to clearly state your need? Examples: *I will be going to bed at eight pm sharp from now on, thank you for understanding. I will be taking two 15-minute breaks each day to walk the dog. I will be going to my room and closing my door for meditation time, thank you for not interrupting.*

Follow through, while managing backlash. If there is backlash—grumbling, criticism, teasing, toxic silence, or lack of support and encouragement (these can be just as hurtful as overt disapproval)—check in with yourself to notice how you feel. Managing backlash starts with you. Don't let it prevent you from meeting your needs. Maintain your boundary. Then, hold your feelings with absolute compassion, welcome this pain (or whatever you are feeling) as part of your healing. Stay in your body, holding the feelings as long as they need you to. Remain curious.

Option to openly address the backlash. This requires creating a boundary to protect who you authentically are (next practice). Remember your words are powerful. They help you strengthen the boundary of who you are and what you need. They remind people what you expect from them. Your words might go like this: *I noticed you got quiet when I explained my new early bedtime. I'd love to explore how this makes you feel. However, it is important you understand how vital this is to me and what I need and it's not negotiable.*

Can you apply these steps to needs you've identified for yourself?

Boundaries to protect who we authentically are.

These boundaries can be even more challenging. People tend to understand and feel more sympathy for the behavior changes we establish to address health and wellness. But to create change just because we want to? Who do we think we are?

Sometimes we just need to teach people where our boundaries are. Those who care about us will honor them.

The practice you just did to protect your energy prepares you for this. Identifying what you need, declaring those needs, and implementing change, then managing, and perhaps openly addressing backlash, helps you develop embodied self-awareness with agency. It's part of getting your reps in, of building your embodied self-awareness and personal agency muscles.

It may sound like it's working backwards. But if you can say, "this is what I need, my needs matter, I ask for what I need," well, you're that much closer to knowing who you authentically are. Every time you go through that same process, you expand on that. This is a process of self-development, of personal growth. And it's a lifetime practice. Who among us starts by knowing the totality of who we are?

The practice of creating these self-defining boundaries is essentially about going through life inhabiting our bodies—our feelings, sensations, and energy states—with deep awareness. Further, it's about how when we walk this way through life, we can operate from a core of strength and authenticity. We carry ourselves with reverence for who we are. We can observe and listen without defensiveness. We can speak our truth with clarity. We can negotiate all our relationships with compassionate strength for all the players, including ourselves. And when we make mistakes, we can dust ourselves off and get on with it.

Self-discovery to learn who we authentically are takes practice. Every day. Paying attention with compassion and curiosity. What else can we do to inhabit ourselves, to discover ourselves? Allow me to suggest a simple powerful practice I depend on every day: a daily writing practice.

Daily writing practice.

I've kept a journal since I was a child. My grandma used to gift me small diaries with tiny locks on them every Christmas. They were dated and lined to record daily activities or musings. She kept diaries herself, filling a page or two every single day of her life with the events of the day. I'm not sure she explored her feelings, but daily writing anchored her.

I became a more serious writing practitioner when I read Julia Cameron's *The Artist's Way*.[57] She set me on a course of writing "morning pages," her prescription for capturing creative wisdom through three pages of longhand writing every morning. Morning was key, because that's when we're the least distracted by what's out there in the world, therefore more apt to access our creativity. And, as I discovered, more apt to get the writing practice done.

Morning pages go like this. Show up every day and vomit up (my colorful language, not hers) whatever you're thinking, feeling, experiencing, questioning at that moment, written without stopping—and with no censorship—for three pages. In the beginning, as my stream of whining and complaining hit the page, I was shown how I really felt. Writing things out helped me identify feelings I didn't otherwise recognize. As my practice evolved, I *needed* to write every day. Unloading my feelings lightened me. And it shifted me from someone who complained to someone who came up with creative solutions. I now understand daily writing practice as a safe place where I can be completely myself and as an invitation to my wise inner guidance to be revealed on the page.

Does your writing practice need to look exactly like that to produce meaningful results? Of course not (my answer, not Julia's). And while I started out following Julia's rules, I've very much made the practice my own. Julia's focus was creativity, but mine became safety. Writing is a safe space, an anchor.

Neuroscientists have shown that we literally re-wire our brains through the writing process. It shifts us into neuroplastic growth. It increases creativity helping us formulate new ideas, solve problems, and work through psychological and emotional obstacles. Writing is a powerful tool for self-observation, exploration, discovery, and self-guidance. It helps us know and strengthen who we authentically are.

By writing every day, you create a safe sanctuary you can count on as you welcome all your thoughts and feelings, giving them space and a voice. Through this process you'll forge a deep bond of trust with yourself, helping you thrive through life's challenges as more your whole, true, authentic self. In this way, your daily writing practice becomes a boundary to protect who you authentically are.

---

[57] Julia Cameron. The Artist's Way: A Spiritual Path to Higher Creativity. First edition 1992.

Suggestions for a successful daily writing practice.

Let's begin with a simple writing practice to deepen your self-connection and create sturdier boundaries for who you authentically are.

- *Set a time and show up every day.* Make this a habit you can stick to. If you have just five to ten minutes to spare, that's great. Consistency builds that trusting relationship between you and, well, *you.* It creates safety.
- *Create your writing space and have your tools ready.* Keep your journal, pen, and a timer (to help you maintain needed time parameters) ready to go in a space you designate for this purpose. This is the sacred space that amplifies safety. It helps to have a comfortable place to sit in quiet and privacy. Choose a pen that feels right in your hand. Juice up the space with objects you love (I have a candle and some rocks I love).
- *Try writing longhand.* Writing longhand may have advantages over typing into a tablet or smartphone, beyond generational sensibilities. But if that doesn't work for you, typing is better than not writing at all.
- *Keep your journal private and don't self-censor.* We all tend to self-censor if we think others might peek at what we've written, so privacy is key. For this practice to work for you, it's imperative to tell the truth no matter how ugly or boring or angry or blah you think it sounds. As I've said about my own writing practice, vomit it all up.
- *Watch out for perfectionism and judgment.* Your journal is a sacred place where you can safely be your whole, true, imperfect, authentically human self. Please don't worry about spelling, punctuation, proper grammar, or neatness. I also think it helps to have a simple inexpensive notebook for this purpose rather than a gorgeous expensive journal we might feel compelled to keep "nice." Moleskin journals are just right for the job. They come lined and unlined and in a variety of colors and sizes. Mess them up as you explore your true messy self!
- *Compassionately work with resistance to starting or sustaining your daily writing.* I find beginning anything new befuddling at first. I

may believe in it and feel completely committed to it, but still forget to do it. What? Forget to do a ten-minute thing first thing in the morning? Yep. We're developing new mind grooves. Takes a while. Writing is special. Not just a new practice, but we're revealing ourselves. This can be scary. If you feel resistance, check in with your body. What do you feel? Welcome those feelings. Hold them with compassion. Ask them what they need. Create the safety.

PAUSE AND BREATHE.

Daily writing practice tools to amplify your growth.

Writing is a powerful tool to help us create our lives. In addition to free-form daily writing practice, we can work with specific writing techniques to assist us in whatever we want to achieve. One of my favorites is writing affirmations.

Affirmations are carefully crafted mini stories that declare where we want to be and remind us that our problems can change.

In various iterations, affirmations have been around throughout human history. We've called them prayers, chants, mantras, and devotions. They powerfully meet our need for encouragement, solace, and guidance, while connecting us through time and over space to ancestors and people all over the world.

This too shall pass. I am Divinely guided and protected. I am loved. Shine your light. Om Namah Shivaya (I bow to Shiva; I bow to my inner self).

Affirmations are not meant to wish our way into a better future. They're not rose-colored glasses. Our goal is not to delude ourselves, but to chart our course. Affirmations assist us.

GUIDELINES FOR CREATING EFFECTIVE AFFIRMATIONS.

- *Create a positive, present-tense affirmation to articulate your goal.* This makes your affirmation "sticky," mobilizing the resources you need to bring it to life. It affirms the direction you are headed (forward, into needed change), the possibility of change (away from the perception of being stuck), and attracts the help you need as your new mind grooves develop. Don't worry if your goal seems unattainable. It's *your* goal. Shoot for the stars.
- *To make affirmations extra "sticky" attach a gratitude statement to it.* Gratitude grounds us in our bodies. It opens the heart, engages all the senses, and supports brain function. Declaring your goal with gratitude expands your internal creative resources for moving you toward your goal.

Practice.

Declare your goal. Keep it present tense (this affirms the goal is already developing), positive (this focuses on the goal rather than the problem), and attach gratitude (this makes it more "sticky," to activate all your supportive resources).

I am grateful for my radiant new energy.

I am grateful to receive all the support and resources I need for vibrant new energy.

I am grateful for my new successful writing practice.

Repeat your affirmations several times each day because practice makes progress—those new mind grooves. Write them or read them out loud. Write your affirmations on sticky notes and place them where you'll see them throughout the day. If you want to keep them private, be sure to place them where only you will see them—stick them in a pocket, in your briefcase, or on the dashboard of your car.

As you say your affirmations, let the words wash over you. *Feel* them. See if you can soften any disbelief, judgment, or resistance that might arise.

Boundaries to ask for help with discernment.

Finally, we create boundaries to assist us in asking for help, which makes us active participants in the process.

What if we don't know what we need? We just know we hurt. We feel utterly clueless about what to do.

Asking for help when we don't know what we need can feel wildly uncomfortable, because there's so much uncertainty and vulnerability involved. But it doesn't have to be a position of weakness. We can need help, feel uncertain and vulnerable, *and* navigate all that with discernment.

Discernment is key to our agency. We may not know our needs beyond wanting to feel better or get our lives back on track. We may not know who to turn to. Even if we identify an "expert" for our problem, we won't know what they know until we sit down with them. Even then, will they be able to help us?

With so much uncertainty, what do we do?

First things first. We stay in our bodies. We breathe. We observe our feelings, sensations, and energy states. We let all that guide us as we ask questions.

- Are we ready to receive help?
- Do we like/trust/feel safe with the expert we've asked for help from?
- Does their exploration and assessment of us truly get us?
- Do they listen to us empathically and answer our questions thoroughly and respectfully?

- Do their recommendations make sense, resonate with us, or seem feasible?
- Is their plan for follow up responsive to our needs?

This self-guidance in the face of uncertainty means we don't take any of it lying down. We need help and don't know what we need, but we're not passively participating in this process. We're assessing our readiness and *leading* the process. We're *choosing* our expert. We're *selecting* our strategy. We're *observing* our own outcomes. We're *defining* what success is.

Get it?

The key is this: we enter the encounter in full embodied self-awareness with compassion, curiosity, and agency. We breathe. We notice. Everything we've been practicing.

Let's practice.

- Name one thing you need help with.
- Tell the story succinctly, in just a few sentences.
- Who might you ask for help? If you know, great. Contact them for an appointment or meeting time. Then, follow all the guidelines discussed above. This might feel uncomfortable so remember the drill—stay in your body, breathe, hold yourself and your feelings with compassion, stay curious.
- Don't know who to ask? Can you tap into your network for ideas? Maybe there's someone your trusted friends or family have already vetted.
- Still don't know who to ask? If this is a health concern, you might start with the primary person on your health team—tap into their network. If it's not health related, start placing search terms into your favorite search engine and see what comes up. Be discerning—check in with yourself, what resonates? Frustrated and exhausted when you find nothing? Put it down. Take the rest of the day or even several days off. Come back when you're fresh.
- Through all this, remember: Stay in your body, breathe, observe your feelings, sensations, and energy states. They're not wrong. Let them guide you.
- Keep working it. Remain discerning. If you hit obstacles, rest, be tender with yourself, but don't give up.

LAST WORDS.

I suspect for many of you I've been preaching to the choir. I'm so glad. One, it means I'm on the right track. Two, so are you! But if you're like me, even if we're on the right track, we need reminders every day. And fresh ideas to keep it interesting, to go deeper into our practices, and to remember we're never alone.

What if we forget to practice? Forget to stay in our bodies? Forget to breathe? Forget to circle back to what grounds us in our own experience and authenticity?

You will forget sometimes. We all do.

But here's another reminder to help you, circling back to our agreements to keep things simple, small, and slow. To breathe into yourself with compassion. This is what shifts you back to present time, back to your body, back to yourself. Whether you're new to presence practices or an old pro, allow for gentle shifts, don't insist on immediate success or drastic changes.

And every second you're curious or gaze upon yourself with compassion? Every time you pause and allow your needs to matter? Every time you appreciate the ordinary everyday moments that you're alive? That's present time. Build on that.

Presence is the path. It's the practice. And presence is our prize.

Because everything worth anything occurs right here in present time. In our bodies. In our experiences. In our awareness. Not 'out there,' but 'in here.' *Always* 'in here.'

And beyond that? It takes a hell of a lot of presence to activate our healing-the-verb and reveal our most sparkly wholeness.

THREE PROMISES.

Make these simple. Small but fierce next steps. Don't overthink this. Be gentle.

1.
2.
3.

CHAPTER SEVENTEEN
Second *Un*Broken Core Resilience Steppingstone:

BALANCE.

I trust the wind. I grow strong roots. I flow with ease. Like a sturdy tree.

W hat *is* balance?

Is it a perfect schedule, perfectly organized, with perfect vigilance to all our desires, wants, and needs? Is it the grind of perfect lives perfectly executed?

Or is balance that place smack dab in the middle where we land once we've gotten *all* our shit together? A life devoid of highs and lows. No struggle, overwhelm, or chaos. Is *that* balance?

Would we *want* that?

How about this instead?

What if balance is about being sturdy? About trusting ourselves to manage the challenges and uncertainties of life? The work, the unexpected hurdles, the catastrophes, the joys, and the daily chores? What if balance is planting our feet and holding our center even when our lives are hard, to not just manage the challenges and uncertainties, but thrive through them, grow from them, strengthen because of them?

What if being sturdy and trustworthy isn't about perfection, vigilance, or success at all? Certainly not about having all our shit together. But about flow. And not just *any* flow, but flow that is anchored in a consciously, robustly, tenderly curated core.

And what if this core is a place inside us? *All* of us. A place we can touch, feel, and tap into at will. That we can develop. That we can learn to trust, lean on, turn to for support, hold us in our storms, draw strength from, and feel safe in. To count on in all our arenas, to help us up when we're knocked down, to hold us steady when we're overwhelmed.

Like a sturdy tree.

That's what I think balance is. Sturdiness.

I'm always stunned by how the magnificent Midwestern oaks bend to unfathomable lows in the ferocious winds of summer storms, then recover to full height leaving only a few branches on the ground. Or how they split in two but heal nonetheless, to once again gently, effortlessly sway in the breezes of calm sunny days.

What do trees have that let them bend so far, under so much force, without breaking, then effortlessly stand back up?

They trust the wind. They grow strong roots. They flow with ease.

Trees don't resist their dynamic equilibrium. They don't deny Earth's laws . They don't worry about looking like they have all their shit together.

We have a lot to learn from trees.

What if *we* learned to trust the wind?

What if *we* trusted ourselves to bend and shake and sway in the wind, knowing we'd eventually land on our feet?

We'd strengthen our roots. We might live with greater faith in what's to come. We'd take more risks and live more life. We'd learn to flow with greater ease. We'd discover the secret of trees also belongs to us.

The sturdiness of trees is in how they're built.

Trees harness Earth's law of elastic energy, converting the kinetic energy of wind into elastic potential energy they can use. Elastic energy allows their trunks to stretch and compress and bend deeply so they can sway in the wind without breaking, then stand up straight again. The more they're challenged by the wind, the stronger their trunks become, the more elastic energy they hold, and the deeper their roots grow. Trees use Earth's energy to create resilience.

That's balance. Elasticity. Resilience. Sturdiness.

Not magic.

As humans, we have the same potential. Human resilience is an equilibrium of strength, energy, adaptability, *and challenge.* We grow our resilience through the risks, uncertainties, and ambiguities of life. We become sturdy. We learn to flow with greater ease.

For this *Unbroken* core resilience steppingstone, *Balance*, we'll anchor our flow through a consciously, robustly, tenderly curated core. A trusted center of balance. Like a sturdy tree.

How do *we* trust the wind?

Through a real life lived. A life we're consciously present for. Even with— *especially* with—challenges, uncertainties, and endless chores. We let ourselves fall *out* of balance. Sometimes *I* don't know what balance is until I've been smacked down. But we stay in our bodies. We get back up. We convert the kinetic energy of our fall into elastic energy we can use and grow from. We pay attention to our feelings, sensations, and energy states. We hold ourselves with compassion. We stay curious. And by staying present for it all, even when it hurts, even when we're exhausted and overwhelmed, we get it all. Balance takes us straight to grace.

What's our first move?

We tell our new story: *I trust the wind.*

We stop calling it failure. We flow even when it feels nothing like flow. But our flow has an anchor we can trust. We trust our progress, we trust ourselves. We trust life. Even when it feels like we can't trust, we *choose* trust. We practice the new story.

BALANCE IS IN THE BODY.

I think it helps to work with balance as a literal place within the body, like the large trunk of a sturdy oak.

It makes sense after everything we've learned. We're body-mind-spirit-emotional-community-planetary beings. Of course, balance is in the body, not just an abstract idea meandering through our minds.

In humans, balance is exactly where you'd think it is. In your core, between the naval and solar plexus, beneath your ribs. You can place your hands there right now. Flex your abdominal muscles just a bit by bending slightly forward into a little crunch. That's your core, your center, the geographical balance point of your body. It's your version of a trunk. From where you can bend over deeply then rise back up. It's where you transform the energy of challenge into growth.

This part of your body is filled with things you depend on to survive and thrive. Your adrenal glands are there, directing all the business of your energy needs. The largest blood channel, the aorta, passes through your core to deliver freshly oxygenated blood to your entire body. Your spinal cord runs through your core to innervate your body and serve as the main thoroughfare for all the communications between your brain and every part of you. Your Autonomic Nervous System (ANS) is centered there, keeping you safe. Your guts are in there, providing you with nourishment, protecting you with critical immunity, housing your microbiome, and delivering your gut feelings. And around all that? Fiercely protective connective tissue that surrounds and connects all your organs and powerful muscles of your abdomen, sides, and back.

So much power runs through this core of your body in the forms of structure, function, and energy. Anchoring your flow. Connecting your parts. Running your show.

Here's what you most need to know. This isn't just about appreciating how much goes on in your core, amazing as it all is. It's also to show you how you can protect it, engage with it, learn from it, and strengthen it. Just like everything we've talked about so far, your core is there being amazing in service of you whether you pay attention or not. But consciously tended to? With your full presence? We're talking incredible strength. Gorgeous balance. Resilience and sturdiness you can trust through any storm.

Balance is about *trusting yourself in the face of challenge.* A strong core helps build that trust. It anchors your gorgeous flow.

PAUSE AND BREATHE.

Connect with your core.

Let's find the center of our bodies, our core of balance.

Place your hands over your midsection, between your naval and solar plexus, just beneath your rib cage. Press firmly, hands side-by-side or one on top of the other, let your core know you're there. This is you. Your center. Your strong core of balance.

When we feel out of balance, we don't like the equilibrium we're at—the pain, discomfort, overwhelm, fatigue, feeling stuck, whatever it is. This is the language of our bodies telling us what they need, the dynamic equilibrium where our present circumstances have brought us.

If balance is about trusting ourselves in the face of challenge—trusting the wind—how do we get there?

We tap into our core.

In ancient Middle Eastern Vedic tradition, the core of the body, located between the naval and diaphragm, holds the emotional energy of personal power. This third "chakra" in the Vedic energy anatomy system is closely aligned with the centrally located 'self-esteem' sector from 20th century psychologist Abraham Maslow's hierarchy of emotional and developmental needs. Both traditions localize personal power to the center—the core—of human experience and the human body.[58]

---

[58] More on this relationship in: Karyn Shanks MD. *Heal: A Nine-Stage Roadmap to Recover Energy, Reverse Chronic Illness, and Claim the Potential of a Vibrant New You.* 2019. Chapter Nine: Flow (Trust Your Emotional Wisdom).

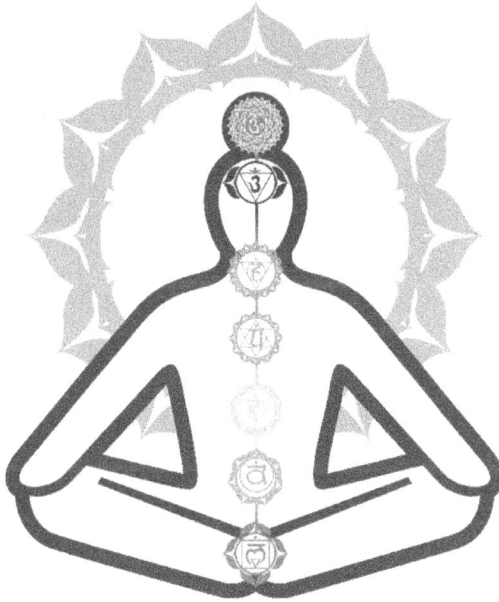

Vedic Chakra System

CROWN
Connection to Divine, Universal Intelligence

THIRD EYE
Wisdom, Discernment

THROAT
Verbal Expression, Listening

HEART CENTER
Love, Compassion

SOLAR PLEXUS
Personal Power, Self-Worth

PELVIS
Creativity, Pleasure, Personal Boundaries

ROOT
Survival, Belonging, Nourishment

Maslow's Hierarchy of Needs

Self-Actualization
Personal Growth, Peak Experiences, Self-Fulfillment

Self-Esteem
Dignity, Respect, Achievement, Independence

Love & Belonging
Friendships, Intimacy, Family, Connection

Safety
Security, Health, Personal Well-Being

Physiological
Food, Water, Sleep, Shelter

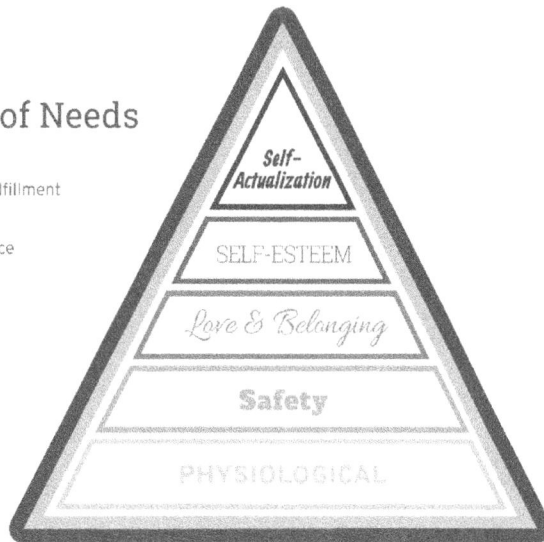

Now that you've found your core, let's work with it to bolster personal power. This amplifies balance—trusting yourself in the face of challenge, trusting the wind.

Breathe: With hands over your core, let your core know you're there, and breathe. Breathe into the core of your body. Just notice, welcoming whatever is there.

Use your powerful words: I honor my whole true authentic self. I trust who I am. I have faith in my strength to do what best serves me and those I love. I can weather any storm. I hold who I am with compassion, reverence, and curiosity. This is my source of strength. My anchor.

Move: Engage your core in everything you do. Feel its strength to hold you. Stand and move from the strength of your core center. Stand tall with hands on hips and shoulders back, rising out of your core. Build fire here with abdominal crunches, leg lifts, sitting v-ups, or boat pose (for yogis). Resist spending time in postures that keep you folded forward, sitting, or covering your core with your arms.

WHAT HAPPENS WHEN YOUR CORE IS WEAK?

Think of all the amazing things running through your core: the adrenals, aorta, spinal cord, and guts. Bones, muscles, connective tissue, organ support tissue, and countless blood and lymphatic vessels. What do you think happens to them when your core is weak? When you sit a lot, slouch, bend for hours over your devices, or hold yourself in collapsing postures (trees would never!).

You bend, compress, and weaken them. You ask them to take on shapes they were never meant to take. You ask them to hold you up even though they're not strong enough. If your core is weak, you can't hold yourself well in supportive postures. If you fall, you may not be able to get back up. You might break.

When you sit on your blood vessels for hours every day, they learn. They *stay* bent. It's the law of least resistance. Same with muscles, connective tissue, lymphatic channels, nerves, and all the supportive structures of your internal organs.

What happens when your core structures stay bent?

They get weak and change function. Blood and lymphatic flow stagnate. Tissues no longer receive the rich nourishment of blood, and fluids can't drain properly. Bones and muscles become weak. Organs move where they're not supposed to be. You can't stand up straight or hold your head where it's supposed to be. You land in a world of hurt and dysfunction.

It's just like when your garden hose kinks. The water stops flowing. If the hose stays bent, it becomes harder to unkink, harder to maintain the flow. (And by the way, those "anti-kink" garden hoses? They're just built with thicker walls, meaning stronger cores!)

What does this new shape and function say to your genes?

You guessed it: "We're in big trouble here."

As a result, your genetic expression shifts in response to the danger, ramping up survival biology to rescue you. Your immune system upregulates inflammation and your adrenal glands pour out cortisol. Your brain jumps into the action, saying "Our core is weak, we can't stand up straight, our core biology is dysfunctional, we can't defend ourselves, we're in danger," shifting you into sympathetic nervous system dominance, keeping you more stressed, vigilant, and scared.

We depend on a strong core we can trust to hold us through our storms, so there's a lot to lose when shape, strength, and function fall off. We lose resilience. We lose sturdiness. We *feel* weak, we *feel* unstable, we *feel* incapable. We no longer trust ourselves.

With so much at stake, why aren't we more concerned?

We tend to view the evolution of shape change and organ dysfunction of the human body as a "normal" part of aging. Because that's the prevailing narrative, isn't it? It's a narrative that has evolved in a population of folks who are disconnected from their own bodies. But it's *not* normal. We are not designed to become bent over, weak, chronically ill, and dysfunctional as we age. That happens because of lifelong habits, nothing more.

The conveniences and stresses and belief systems of our modern lifestyle have disconnected us from our cores and the gigantic potential of our human bodies. Therefore, we're no longer strong and we can no longer trust ourselves to take on the strenuous upright life we were designed for. We're no longer anything like the sturdy oaks who trust the wind.

WHEN OUR CORE IS WEAK, WE FEEL LESS SAFE.

A weak, bent core is not just a physical problem. If your core is weak, if you can't hold yourself in supportive postures, if you can't bend in the wind, what else happens? What do you *feel*?

You won't feel safe.

You won't trust the wind or grow strong roots.

Research links core strength and activation to experiences of personal empowerment, confidence, personal agency, the ability to speak one's truth, and improvement in personal outcomes.[59] This is important. And it aligns perfectly with what the ancient Vedic mystics taught—that an activated core leads to personal power and resilience.

How can we unwind our bent, compressed, weak cores and learn to trust the wind? How do we create flow with an anchor to become sturdy again? To trust ourselves in the face of challenge?

First, breathe. Get into your body. Be present. Hold everything you feel right now, hold yourself with fierce compassion.

The truth is hard, isn't it? We resist. We take it personally, like we're being chastised. But we're here to know the truth. We're here to heal. So, we breathe and hold and stay curious about everything.

Then we do something about it. We get back into our bodies. We exercise our self-awareness with agency.

Consider the following suggestions while remembering the core principle of simple, small, and slow. Don't do it all at once. Choose a few things to start slowly on, then get to work, commit to it, expand into it.

---

[59] Amy Cuddy. Presence: Bringing your boldest self to your biggest challenges. 2015.

UNWIND OLD HABITS, STRENGTHEN YOUR CORE, THRIVE THROUGH LIFE'S CHALLENGES.

Nothing helps you find your balance like a strong, flexible, ready-to-engage core. This is the balance point of your body, and like a compass rose, it is ready to guide you through the challenges life puts before you. You are a mind-body-spirit organism with mind-blowing intrinsic genius. Let's unleash it now.

Your core strengthening program contains:

- Unwind old habits that hijack your core strength.
- Begin new practices to strengthen your core.
- Tap into your strong, resilient core to help you thrive through life's challenges.

Unwind old habits that hijack your core strength.

This part is simple. Sit less, stand more, and move often.[60]

We're the culture of sitting, aren't we? We're increasingly aware of the problems this poses, and that's a baby step in the right direction. Let's take it further. Unless you work construction or are a landscape gardener, this lesson is for you. As a physician-consultant and writer, it's absolutely for me! My job requires a lot of sitting. I use a sit-stand desk, but I still sit too much for how I was built—for how we're *all* built. So, I'm right there with you.

The following is a list of habitual postures that keep us compressed, bent, and weak. See if you can slowly merge out of these. Start with a few minutes at a time. Avoid too much change here all at once—that could hurt! You'll be using your body in new ways. Like any new exercise or posture, ease yourself into it.

- Sit less and move often.
- Avoid all continuous static postures.
- Hold your torso upright and avoid all head-forward postures.

---

[60] Katy Bowman. Move Your DNA. 2015.

Sit less and move often.

Slowly work toward sitting no more than fifteen minutes at a time, and not more than thirty minutes every two hours. Use a sit-stand desk so you can vary your posture during your workday. You can create one by simply placing a stack of books or a cardboard box on your desk—place your laptop at a level you can comfortably use while standing, keeping your neck aligned with your spine and chin slightly tucked. Create a midway posture using a stool to rest your leg, moving back and forth between legs. Whatever you're doing in your seated position, try to vary and interrupt your position frequently.

Avoid all continuous static postures.

Sitting isn't the only problem. Prolonged postures of any kind are harmful. The goal is to create fluid changes in movement and posture throughout the day. When you sleep, you automatically move. Your body doesn't like continuous postures so it will move on its own when you're not aware of it. Come up with a bunch of reasons to move during your day, and not just workouts and planned walks. We want to break up the continuous postures that are a part of many of our workdays as well as when we're relaxing. If it helps you remember, set reminders on your smart watch or phone.

Some examples of reasons you can use to move: bathroom, water, and food breaks, short dog walks, small chores such as laundry or dishes, walk outside for a breath of fresh air, and so on. Give yourself permission to step away from your work or other activities to make time for these kinds of restorative movement.

Hold your torso upright and avoid persistent head-forward postures.

Whether you are sitting, standing, or somewhere in between, focus on holding your torso upright, without slouching or bending. Stand up straight, stick your heart out, slightly tuck your chin, and take deep breaths into your entire torso.

Karyn Shanks MD

Take extra care to avoid persistent head-forward postures. To single out the most common one, don't look down at your phone. Notice people using their phones in public, whether they're sitting, standing, or walking. They hold the device in their hands at about waist level (to avoid the effort of holding it high) and bend neck forward with head down (sometimes as far as ninety degrees!) to look at it. They often hold themselves this way for extended periods. This puts enormous force on the neck (our heads are heavy) and its core structures while compressing, bending, and weakening the central core.

For reading, gaming, or any device-related activities that go on for more than a moment, use your arm strength to hold your device directly in front of your face so your head does not have to bend down, or place it on a stand that is elevated enough to look straight at it. See if you can do some of this activity standing rather than sitting. If you're out walking or crossing the street, put your phone away, keeping your head upright to observe what's around you and stay safe.

Begin new practices to strengthen your core.

In addition to unwinding old habits that weaken the core, it's important to work on actively strengthening your core. Two of the best ways to accomplish this are by walking more (any movement while in an upright position engages and strengthens core muscles) and participating in a core strengthening practice, such as yoga, Pilates, or strength training.

If you start a new practice, such as yoga or strength training, consider what you need to keep from hurting yourself. Start out slow and seek out guidance for your level of fitness. Ideally, work with a professional who can personalize your practice to you and your needs. They will be able to assess you carefully and address weaknesses while building strength in a safe way.

Can't fit that into your schedule or budget just now? No problem, check out a video or online course for beginners or try the simple movements below.

These are some simple core strengtheners you can add to your current strength practice. They're safe enough for beginners with no prior exercise experience, but if they're too hard, or you find yourself hurting after trying them, seek assistance from an exercise professional or physical therapist.

- *Gentle crunches.* Lie on your back with knees bent, feet on the ground, arms crossed over chest. Keeping head and neck aligned, elevate head just enough off the floor to feel your abdominal muscles engage. Hold for a second or two, release, and repeat. Do three sets of ten to start.

- *Hip bridges.* After your crunches, lift your hips up off the ground, feet flat on the floor, hip distance apart, arms up overhead. Squeeze your butt. Hold for 10 seconds. Repeat this 3-5 times.
- *Elbow plank pose.* These can be done on knees or toes. Set your forearms directly under shoulders and lift yourself up off the ground on knees or toes. Keep your back straight or slightly flexed so your abdominal muscles feel engaged. Hold for 5-10 seconds at first, then release. Repeat three times. Over time, increase the length of the hold before releasing.

Once you've got these going strong, here are some more advanced core strengtheners.

- *Full sit-ups.* You'll often hear trainers say sit-ups are bad for your back. This is true when the core is weak. That's why we never start with them. You've been doing your crunch, hip bridge, and elbow plank practice and it's getting easy peasy because your core is becoming strong. Lie on your back with legs straight out in front of you and arms crossed over your chest. Engage your core first by lifting your head off the ground like you did for the gentle crunch. Once your core muscles are turned on, sit all the way up. Keeping your core engaged, lay all the way back down. Don't flop down, rather let yourself down slowly on a 5-count. Repeat this 5-10 times.
- *Hip bridge single-leg extensions.* Now that the hip bridges are too easy, let's take it up a notch. After your sit-ups, lift your hips up off the ground while engaging your core. Hold for a second or two. Then, while holding your core as stable as possible, lift one leg up into an extended position about 45 degrees from the horizontal (halfway between horizontal and straight up). Squeeze your butt and keep it up as high as possible. Set your leg down while maintaining your bridged core. Then, lift the other leg in the same way. Keep your core and butt fully engaged the entire time. Do 5-10 reps on each side.

Karyn Shanks MD

- *Downward dog into full plank pose.* This is your prep for full straight arm plank but is more advanced than elbow plank. Begin standing. Bend down and plant your palms on the ground a few feet out from your feet. You'll look like an upside-down "v." Your heels will likely come up off the ground. This is downward dog pose. Stay in this position for a few moments, gently stretching your calves one at a time. Then carefully walk your hands out and allow your torso to become straight. Keep your core engaged. This is full plank! Stay here for a few seconds, then walk your hands back until you are in downward dog again. Go back and forth between downward dog and full plank poses slowly and gently. Get a good stretch and core activation.

Tap into your strong, resilient core to help you thrive through life's challenges.

How do we trust our own wisdom as we put it into action, standing in the various arenas of our lives?

Our core must be strong—*literally* strong—to hold us securely in space as it moves us with strength, steadfastness, surefootedness, and grace through our lives. This equilibrium of balance supports us physically, emotionally, cognitively, and spiritually. It helps us feel safe.

Social psychologist Amy Cuddy showed how activating the core of the body through "power poses," (made famous in her popular TED talk) leads to greater confidence, sense of presence in the body, and ability to speak one's truth.[61] You don't even have to be standing to reap the benefits—her work extends to those in wheelchairs, unable to stand or walk. Even *imagining* oneself in a personal power stance leads to the same sense of personal empowerment.

If you stand in a power pose, it's clear how active the core must be. It completely unwinds the bent over postures that lead to unsupportive shapes with decreased strength and altered function. The brain receives different signals when one moves from the persistently compressed bent shape to the upright core-engaged shape. The brain state shifts from danger to safety, from

---

[61] Amy Cuddy. Your body language may shape who you are. TED talk. 2012.

sympathetic nervous system dominant to increased parasympathetic ventral vagal safety-wellness-alertness.

So, tapping into physical core strength shifts the language of the body and brain, leading to the emotional-psychological strength Dr. Cuddy observed as personal empowerment.

Let's go there right now.

PAUSE AND BREATHE.

Tap into your strong core.

Stand with your feet slightly more than hip distance apart. Allow a gentle bend in your knees. Gently rest your hands on hips. Breathe. Feel your feet on the ground. Let your hips sway gently from side to side. Not too much effort. Stay loose. Let your shoulders rest in their sockets. With a great big breath, let your chest expand and your heart open. Close your eyes or look up toward the sky.

Send your attention to your core, the space between your hands as they rest on your hips. As you sway (like that sturdy oak in the breeze), your core is holding you in strength. Breathe into your core, the space between your hands, breathe out (with vigorous sighs if you need to) whatever needs to be released—pain, suffering, stories that no longer serve, whatever it is.

Inhale new energy. Exhale the old, the past, what's no longer needed.

Continue to breathe in this fashion, connecting to your core, allowing your strong engaged core to move and stay flexible as your hips sway. Take as many breaths as you need.

Use your powerful words.

I'm right here. In my body. Held by my core of strength and wisdom. I am held, I can hold.

I am supported by my breath, my present moment awareness, my body with its gentle movements, and by the strength of my own sturdy core.

My core holds me as I stand in the arena of my life to face all the challenges that come to me.

I trust my core. I trust my strength and wisdom. I trust that I will always land on my feet. And when I don't, I'll always be able to get back up.

Like a sturdy tree, I trust the wind. I grow strong roots. I flow with ease.

Now, holding this truth of you within your core, what is your next small step to honor and support what you need to heal, to shift your equilibrium, in any arena of your life?

What does the wisdom of your core suggest to you? Ask it.

Let this be simple, small, and slow. Don't overthink it.

Your answer may be some next step to take. Or it may be to simply enjoy and affirm this strength within you.

Final lesson for the intr

FINAL LESSON FOR THE INTREPID: UNWIND VIGILANCE, COMMIT INSTEAD.

One more thing about balance.

We said balance is about being sturdy and trusting ourselves to manage the challenges and uncertainties of life. More than manage them, but thrive through them, grow from them, strengthen because of them.

Being sturdy and trustworthy isn't about perfection, but about flow. Flow that has an anchor and a consciously, robustly, tenderly curated core.

Here's the hardest part of creating flow with an anchor, flow we can trust.

We have to allow it. Allow the anchor. Allow the flow.

Allowing leads to experience. Experience is the only way to build trust.

For balance, we must trust our anchor. Trust our flow. Trust *ourselves.*

So, how do we build that trust?

Let yourself fall *out* of balance.

Falling out of balance is the only way to know what balance *is.* To know it where it counts. In your body. In your lived experience.

Falling out of balance is going to happen regardless. So, what happens when we don't allow it, don't trust it, don't trust our bodies, don't trust ourselves?

We make life harder. We live scared.

Stop working so hard. Release the vigilance.

The word vigilance is derived from the Latin, vigilare: to keep awake; to stay alert; to watch; to guard.

Vigilance says, "I must do it all just right, I must pay attention every second, I must be perfect in everything I do, I must be perfect in my healing, I must not look away for a moment."

What does that sound like to you?

To me, it sounds like fear and unworthiness, the strategy of a traumatized person who's scared to be wrong, to make mistakes, to fall, to be vulnerable. To be anything less than perfect.

Vigilance was a genius strategy that kept many of us alive at some time in our lives. But it's gone on too long. It no longer serves. It activates survival biology, keeping us scared and on guard, not in our flow.

Commitment says, "Yes, I see what needs to be done here, I flow with tenderness for how I hurt, I trust my own process and the pace I most need, I'm gentle with myself as I learn new things, I am exploring the conditions for my healing with curiosity, I protect but allow my vulnerability, I flow with ease and grace."

Commitment allows us to fall. To make mistakes. To be vulnerable. Commitment understands that these are strengths.

Karyn Shanks MD

Commitment is self-love. But don't underestimate commitment. It can be fierce. It can be relentless when it needs to be. But it allows us to rest. It understands the necessity of falling. It's tender toward our vulnerability.

So, balance is also about commitment to our growth. Commitment to our healing.

We trust the wind. We grow strong roots. We flow with ease.

How?

We shift. Small, easy steps made softly, with tenderness.

Where do we begin?

First breathe. Vigilance makes it hard to breathe. It tightens our muscles while weakening our core. It keeps us scared and hunched over and afraid to move, afraid to take a chance. Breathe slowly and deeply. Rest. Be in your body. Stay curious.

Then, whatever you call vigilance (*trying hard, doing my duty, keeping it all together, going after my goals*, and so on), can you feel it in your body? The urgency of it? The tightness? The conviction that overrides everything else? Stubbornness? Resistance? Fear? Whatever it is, don't try to change or fix it, but hold it with tenderness and understanding. Send it your breath. Tell it, "I see you, I hear you, you matter."

Be so tender and reverent toward your vigilance for how it has kept you safe. Gently acknowledge how it is no longer what you need.

Acknowledge the deep mind grooves you've created dedicated to vigilance, keeping it alive long past its usefulness. Gently explain how you are shifting into a new way of being. Out of vigilance into commitment. Out of perfection into authenticity. Out of tightness into flow. Out of survival biology into ventral vagal relaxed, alert wellness. Out of weakness into robustness.

Then, commit to a daily practice of shifting, of paying attention. Use the presence practices we just learned along with your core strengthening practices.

It's no longer about having to muscle through, but instead gently shift, nudging ourselves into balance, into sturdiness, into flow that has an anchor, flow we can trust to hold us and tenderly pick us up after we fall.

LAST WORDS.

We can finally breathe. That's enough. Rest. Breathe. Be present to it all. No longer needing to prove anything at all. Not to me. Not to yourself. Not to anyone.

It feels like a lot of work sometimes though, doesn't it? Unwinding our vigilant approach to life, to healing, to standing on our feet.

Bravo for all you've accomplished. Bravo for getting this far.

When you're ready, join me for the next *Unbroken* core resilience steppingstone. I'll give you a hint: it's all about the rest we deserve but often don't allow ourselves. Sometimes resting is the hardest thing of all.

THREE PROMISES.

Fall, breathe, get back up? Go for it!

1.

2.

3.

CHAPTER EIGHTEEN

Third Unbroken Core Resilience Steppingstone:

REST.

I work, but I also play. I find ways to play while I work, braving disapproving glances as I do. I play with abandon, with joy, without apology. As evening comes, I let my day go. I revel in the darkness. I relax and sleep deeply.

IT'S TIME TO REST.

My client, Chelsea, was sick with persistent fatigue, burnout, joint pain, and upset gut. She had many responsibilities to tend to at work and a young son to raise on her own while her husband was deployed. Could we launch a new food plan, change her job, and get her to bed earlier? No! Much of our first visit together was exploring an entry point to healing that would allow her to rest, soothe her exhausted nervous system, and reconnect her to herself.

Her first prescription was to sew. She had an entire room in her home dedicated to sewing. She was a master seamstress and could sew in her sleep. She could lose herself while sewing. So, that's what she did. After putting her baby to sleep in the evenings, she sat down to sew. As she did, night after night, she unwound. She sewed and cried. She sewed and felt. She sewed and thought.

After a few weeks, she had her life figured out. She quit her job. Started food planning, shopping, and cooking healthier meals. Another job came along that she loved. She slept better. Her energy recovered. Her gut healed. Miraculous? No way. She rested, reconnected, tapped into her own wisdom.

Another client once told me after a long and hard, but highly successful journey of recovery from chronic complex illness, "Healing is *not* for sissies."

What was she saying?

Healing can be hard. It's not as hard as suffering, but real healing, healing-the-verb, *is* hard.

My client also said, "but it's not as hard as being sick, out of options, and with no hope."

It's *all* hard.

So, guess what?

It's time to rest. *Really* rest.

Sit or stand right where you are. Gently close your eyes. Notice your breath without trying to change it. Allow yourself to sigh. For this moment, let go of your day so far. Let go of your to-do list. Allow yourself to be. Right here. No effort. Just rest.

There. That was you on pause. For the briefest moment of rest. How do you feel?

Pauses like that can make me teary. It's the tenderest thing we can do for ourselves when we work so hard. Rest feels sacred.

How do you feel about rest?

Is it something you're able to make space for in your life? Can you sink into rest? Like our children or my dogs, play hard, then rest hard? Without apology?

Or, like so many of us, do you bypass rest? Skimp on sleep? Nap only when you are crisis-level exhausted? Do you make room for pauses or play scheduled into your busy life of chores, work, duty, and checklists?

One of my mentors, Trisha Hersey, teaches that rest is a portal to the Divine within us.[62]

What's she saying?

---

[62] Tricia Hersey. Rest is Resistance: A Manifesto. 2022.

That rest isn't passive? Doing "nothing" isn't a waste of our precious time? A portal?

As a culture of doers constantly doing, many of us have forgotten how to rest, sleep, play, and place ourselves on pause. We've disconnected from parts of ourselves we lose to fatigue, distraction, overwhelm, and our cultural imperative to grind. We don't reflect. We don't meander or putter. We don't restore ourselves. We've traded access to the inner divinity for life's hustle.

What happens to your body when you hear or say the word, "rest?" Check in right now. What do you notice in your body as you consider the notion of rest, napping, deep sleep, play, or taking pauses throughout your day?

Me? It used to take me straight to fear. Thinking about rest made me feel anxious. I couldn't sit still, even to get the sleep I knew I'd suffer for if I didn't get enough. But to sleep when the children needed me? When my husband wanted me? When there were dishes to be done?

For me, being awake was about proving myself to everyone, including myself.

No more. While I'm still very much a work in progress, I now sigh and purr as I take my many breaks, close my eyes, sit down for meditation, or slide under my covers for yet another early bedtime. Not resting is not an option for me anymore. But I've had to work hard (I know, an oxymoron!) to change my relationship to rest and discover where that portal leads me. Rest has become sacred. It's been a profound part of my recovery from vigilance and perfectionism, into greater resilience. Rest connects me to present time, to my body, to what I know, to my Divinity. Rest celebrates me, celebrates this precious life. It supports my being over doing.

Why does rest make us squirm?

We're not talking about lazy gluttonous avoidance of our most precious responsibilities here, are we? The children need to be fed, dogs walked, and chores completed. No, we're talking about letting go, laying our weary bodies down, pressing pause, stopping the doing, landing in our bodies in present time. Giving ourselves permission to rest, restore, and rejuvenate.

And here's the key: we rest in ways that fit us, fit our needs, fit into our lives, accomplish our goals, feed our souls. This is not a prescription. I'm not here to prescribe to you, I'm here to encourage you.

Okay, how does *this* feel in your body?

Rest just because. Rest for pleasure. Rest for self-love. Not just to fill an empty tank. Not as a last resort to exhaustion. Does *that* make you squirm?

I think there are three primary reasons we're uncomfortable with rest.

First, rest is quiet. We're alone. We feel things. We let go of the doing that helps us feel safe and distracts us from our feelings. Many of us don't feel safe within our quiet, solitary, feeling spaces.

Second, we live in a culture that condemns us for taking time off. We're taught rest is lazy. We're rewarded for what we do, not how we rest. The more doing, the higher the rewards. This cultural trauma leads to our feeling best 'out there,' working hard to "succeed," "make a living," be "productive," "achieve," and "burn the midnight oil," subjugating our needs to do so. Exhaustion and overwhelm are the badges we wear to prove we're worthy of our culture's highest accolades.

Third, so many of us are stuck on the worthiness train. We stay vigilant. We work hard to stay awake. We keep a constant eye out for evidence we're worthwhile humans/parents/siblings/spouses/friends. Our favorite strategies are perfectionism and people pleasing. But they're never enough. *We're* never enough. So, we *can't* lay down or close our eyes.

In these ways, rest has been stolen from us. And as Hersey would say, our *Divinity* has been stolen from us.

Here's what's true. As humans, we *need* to rest. We need deep sleep. We need to play. We need to laugh. We need to wander and wonder. We need to access that portal to our Divinity. As both a sacred and biological need, rest is non-negotiable. And when we *do* negotiate less rest, the consequences are huge.

So. This may be your hardest steppingstone. But it may be the most essential. What finally shifts you out of sickness and suffering. Out of vigilance. Out of disconnection. Into your equilibrium of resilience. Into your potential and possibilities.

The equilibrium of resilience *demands* we rest. There are no shortcuts or bypasses.

We might live in a loop of over-work and vigilance interspersed with "retreats" to revive and rest. I'm not saying retreats are bad. In the context of over-work and self-neglect they're necessary. But we wouldn't need to crash land in our vacations or live from retreat to retreat if we made space for quiet presence and restoration in our daily lives. We wouldn't need to bypass the sources of our fatigue and unhappiness and lack of fulfillment in our daily lives. And we might just heal from persistent fatigue, pain, or chronic illness as we create a sustainable equilibrium of resilience. I see this happen in my clients all the time.

Instead of the bypass and temporary fix, here's what I propose. We're going to tenderly, patiently, courageously lead ourselves back to rest. We're going to access that portal to our Divinity.

How?

How do we give ourselves permission to enter the sacred portal of rest? To lay down our vigilance? To prioritize our needs? To shift into being rather than doing? To honor our flow? To sleep deeply, rest, and play? To wander and wonder?

Like always. Tenderly, patiently, and courageously. We lead ourselves back to rest, taking the baby steps that are sustainable, that shift us the most. We take our rest in micro-doses. As we do, we pay homage to the signatures of trauma we bump into. They're there. They *will* find us. And when they do, we welcome them. We welcome the sensations, feelings, and experiences that arise, holding them all with compassion, knowing the discomfort is temporary. The discomfort is part of our healing. The deepest healing. In the welcoming and compassion, we create safety. When we're safe, we can finally rest. What we've been running from is what finally heals us.

The first steps are the hardest but most powerful.

PAUSE AND BREATHE.

Small steps to big shifts.

How do we prove to ourselves healing isn't rocket science? What shifts us the most can be the smallest things we do.

What small things can we do right now to help us rest?

Even the small things can overwhelm us. With lives filled to capacity, how do we create more space for what we need?

Most of us have abundant opportunities to create time and space by letting some things go. Things that no longer serve. Things that waste our time and sap our energy. Things we do obsessively without realizing we're hooked.

Recognize any of these?

- Excessive e-mail checking.
- Social media scrolling.
- Phone notifications.
- News sources.
- Playing games on your phone, tablet, or computer.

These are all attention gobblers that were designed to be addictive.[63] Literally. And now it's become a part of our culture to always be available to others by phone or email, to respond to notifications instantly, to constantly be plugged in. Even when we're driving. Even when we're in line at the grocery store. It's insane, isn't it? It's exhausting and depleting and maddening. We all know it and feel it. How do we get off that train?

Boundaries.

We've touched on boundaries before. Boundaries help us say "no" to activities that are distracting and time-wasting.

Scary, eh? Tell me about it. But it's so necessary. And guess what? Everyone wants these boundaries, but we're scared to set them. So, what happens when you and I do it? When we cut back on checking messages and responding on a dime? When we turn off notifications?

---

[63] Catherine Price. *How to Break Up with Your Phone: The 30-Day Plan to Take Back Your Life.* 2018. Eye-opening description of this here.

People grumble, don't they (they're used to having us on command!)? But soon, they're doing it too! We gave them permission to do the scary thing we just did.

Set personal protective boundaries around the social electronic attention gobblers to create more space for rest. Here are a few suggestions:

- Check email just twice daily. Set the time. Let everyone know. Stick with it.
- Turn off your phone when engaged in other things—while driving, sleeping, shopping, or out on a walk. Be fully present to what you are doing.
- Take a social media fast regularly. A day or two won't kill you. Then put strict limits on the time you scroll through your feeds. Set a timer.
- Take a news fast. A few days, a week. The world doesn't change that much. If something big happens, you'll hear about it some other way.

Then, stay curious.

How does it feel to create boundaries and free up your time and attention?

Hard at first? Scary? Then what happens?

THE SCIENCE OF RESTORATION.

I've witnessed countless times how optimizing sleep and restful activity has led my chronically sick clients to complete recovery, often with few other adjustments of their terrain. Sleep and rest are *that* powerful. Restorative practices help people relax, renew energy, and relieve lifetimes of suffering from chronic conditions that could not be "fixed" with conventional approaches. Restorative practices help people reconnect to themselves, so they know what to do, like Chelsea. There's hard science to back this up. Sleep, rest, and play shift genetic expression to activate healing processes that help get people unstuck.

The science is clear and deep. What do we get through shifts in genetic expression and biological function via sleep optimization, rest, play, and restorative practices? There are many tremendous resources on the science of sleep and rest that I've included in my *Resources* section for you to refer to. We'll briefly touch on the highlights here.

SLEEP.

Sleep is powerful medicine. There are few aspects of our terrain as necessary to energy and healing. Sleep allows us to power down, repair, replenish, and renew, providing deep recovery of energy, wellbeing, and myriad human processes our organism needs to thrive—biological, cognitive, emotional, creative, and spiritual.

We all struggle with sleep from time to time. For those of us who have suffered from insomnia, we know the cruel exhaustion that can occur. We also all know the solace resulting from *good* sleep—the clear head, the feeling of lightness, the brighter perspective. For so many of my clients the last remaining hurdle to their recovery, the thing that keeps them stuck in fatigue, brain fog, and chronic illness, is not sleeping long enough or well enough.

Persistent sleep deprivation can lead to exhaustion, burnout, cognitive dysfunction, loss of productivity, mood and behavioral problems, and exacerbation of every conceivable illness. Even mild forms of sleep deprivation are important players in persistent illness, contributing to dysfunction and suffering brought about by excesses of stress, inflammation, chronic infections, toxicity, fatigue, injuries, and mood disorders. Restoring healthy sleep leads to repair and renewal.

What does sleep do for us?

While sleep is highly complex, there are four foundational functions that lead to its profound restorative properties:

- Energy conservation and renewal.
- Detoxification and cleansing of the brain.
- The circadian rhythm's regulation of physiology.
- Memory consolidation and dreaming.

These functions are critical for shifting into an equilibrium of healing and resilience, leading to:

- Better energy.
- Less pain.
- Fat loss.
- Improved cognition: focus, memory, learning, intellectual function.
- Better physical and mental performance.
- Less inflammation.
- Improved mood and wellbeing.
- Better emotional resilience.
- Improved resilience to infections.
- Accelerated recovery from chronic illness.
- Reduced "stress," greater sense of calm and relaxation.
- Lightness of being, joy, resilience.

Assess your need for more sleep.

How do we know if our sleep is good? If it meets our needs?

There is no one-size-fits-all prescription for sleep. Our needs are vastly individualized and can change over time. The specifics—number of sleep hours needed, best time of the night to sleep, best wakeup time, and so on—are unique to each of us.

To decide if your sleep is dialed in well, ask yourself these four simple questions.

- Are you waking up in the morning feeling refreshed and restored without the need for stimulants?
- Does your sleep schedule align with the solar cycle of light and dark? Are you awake during daylight and asleep when it's dark?
- Is your sleep mostly uninterrupted?
- Do you feel a strong urge to fall asleep during the day?

The first question is the most important. If you feel refreshed and restored on most mornings, your sleep quality is probably good. The typical adult needs an average of eight to nine hours of sleep each night. But if you feel energized and ready to go without the need for an alarm to wake you up or stimulants to keep you awake, you're probably getting what you need whether you're sleeping six hours or ten.

To receive the most benefit from sleep, it's best to sleep when it's dark outside and expose yourself to natural light during the day. Sleep is part of our body's built-in circadian rhythm which aligns with the solar cycle of light and dark. This cycle guides the expression of "clock genes" that control many key areas of our physiology, including sleep, itself. When this relationship is disrupted, so is our health.

If you have the overwhelming urge to fall asleep during the day, it is highly unlikely you're waking up refreshed. I'm not saying it's impossible, but daytime sleepiness is a strong sign something's off with nighttime sleep. And if your sleep is interrupted half a dozen times to use the bathroom or get more comfortable, you're probably also losing out on sleep quality.

Both sleep and sunlight deprivation are associated with health problems, including high blood pressure, insomnia, hormone imbalance, fatigue, weight gain, difficulty losing body fat, inflammation, poor immune resilience, cognitive dysfunction, mood problems, and dementia.

Optimize your conditions for sleep.[64]

Creating an environment conducive to the best sleep will support everything else we do to allow ourselves to settle into more rest.

I'm going to provide you with a list of the top ten ways to optimize your sleep, considering both behavior and your physical environment. Start with these. For much more detailed information, refer to chapter five in my book, *Heal: A Nine-Stage Roadmap to Recover Energy, Reverse Chronic Illness, and Claim the Potential of a Vibrant New You*, or any of the other excellent sleep references in my *Resources* section.

---

[64] Karyn Shanks MD. *Heal: A Nine-Stage Roadmap to Recover Energy, Reverse Chronic Illness, and Claim the Potential of a Vibrant New You.* Lots of good details in Chapter Five on creating good sleep.

1. *Make good sleep a practice.* Set the routine for going to bed and getting up and stick with it. Your brain likes to establish regular rhythms for sleep, like everything else (those neural grooves we've talked about).

2. *Boost natural outdoor light exposure during the day.* View five to fifteen minutes of early morning light upon awakening to optimize cortisol support of wakefulness and set the internal clock for nighttime melatonin. Keep your daytime spaces well lit. Then, go back outside in the late afternoon to view the red and orange hues of sunset. These practices help entrain your biological circadian rhythm and help you sleep at night.

3. *Turn down overhead lights after sunset.* After your late afternoon sunset viewing, keep lights low for the remainder of the evening. Avoid light-producing electronics (computers, phones, and TVs) within two hours of sleep time.

4. *Sleep in a pitch-dark area.* Use blackout shades or curtains, remove all electronic devices with lights, no matter how small. A single photon can interfere with sleep.

5. *Sleep in a cool room with plenty of blankets for comfort.* The exact temperature will depend on what is comfortable for you, but sixty-five degrees is about average. There are also cooling mattress covers available to help accomplish the need for a lower body temperature to optimize sleep.[65]

6. *Make your bed as comfortable as possible.* Assess your mattress, pillows, and covers. Make sure you feel completely comfortable as you nestle in to go to sleep. Address any sounds that could interfere with your sleep. Consider the use of soft earplugs or white noise.

7. *Let go of your day; relax.* Write down your to-do list for the next day to "unload" your mind. Engage in downtime and relaxing activities before getting into bed. Meditate. Do a guided relaxation or yoga nidra.[66] Meditation at any time of day will help improve your sleep.

---

[65] The eight sleep "pod cover" cools and warms, is programmable, and tracks sleep quality throughout the night. www.eightsleep.com.

[66] You can find many variations of yoga nidra for relaxation and sleep. Free apps include Insight Timer, www.insighttimer.com, Aura Health, www.aurahealth.io.

8. *Avoid alcohol.* Any quantity of alcohol can interfere with sleep. Some folks are particularly sensitive to this effect. If you're not sure how alcohol affects your sleep, try a period of at least four to six weeks of complete alcohol abstinence to see if your sleep improves.

9. *Eat well, hydrate, and support your microbiome.* This may seem like three things, but they go together. You'll find more detailed information about healthy eating and hydrating in the *Nourish* steppingstone. Healthy eating and hydrating support body and brain to optimize everything, including sleep. The addition of fermented foods and probiotics support the microbiome, which plays a key role in brain health and regulation of sleep.

10. *Limit stimulants such as caffeine to early-midmorning.* Caffeine helps override the perception of tiredness that helps drive sleep at bedtime. It's half-life (the time it takes the body to get rid of half of a dose) is five to six hours. So, if you drink coffee at noon, half of the caffeine is still in your body at six. The stimulant effects of caffeine plus its effect of increasing stress hormones and delay of melatonin secretion all interfere with sleep many hours later.

What to do if restorative sleep eludes you.

You've done everything. You've eliminated caffeine and alcohol. You turn off electronics two hours before bedtime. You meditate daily and quietly read before turning off all lights. You're in bed for ten hours. Your sleep environment is perfect. You're comfy under your covers. It's pitch black and quiet. You feel relaxed and ready to sleep. But sleep doesn't come. Or you go to sleep but wake up a dozen times throughout the night. Sometimes you can't get back to sleep for hours at a time. Dang it. What to do?

After months of frequent awakenings in the middle of the night, I once told my own therapist that I just couldn't sleep despite doing all the 'right' things. So vigilantly. Using my best practices to "soften," "release," and ease my mind. Sometimes they worked but other times they didn't, leaving me exhausted and frustrated. She said to me, "Karyn, that's soul time. Don't try to fix it, ask yourself what you need. Be so tender." To really drive home her point, she said, "Karyn, what would you say to one of your patients?" I got it. Would I try to "fix" them, and ask them to be vigilant? If that's not the advice I'd give them, why would I treat myself differently? I learned how tenderness and concern for parts of me asking for my attention was not just kinder but helped me get more sleep because I stopped trying so hard.

So, here's what I have to say to you that I learned to say to myself. First and foremost, be very gentle with yourself. Lying there in the middle of the night, you are your most vulnerable. What you say will leave its mark. Don't blame yourself. And what is frustration to your sleepy vulnerable parts in the middle of the night, if not blame? Be tender. Hold your sleepless self with compassion and curiosity. Ask, "what do you need?" Literally ask. Then, if you've dialed in the "excellent sleep practices" listed above and sleeplessness continues or you feel persistently tired and unrestored in the morning, ask for expert help. There may be more than "soul time" needs asking for your attention.

Ask for help with sleep.

There are many health problems that can make sleep difficult. It is important to explore these with a trusted health practitioner.

There are common problems that can be revealed through comprehensive history taking by an expert who knows what to ask. Daytime fatigue, falling asleep, and headaches can indicate sleep apnea, especially if you snore. Snoring indicates obstructed breathing even in the absence of apnea (significant pauses in breathing) and can decrease sleep quality resulting in fatigue. Snoring, even in the absence of apnea, has also been associated with an increased risk for earlier mortality and coronary artery disease.[67]

Lab tests can help sort out physiological issues that affect sleep quality: thyroid and adrenal function, nutrient levels, iron stores, and indicators of inflammation.

You may need a sleep study, either a home overnight oximetry test or a more extensive sleep test performed at a professional sleep lab. Home oximetry tests detect drops in blood oxygen during sleep that could indicate sleep apnea, obstructed breathing, or respiratory problems. In the sleep lab test, specialists monitor the quality of your sleep, oxygen levels, movements that may lead to arousals from sleep, quality of your breathing, and in some cases, brain wave activity. I order sleep studies routinely for my clients who

---

[67] Imre Janszky MD PhD. Heavy Snoring is a Risk Factor for Case Fatality and Poor Short-Term Prognosis after a First Acute Myocardial Infarction. Sleep. 2008.

have persistent fatigue, or if they had symptoms suggestive of a sleep disorder, such as sleep apnea or periodic limb movement (PLM).

I had a client once with persistent severe fatigue and muscle pain even after a thorough exploration of possible causes. Though she did not snore, had not been observed to have apnea episodes, and was not aware of waking up in the night, I ordered a sleep study for her at a professional sleep lab. Testing revealed extensive limb movement throughout the period of sleep that was associated with frequent arousals from deep sleep. Treatment completely reversed her fatigue and muscle pain.

Bottom line: always consider sleep problems when persistently fatigued and always ask for expert help when you can't figure it out on your own. And if one expert can't help you, move on to another.

Safe supplements for sleep.

Talk to your trusted healthcare advisor about what might be best for you. The following are commonly available over-the-counter supplements that are safe to use for trouble falling to sleep or staying asleep when more serious problems have been ruled out.

- *GABA:* a naturally occurring amino acid that calms the brain. A typical dose is 400 mg taken at bedtime. Consider using this if you feel restless or anxious.
- *5-HTP:* a naturally occurring amino acid that the body will use to synthesize serotonin and melatonin, both important for healthy sleep. A typical dose is 50-150 mg taken at bedtime.
- *Inositol:* a sugar alcohol that is involved in the regulation of serotonin and melatonin. A typical dose is 900 mg taken at bedtime.
- *L-Theanine:* an amino acid found abundantly in green tea that calms the brain. A typical dose is 200 mg taken at bedtime.
- *Magnesium threonate:* a form of magnesium that easily crosses the blood-brain barrier, thus helping the brain with numerous processes, including energy production, cognitive activities, and restful sleep. A typical dose is 2 grams (yields 145 mg magnesium) taken at bedtime.
- *Melatonin:* a hormone involved in regulating the sleep-wake cycle. A typical dose is 3 mg taken at bedtime.

- *Phosphatidyl serine:* a fatty acid involved in protecting the brain from the potentially toxic effects of high cortisol production associated with stress. A typical dose is 150 mg taken at bedtime.
- *Omega-3-fatty acids:* fatty acids derived from fish, algae, and present in pastured meat, poultry, and eggs, important for cell membrane support and regulation of inflammation. Essential for healthy brain function, including sleep. A typical dose is 2 grams of a combination of EPA and DHA taken daily with food.
- *Botanicals:* Many herbs and plants have relaxation properties that help with inducing sleep including chamomile, passionflower, valerian root, skullcap, magnolia, and lemon balm. These are commonly found in various combinations for sleep support. They can also be obtained as fresh dried herbs for tea used at bedtime.

BEYOND SLEEP—REST, PAUSES, AND PLAY.

Sleep can save your life, but rest, pauses, and play will make your life worth living.

As we keep saying, we've unlearned what once came naturally. Like our children, we too were fully engaged every waking moment with our own spontaneous agenda. We were free, creative, and exploding with curiosity, experimentation, and growth. And we had so much fun doing it, didn't we? After play, we dropped into little heaps right where we were, without a care or worry, to take our needed rest. We may not have been able to articulate what we needed, but we certainly claimed it.

Then, we morphed from spontaneous little geniuses into overworked, regimented, exhausted adults, desperate for rest, pauses, and play.

Aside from being opportunities for fun, what do we know about the benefits of rest, pauses, and play?

- Autonomic nervous system (ANS) regulation—shift into ventral vagal social engagement and relaxation.
- Enhanced growth and learning.
- Better brain function, including support of memory and cognitive abilities.
- Support of mood and wellbeing.

- Greater creativity and problem-solving abilities.
- Better sleep.
- Decreased inflammation and improved immune resilience.
- Improved self-awareness.
- Enhanced empathy and compassion for others.
- Improved energy.

How do we remember our childhood patterns to gently shift back to rest, pauses, and play?

Some of us just need permission and the rest is easy. Heck yah, bring on the rest! For others, it's not as simple. We bump headfirst into the worst trauma of our lives. I did. The worthiness train I spoke of earlier? I was on that train. I was one hundred percent committed to being on that train. I wanted to look, feel, and *be* successful. A successful human, doing successful things, feeling successful. For me it was a collision of early life trauma with cultural trauma. Of letting others define my worth and working my ass off to prove my worthiness.

What did I do to get off that worthiness train?

I willed myself to feel it—the fear, sadness, and loneliness that hid beneath the story of unworthiness. I learned to have compassion for the parts of me that felt that way, and to legitimize their experiences and explore them with curiosity. I had a lot of help doing this. I explored many books and resources on trauma and how to heal it (I'll include many of my favorite sources in the Resources section) and have worked with trauma therapists.

Healing trauma was one of the keys to my learning to rest. It was also much easier once I experienced the incredible benefits of rest, such as more energy, better mental clarity, and greater zest for life.

WHAT REST, PAUSES, AND PLAY MIGHT LOOK LIKE.

Naps.

Total shut down. Sleep during the day. Remember though, your dynamic stillness isn't passive and it's not neglectful. Naps don't have to mean you're exhausted or *must* nap. They can be joyful, indulgent timeouts.

Active Pauses.

Active pauses temporarily shift us out of our routine. They take many forms. Breaks from hard work and deep focus. A pause for a single conscious breath. A loud sigh. A walk across the room or around the block. A break to hug the dog or take them on a short walk.

A favorite of mine is when I luxuriate in the sensory experience of handwashing between clients. I breathe deeply as I enjoy the warmth of the water on my hands and smell of the lavender in my hand wash. I let go of the work I just completed, landing in present time.

These pauses shift us. They refresh and renew and invite inspiration, insights, new ideas, or solutions to our problems.

Play.

Play can be anything we do for sheer enjoyment. Play can have rules and structure, and can call on our skills and accomplishments, but most importantly, it's fun. We pretend, imagine, or improvise. We get lost in something we're good at. We become completely focused on the moment of high competition. We flow. There may be time limits, but the process is time expanded—we're not aware of time. When we play, we're fully engaged in the moment.

Puttering.

Puttering is action with a purpose, but without limitation of time, sequence, or endpoint. We can putter at most anything, from fixing things in the workshop, to rearranging furniture, decorating a room, or sorting through closets. Done without time stress, puttering releases us from ordinary time, landing us in our flow.

Puttering can be the key to finding solutions to our problems. We set the problem aside, enter the present-moment awareness of our project and ideas flood in while we're not actively searching for them. Puttering gets us out of our own way.

Laughter.

Laughter is the best timeout known to humankind. It captures our lightness and wisdom about what may be otherwise inexpressible. The author Anne Lamott calls laughter "carbonated holiness." Laughter transports us out of ordinary time and place. It gives air to our suffering, strengthening us with its waves of understanding and wisdom, and connecting us with those who laugh with us.

Laughter has many health benefits. Dr. Norman Cousins famously credited reversing his autoimmune disorder to daily doses of laughter.[68] Laughter reduces stress hormones levels and inflammation. It makes us feel happier. It helps us breathe. It releases strong emotions.

Laughter helps us avoid taking ourselves too seriously. Our work is important, but we're all works in progress, and we're hilarious!

Creating Art.

Creating art is puttering, play, and creation in total present-moment engagement. Art is flow. Art is anything we set aside time and space to create for our pure enjoyment (even art created from a bedrock of enormous skill)—painting, cooking, gardening, party planning, organizing . . . it's all art. It all pulls us out of ordinary time, engages our present-moment awareness, and provides necessary pause.

Meditation.

Meditation is any form of quiet contemplative activity, still or active, that cultivates self-awareness: of being in our bodies, connected to present time, and aware of our sensations, feelings, and energy states. Meditation "rests" us from the past (regret, grief, rumination) and the future (worry, fear, vigilance), soothing our nervous systems, enhancing safety. As compassionate observers, we hold ourselves and everything around us with curiosity, releasing judgement, opening to possibilities.

REST IN BABY STEPS.

Sleep, rest, and restorative practices are not passive.

They may be silent, slow, and still. We look like we're doing nothing. But just like the Earth in winter, still and cold and silent, we are incredibly alive beneath the surface. Without winter, there would be no spring. The lifeforce of

---

[68] Norman Cousins. *Anatomy of an Illness as Perceived by the Patient: Reflections on Healing and Regeneration.* 1980.

trees and plants and animals depend on winter to emerge in their fullness after the final freeze.

We are not passive when we rest. Not doing nothing. Not unproductive.

And rest is devastating to bypass—there's so much to lose.

Rest takes practice. Baby steps. Like any practice, you're getting your reps in, your hours. And with each rep and hour, you're stronger, more resilient, it comes more easily.

You've created space for this practice (see the last *'Pause and breathe'* practice). Now, use that space. Start by pausing for just five minutes per day. Micro-dose your rest. Stare out the window noticing the trees and birds. Take slow deep breaths and big ol' sighs. Lay down on the couch. Add five minutes to your sleep time. Optimize your sleep conditions. Gradually work your way up, calibrating to how you feel.

N*otice* how you feel. Realize how rest, just like we said about healing, is not for sissies. No joke, my friend. For many of us, rest is insanely hard. So, hold on. Be tender with yourself. Stay relentlessly curious.

LAST WORDS.

Let's use our powerful words.

Rest is how I expand into myself. Not work, not struggle, not achievement, not denying my needs. Not doing, not crashlanding into my bed or vacation or mountaintop retreat.

My challenging life is punctuated by pause. It envelops me with softness. It holds me in the deepest sleep. I grow from challenge but emerge into my fullness through the subterranean passages that contain my genius.

Rest is how I rise.

THREE PROMISES TO MYSELF.

Land here for a moment. Breathe. Sigh it out. What three promises can you make right now that support you in rest? Gently, now.

1.
2.
3.

CHAPTER NINETEEN
Fourth *Un*Broken Core Resilience Steppingstone:

MOVE.

... I move and breathe and have my being.

—Acts 17:28.

All human experience is linked to movement. Think about that for a sec. If not for movement, why have bodies? Movement is living. Movement is the pulse of all Nature, all her parts and processes. From subsistence to safety to energy, movement is what gets us there. We move to find shelter, food, and warmth. We move through our chores and relationships. We move to raise our children and build our communities. We move to create and express our genius. Our bodies are always moving. Even when we sleep. Even when we're not aware. Movement is the crux of our survival, the crux of all our connections, and the crux of the quality of all our experiences.

Why's that important?

Well, for one, we love our moving bodies, don't we? They're where we live, breathe, feel, connect, and create. That's enough, isn't it? Because our connection to our bodies is *everything.* It's what we keep saying—how by fully inhabiting our bodies and experiencing their sensations, feelings, and energy states, we connect to everything worth anything.

Movement is key to our equilibrium of healing. It plays into all the equilibria we experience—of illness, suffering, energy, safety, and resilience. And our movement is, well, mobile. We have control over it. We can shift it. By shifting it, we shift all the equilibria of our human experience. In this sense, movement is one of our most powerful tools for inhabiting our potential and possibilities.

Many movements we can see. The blinking of our eyes. The rise and fall of our chests as we breathe. The subtle movements as we sleep. The countless movements of our days doing all the things we do. And there are innumerable infinitesimally small movements we can't see that we couldn't possibly live without. Like the movement of electrical impulses along our nerve fibers. The movement of atoms and molecules across our cell membranes. The movement of blood and body fluids through their various channels. The movement of digested food molecules through intestinal wall, into portal vein or lymphatics, to all the relay centers of their myriad destinations, running all the business of our bodies.

It's all movement. All human experience and function and evolution is based on movement.

So. If movement is a given, why does it need to be an *Unbroken* core resilience steppingstone? Doesn't it just happen?

Short answer? Yes, movement will just happen. But like any dynamic equilibrium of the human experience, it will happen to our detriment if we're disconnected from our bodies and unaware of what we need.

What do I mean?

The movement we personally direct will affect all the infinitesimal movements we cannot see. They are linked, like the strength and function of our core we discussed in the *Balance* steppingstone. How we move and hold ourselves in space has everything to do with how our bodies function. And how our bodies function at the level of those infinitesimal movements we cannot see has everything to do with how we're able to move and hold ourselves in space.

How about energy? Our lifeforce? Movement directs energy. The more we move, the more energy we're capable of creating. Movement depends on muscle function. Muscle function depends on muscle growth, strength, rest, and repair. All of this requires energy. Movement drives mitochondrial function. Recall how mitochondria are our powerhouses for energy production. Increases in movement drive both the number of mitochondria we have in each of our cells as well as the ability for each mitochondrion to make energy. And the reverse is true—less movement leads to fewer mitochondria with reduced function, meaning *less* energy for you to experience and enjoy and depend on.

How did this complex relationship of movement, function, and energy come to be?

Consider the earliest humans who, adapting to their upright lives and big brains in complex environments, had to move a lot. They moved all day. That movement varied greatly from upright walking and running to stooping and squatting and everything in between. They moved under heavy loads. Early humans moved to survive, securing shelter, food, warmth, and community. They hunted, foraged, cooked, and raised their young. Over hundreds of thousands of years of human evolution through all the ancestral lineages of the planet, the human genome became highly specialized for movement—all day long, highly varied, under heavy loads. To support the energy needs of our hard-working ancestors, the genome evolved to link strength with energy production.

Today, movement is more optional. Recent human history has rapidly transformed the human lifestyle through greater ease and convenience in just about everything. Consider what the modern human lifestyle consists of:

Ultra-convenience. Not just cars and planes and one-stop-shopping, but escalators, elevators, automatic doors, and Amazon! No need to walk, use your arms, or even step in and out of your car.

Ultra-comfort. Comfy beds, comfy pillows, comfy couches, and comfy shoes. No need to squat, let your feet touch the ground, or sit on the floor.

Ultra-dependence. Dependence on industrialized food, manufactured clothes, and mass-produced household goods.

And that leads to ultra-specialization of our skills. Who grows their own food, makes their own clothes, fixes their own tools and appliances, or walks to work anymore?

The human lifestyle of ultra-convenience, ultra-comfort, ultra-dependence, and ultra-specialization should give us more free time and shelter us in optimal safety. But it also drives us to work more, buy more, and waste more time. So, we sit too much, move too little, eat too much, and are deprived of sleep, rest, and play. But it's what we know and hard to feel. We don't register the mismatch.

But the human genome hasn't changed to match our more sedentary modern lifestyles. So, what happens when the human genome, evolved for optimal human function and robustness through the imperative of movement, suddenly (evolutionarily speaking) collides with massively reduced movement due to comfort and convenience? Mismatch is an understatement.

What's the outcome?

Nothing short of disaster. Lost strength. Lost energy. Lost function. The loss of challenging movement in the human lifestyle is at the heart of the global pandemic of human chronic illness and suffering.[69]

I love so much of the modern world I live in. But there's tragedy in it as well: lost human potential, suffering on a massive scale.

But we know what to do now.

Shift. We begin to shift. We bring movement back. We recreate the imperative of movement in our daily lives, so we become better aligned with our movement-optimized genetic expression. We renew our energy. We rise out of suffering and chronic illness. We recover our lifeforce, our resilience, and who we're meant to be. And as you'll see, we don't have to return to the stone age to do it.

That's why *Move* is an *Unbroken* core resilience steppingstone. Movement is one of our essential paths back to healing, flow, and our sparkliest wholeness.

PAUSE AND BREATHE.

Let's begin our practice right now.

Wherever you are right now, stand up. If you can't stand, sit up straight and engage your core. If you can't sit up, tuck your chin just a bit and engage your core. If you're standing, allow your attention to

---

[69] Frank W Booth et al. *Lack of exercise is a major cause of chronic diseases.* Review. Compr Physiol. 2012.

Frank W Booth, et al. *Role of Inactivity in Chronic Diseases: Evolutionary Insight and Pathophysiological Mechanisms.* Physiological Reviews. 2017.

drift down to your feet. Feel the ground beneath you, noticing how it supports you. Place your hands on your hips, tuck your chin, engage your core, and take a few big breaths in and out. Notice the rise and fall of your chest. Notice the blinking of your eyes. Soften your knees and let your hips gently sway. Let yourself move so gently.

Gently. This is how we shift. This is how we shift from sitting to standing. And how each of us in our own way can transition with gentle embodied conscious awareness to a life of more vigorous movement we were designed for.

All day long. Highly varied. Under heavy loads.

Did you feel how gentle our first practice was? Don't let movement scare you. We're not going to start running or doing three-hundred-pound deadlifts just yet (unless you're already doing them!). We're shifting, beginning where you are, gently.

Here's where we're going in our *Move* steppingstone practice:

- Gently shift out of prolonged postures and bent compressed shapes.
- Gradually add variety to your ordinary daily movements.
- Gradually add loads to your ordinary daily movements.
- Beyond ordinary daily movement: exercise and strength training.
- Incorporate movement-responsive rest and recovery into your more active life.

Think of movement as an extension of your embodied self-awareness practice. Because it is. And the more present you are in your moving body, the more you feel, the more you stay curious about your experience, and the gentler you are in your approach? The greater you'll shift. The more you'll access your potential and possibilities.

This is where we start, gradually working up to "all day long," then "highly varied," and "under heavy loads," with rest periods sprinkled in between for recovery. These are important attributes of the most robust and healthy humans. And they're necessary to reverse chronic illness and rise out of suffering.

But we start where we're at. Many of my clients are in the rebuilding stages after severe or prolonged illness. They're shifting and moving very differently than everyone else. They shift more slowly and cautiously. This is important to their continued healing and safety. Getting up to shower, spending more time sitting up in bed versus lying flat, walking across the room to grab a bottle of water are all ways they may progress. Gradually adding steps, standing to fold laundry or chop veggies, stooping to pick a few weeds out of their yard may be heroic achievements for someone in recovery. Make this process yours. Stay in your body. Be gentle. Celebrate every success.

GENTLY SHIFT OUT OF PROLONGED POSTURES AND BENT COMPRESSED SHAPES.

Prolonged postures mean you're not moving.

We began this practice in the *Balance* steppingstone, by unwinding old habits that hijack core strength, such as prolonged sitting and slouching over our electronic devices. We started out gently, didn't we? Gradually releasing our continuously static, bent, and compressed postures. Slowly beginning new practices to strengthen us, first through holding our bodies more upright and aligning our necks with the rest of our spine, second by engaging in core strengthening exercises.

Think of it this way. Whatever you ask your body to do the most, it will adapt to that shape and level of energy expenditure. If that shape is sitting and slouching, your body adapts to a bent compressed shape with sedentary energy. Your body will lose function, strength, and energy. If that shape is varied, upright, and moving most of the day, your body adapts to open balanced shapes with active mobility, optimizing function, strength, and energy.

So, we begin by coaxing your body out of unhealthy adaptation by unwinding your most habitual shapes, gently shifting, gradually moving into a variety of shapes.

You've already begun practicing improved shapes through a varied movement lifestyle:[70]

- Sit less and move often.
- Avoid all continuous static postures.
- Hold your torso upright and avoid all head-forward postures.

GRADUALLY ADD VARIETY TO YOUR ORDINARY DAILY MOVEMENTS.

You're unwinding your body's bent compressed adaptations to prolonged sitting. You're venturing out of continuous static postures. You're realigning your spine and holding your head high. Your upright core is stronger and you're moving more. Your blood and lymph are flowing better. Your tissues are recovering more readily, as they're more nourished and oxygenated. Your muscles and bones are already stronger. Your body is upregulating mitochondrial function and making more energy. You may not be able to feel it yet, but I assure you that's all happening.

You had to do all that first to prepare for what's to come. Because what do you think happens to a bent compressed shape with low energy and a weak core that goes directly to the gym? You got it. It gets hurt. Maybe not today or tomorrow, but when the loads and demands expose the vulnerability? You take many steps back. That's *not* what we're after.

Let's make a distinction between movement and exercise. Sure, exercise consists of movement, but the two are not the same. Exercise is a defined period of movement that's intentionally ramped up—faster, more complex, under heavier loads. For many people exercise is the bulk of their daily movement. And the main reason people get hurt as often as they do when they work out is because they only move when they exercise. They haven't unwound their bent compressed shapes and weak cores (even if they do core exercises!). Look around you at the gym or at people you see jogging down the street. Observe their neck-spine alignment, how their shoulders are placed,

---

[70] Review the section "Unwind old habits that hijack your core strength" in the second *Core Resilience* steppingstone, *Balance* for the details.

and the angles between their legs, hips, and back. If you look carefully, it's like they're still partially sitting, isn't it? And this makes them more vulnerable to injury.

While there are health benefits to exercise, huge benefits when it's done correctly, it can't make up for the detriments of being sedentary the rest of the time. We'll address both, starting with the most important part of your movement regimen—normal daily movement that's varied and interesting as you go about doing what you do.

So, first we unwind. Then, from our unbent decompressed open flowing gorgeous body, we can safely make it more interesting. Already moving more (we had to as we shapeshifted, didn't we?), we'll add variety to our movement. As we add variety, we'll be moving more and progressing function, strength, and energy.

Let's see how easy we can make this. 'No pain, no gain' is *not* our motto here. Gentle, kind, consistent, and committed is what shifts us the most.

Our capabilities and interests are on a wide spectrum, so as we proceed, carefully consider where *you* are, honor that, move from there.

HOW TO MAKE ORDINARY DAILY MOVEMENT MORE VARIED AND INTERESTING.

Consider what you do in a typical day. What part of that day keeps you in a stationary position? How can we break that up to add variety and more movement?

I have a job that requires me to focus for long stretches of time. Whether I'm working with clients, researching a topic, or writing, I'm tethered to one place for at least an hour at a time and often more. This is a common situation, so I'll tell you some of what I do.

I use a sit-stand desk so I can move seamlessly between sitting and standing, and I do so frequently. When I sit, I fidget (comes naturally). When I stand, I fidget as well and frequently step away from my desk to walk around the room. Every half hour or so, I take a longer break. I walk out of the room. I have small things planned to do—eat a meal, water plants, feed birds, let a dog out, get the mail, do laundry, and so on. So, rather than do all these small chores at once after my workday, I sprinkle them through the day. They get me purposefully moving in a variety of ways throughout the day, and they take just a few minutes so don't derail my workflow.

There are added benefits of this routine. I get my chores done early and have more free time in the evening. I also feel better, I'm able to focus longer, and my mind is more creative for taking breaks.

When I'm working with clients, I can't just get up and walk away. I've made peace with a sedentary position during consultations. It helps me stay focused on my client and is the most comfortable position for me to take notes in. As soon as our work is complete, I'm up and moving for chores between clients. I know some folks who do "walk and talks" with clients. That's great when it works. I find notetaking is key to my work with complex clients (wish I had an amazing auditory memory!) so my work is centered around writing space.

When I'm working it's important that I alternate between sitting and standing. Standing is important for a less bent compressed shape and stronger core, but standing without moving can become a problem too. Blood flow depends on muscle contraction throughout the body, especially in the legs. Prolonged standing causes blood to stagnate.

There are under desk treadmills so you can walk while working. I don't have one yet but am intrigued. In researching them for this book, I see the highly rated and well-reviewed versions are reasonably priced, portable, and easy to maneuver.

What else can be done to keep moving?

- Clean out a drawer.
- Sort a shelf in a closet.
- Stoop down into a full squat to pet the dog.
- Begin prepping your evening meal.
- Walk and talk for calls during your workday.

Can you name three more small chores or activities you can easily insert into your daily routine?

Can you also name three ways you can modify your work to accommodate more movement? Keep these activities small, simple, and readily doable.

GRADUALLY ADD LOADS TO YOUR ORDINARY DAILY MOVEMENTS.

You've already been loading. Every time you're upright or move from sitting to standing and back again, you're loading. Every time you walk across your house or office, you're loading. It's your body against gravity.

Loading is important to being a healthy human. Not just for strength but for running all the business of the body. For shifting into the healthiest genetic expression to support everything you do. Loading the body engages and strengthens your muscles, fortifies your bones, and keeps your blood moving. It stimulates energy production, supports detoxification, lowers blood sugar, and reduces body fat. Consistent loading through bodyweight movements and carrying heavy objects has a positive effect on every aspect of your biology while making you stronger. Stronger *feels* good. Inhabiting a strong body helps us feel safer, more capable, and confident.

How do we load?

Initially, see how you can add load by using our own body weight. You know how to do that. How can you maximize loading through your normal daily routine?

- When you get up from a chair, see if you can do it without using your hands for support. Work up to this.
- Find reasons to go up and down your stairs more frequently.
- Sit on the floor. This not only gets you into a new shape, but it also requires you to get back up. Work toward doing this without holding onto anything for support.
- Squat all the way down to pet your dog.
- Squat all the way down to pull weeds. Move in and out of that squat.
- Fold the laundry standing up.
- Sweep or mop the floor using your core strength.
- Take breaks from work to walk around your house or yard.

Can you come up with three additional ways to load using your own bodyweight in the course of your daily routine?

Then can you come up with ways to *add* load to your bodyweight in the course of your day? How about these?

- Use your core strength to carry the groceries into the house.
- Pick up your pet or child, using your entire core to do so: activate your quads (thigh muscles) and glutes (butt muscles), then carry them in a strong upright position.
- Pack those unwanted items in a box and carry it out to your car for a donation drop-off.

Can you come up with three more?

BEYOND ORDINARY DAILY MOVEMENT.

You may already be a gym rat. That's awesome. Adding more movement into the course of your day to unwind bent compressed shapes and add core engagement will totally up your game, adding strength, endurance, and resilience to injury. Don't be surprised if you're tired or your gym metrics fall off as you initiate upping your home/work movement game. All movement has something to contribute to your strength, mobility, and overall function.

Even for those of us with active lives, the movement patterns of our typical days will never be what our remote ancestors were adapted to (what shaped our genome), so strength and endurance training are excellent ways to make us even stronger, more energetic, and resilient. They can also be great fun. Incorporating both strength and endurance training into your exercise repertoire is ideal as they lead to different forms of physical adaptations that lead to longer, healthier lives.

There are many fantastic choices for strength training and body conditioning readily available to all of us. I won't go into detail here but there are countless books, videos, programs, and podcasts available for you. I'll include some of my favorites in the *Resources* section of this book.

I have just five important bits of advice as you venture into more challenging movement practice:

- Choose what interests you, then stick with what you most enjoy.
- Variety is the spice of life.
- Try something awkward, unfamiliar, or particularly challenging.
- Challenge your balance.

- Work with a trained professional, especially in the beginning or if you have unique needs in a highly physical environment.

If you don't love it, you probably won't stick with it. Rather than get discouraged if you don't enjoy something, set your sights on trying out a variety of activities, then revel in what you love. But continue to explore. Include things that are new to you or require skills you don't have yet, taking you out of your familiar comfort zone. I like to include balance skills that make me feel ridiculous at first. Until I nail them!

Gradually find a variety of ways to promote strength and endurance. Cross-training keeps things way more interesting and allows you to explore different ways to challenge your body. Over-specialization and repetition can increase the risk of injury.

It can be helpful to work with professionals who can personalize your experience, help you with proper body mechanics, address vulnerabilities and injuries, and provide encouragement as you challenge yourself.

EXERCISE FOR SPECIAL NEEDS, REHAB, AND AGING.

Some exercises don't fit the needs of our bodies. I've talked about my hypermobility. My stretchy ligaments and lax joints don't love many forms of yoga because they emphasize ultra-elongation of the body. My extra-long hamstrings (back of the thigh) became stretched past the point of balanced reciprocal engagement with my quadriceps muscles (front of the thigh), and they were often injured until I figured this out. I learned you can't stretch the bejeebies out of hamstrings that are already long, then ask them to carry a heavy load or run fast or sit for a car ride (even a short one!). It took me years to get my persistently sore, tight hamstring insertions to heal! Now, I modify my yoga extensively to allow for my unique body.

Sometimes working with professionals can help, but even they don't always have the answers. I remember bringing up my chronically injured hamstrings to yoga instructors and being given the side eye. Sometimes pros don't want to admit their specialty isn't for everyone. So, work with a professional while keeping your own sense of agency fully engaged. You know yourself best. If you have special needs or concerns about working out hard, interview teachers and trainers who seem qualified. Find out how they might work with you. If you decide to work with them, understand experience will be your best teacher. Plan to reassess how you feel your needs are being met through working with them from time to time.

Strength and endurance fall off more rapidly as we age during periods of inactivity. Those of us in our fifties, sixties, and beyond must work harder and stay very consistent to maintain strength and endurance and all the health benefits that go with that. The good news is we *can* maintain them as we age. The more active we've been throughout our lives, the easier it is, but it's never too late to start.

If you're in your 'second act,' as I am, I encourage you to stay or become as active as possible to enjoy the greater strength, energy, and resilience that comes with it. The same guidelines we discussed above apply. Find a variety of activities you enjoy and stick with them. Remain active every day. Absolutely work with a professional to help you transition into more movement with greater loading, complexity, and balance. This can be a physical therapist or professional fitness trainer with interest and expertise in programming movement and conditioning in older adults.

INCORPORATE MOVEMENT-RESPONSIVE REST AND RECOVERY INTO YOUR MORE ACTIVE LIFE.

"All day long, highly varied, under heavy loads" may be our motto, but it doesn't mean we don't rest. In fact, rest is as necessary as loading for strength and energy production. It's also our antidote to excessive soreness and helps prevent injuries.

How much rest do we need in the context of movement and exercise, beyond the rest we've already explored?

We need enough. I know that sounds evasive, but the amount of rest needed to recover, restore, and repair is highly variable between each person and each day.

Rest and recovery in an active life can mean many things. This is a topic of much discussion in the realms of professional athletics. Not as much for the rest of us. The following are the key takeaways:

- Dial in your sleep—go back to the *Rest* steppingstone. Sleep is your most important form of restoration.

- Follow the guidelines for becoming more active during your normal daily life—this movement is more important for your health and wellbeing than exercise.
- Add in periods of more intense exercise with rest periods in between. Light to moderate exercises like walking, hiking, playing outside with your kids or dogs, or gentle yoga can be done every day. More intense strength or endurance exercises like gym strength training, intense yoga or Pilates, running or sprinting, CrossFit, or high-intensity interval training should be followed by a period or rest. Three days per week with a rest day in between or an every-other-day schedule works well for most people.
- Take short rest periods *during* intense exercise. Short rest breaks lasting 2-3 minutes between sets of heavy lifting or intense movements are both kind and most fitness professionals agree improves overall performance.
- Every month or two, take a week off from more intense training. This can be done by stopping altogether, while continuing less intense daily activities, or by having a "de-load" week, reducing the intensity and number of reps in the gym.

LAST WORDS.

What happens when we move our bodies with intention? When we inhabit them with tenderness, kindness, and commitment? When we're truly wholly present in our bodies? *To* our bodies?

It's not just the movement we benefit from, is it?

Because we're embodied. We're engaged with present time. We're practicing present moment embodied awareness with focused *in*tention, devoted *at*tention, and profound agency (it takes a hell of a lot of agency to step into the unknown of what we can do).

Once again, we've come full circle. Everything is connected to everything else. So, it's no surprise at all where movement has brought us. Practicing movement isn't just about shifting genetic expression to create physical resilience, to help us shift the equilibrium of suffering, weakness, low energy, and chronic illness. We all know this now, don't we? How we're complex multifaceted beings of body-mind-spirit-community-planetary wholeness.

Which is to say, we're more present. And that presence brings us closer to everything worth anything.

So.

All day long. Highly varied. Under heavy loads.

This is what robust bodies and vibrant curious minds do. What they're capable of. What each one of us is capable of. We carry this potential in our genome. And as we relearn how to live more active and challenging lives well, we reap the enormous benefits of moving in alignment with our potential. Movement is us. Movement is why we have bodies at all.

So, we shift. Gently. With curiosity. Staying in our bodies. We move and breathe and find our being.

THREE PROMISES.

What three promises can I make to myself regarding movement?
1.
2.
3.

Karyn Shanks MD

CHAPTER TWENTY
Fifth *Un*Broken Core Resilience Steppingstone:

NOURISH.

Like your grandma said, you are what you eat (and what you eat eats).

Everything you take into your body is information. The food you eat, the fluids you drink, the medications and supplements you take, the air you breathe, everything that touches your skin—it's all information. Not a single molecule of that information goes unnoticed by your body. They continuously shift your genetic expression, your biology, all structure-function-body-mind-spirit of you. This information is *you*.

How do we use the information of food to thrive? To shift out of suffering and chronic illness? To shift *into* healing?

In this *Unbroken* core resilience steppingstone, *Nourish*, we'll explore food, drink, and supplements and what their specific molecular information says to our genes, turning them on and off, shifting their expression in meaningful ways. We'll learn to use food to direct our gene expression, our biology, and our life outcomes.

What does this mean in terms we can all relate to?

We *are* what we eat (Yah, your grandma knew, didn't she?).

Food is one of the fastest and most powerful ways to shift yourself up out of the mud and into your sparkly wholeness.

How?

First, food has *a lot* to say to your genes. Food is chock full of atoms and molecules your genes want to know about.

Think about it this way. Everything we ingest is either friend or foe. If it's friend, that means it can participate in running the important business of supporting, protecting, and nourishing the body. Good things happen. We want more of that. We want to remember its taste and smell and texture, and where to find more of it. If it's foe, that means it's potentially harmful. Bad things happen. We want to stay away from it. We want to remember how it tastes and smells, what it looks like, and where it grows. Our genes may send out danger signals throughout the body, so our defense systems can protect us from it.

We've evolved into complex beings needing a complex array of molecules to run all the business of being us. Our structure (bones, sinews, cell walls, and so on), function (every bit of our biology), and energy (all the circuits, the chemistry, the transportation). That business is run by a genome that evolved over millions of years of mammalian life on this planet Earth. Fine-tuned by human life, but unchanged in the relatively short timescale of modern humans. Our genome demands a lot of us to run all that business with precision while keeping us safe. We can't fight or hack or override our genomic imperative for nutrition.

We know a great deal about how food can nourish or hurt the body. So, we have many clear nutritional paths at our fingertips to move us toward our genomic imperative for optimal function, wellness, and energy, and to participate in all aspects of healing.

Still, despite its ubiquity, food is often a lifestyle arena people know little about, so it's a huge inroad for education and lifestyle change to support healing.

How did we become so disconnected from food when it's so essential to good health? Our remote ancestors knew all about food. They had to. But the industrial era of food production moved us away from real, nutrient-dense, slow food toward processed, high caloric, nutrient-poor, fast food. And, weirdly, nutrition isn't taught in schools, not even medical school! So, our children don't learn how to eat well—and they aren't fed well in school (catsup is a vegetable?)[71]—and our doctors aren't trained to teach nutrition to their patients.

---

[71] In the Reagan administration's attempt to slash $1.5 billion from children's nutrition funding, school lunch program requirements were altered to allow ketchup as a vegetable, allowing the USDA to eliminate one of the two vegetables mandated to meet minimum nutrition standards, considerably

Karyn Shanks MD

Finally, we can use nutrition to access every cell, tissue, organ, and system of the body. That means we can direct specific nutritional strategies to anywhere in the body to help address any goal or problem. If there's an energy problem, we can employ energy nutrition strategies. If there's a toxicity problem, we have detoxification nutrition strategies for the job. If there's an allergy or chronic infection, we can utilize immune support and anti-microbial nutrition strategies. If we have an inflammation problem, there are innumerable nutritional inflammation-modulation strategies to support us. If there's a sleep or mood problem, there are nutritional strategies for those as well. And so on. You get the picture. Nutrition is an enormous tool in our healing toolbox.

With so much to know about nutrition, how can we keep this steppingstone short but sweet, to pull us out of the mud but not overwhelm? I'm going to give you an overview of the most important nutritional information *everyone* needs to know so you can choose food and supplements to support your foundational needs and address common problems. Then, I'll challenge you to name and create three changes to your eating strategy you can start on today.

Before we get to all that, we need to address the elephant in the room when it comes to our food choices. Hint: they're usually not choices at all! (And it's not your fault!)

THE ELEPHANT IN THE ROOM.

Rather than an elephant, maybe it's more like a hibernating bear who wakes up whenever we get too close. She emerges hungry, grouchy, and scared all at once. Sometimes with a ferocity that shocks us.

Our plan was set. Our expectations for the amazing outcomes established. To shift our body composition, have more energy, reduce inflammation. To feel better. To get our lives back. All our preparations were made with intelligence and precision. It was supposed to be so easy. What the hell happened?

---

decreasing costs. More reading: Amy Bentley. *Ketchup as a Vegetable: Condiments and the Politics of School Lunch in Reagan's America.* Gastronomica. 2021.

We all know who that bear is, don't we? She is all the hungry, grouchy, scared parts inside us that we've soothed and settled and numbed with food. We used food excess and food restriction. We've used certain kinds of food—sugar, fat, salt, a combination of all three—to shift our mood, our feelings, our energy, and sense of control over our lives. They're genius strategies really. We've used food chemistry to alter our own biology. To feel calm. To feel more alive. To feel safe. Food really is powerful medicine.

We're going to approach food like its chemistry. Because it is. And it's the chemical information that shifts our genes, our biology, our bodies, our outcomes. But we'll never forget how we've used food and drink our entire lives. We must tenderly, intelligently, and courageously tend to the myriad feelings and experiences we bring forth—that hungry, grouchy, scared bear—as we change how we eat.

In this way, the practice once again becomes our prize. With food, the prize is twofold. We get to shift our chemistry, biology, and bodies into robustness, out of the mud, out of pain, suffering, and feeling stuck, into our sparkly wholeness. *And* we get to shift the emotional pain that has kept us stuck. To shift it, we must feel it.

So, we'll breathe and stay curious and hold ourselves in fierce compassion as we go.

THE NOURISH NON-NEGOTIABLES.

I call them non-negotiables, but everything is negotiable. And I'll repeat, we're looking for shifts here, not grandstand plays. Take your time. Small, slow steps. Stay in your body.

But if you want the information you ingest to hold you and your genes with messages of healing, to take you to your full potential, there are clear guidelines to follow. I'll call these the "non-negotiables" because you can't negotiate them *and* get to your full potential. You'll have to choose.

The recommendations I'm about to present to you are designed to help you optimize those attributes of food most important for your all-round health and healing. This includes body composition, energy production, and all aspects of core systems biology that determine your health and wellness.

What are these attributes?

Nutrient density.

Nutrients run *all* the business of your body—all structure, function, and energy. Nutrient density includes quantities of *micro*nutrients (vitamins, minerals, antioxidants), *macro*nutrients (fats, proteins, peptides, carbohydrates), and *phyto*nutrients (complex plant compounds that assist body function). It also includes macronutrient *quality*—not all fats, proteins, and carbohydrates are created equally! The optimal food plan dials in all these factors to support your unique needs while avoiding over-consumption of calories.

Microbiome support.

Trillions of microorganisms inhabit our body, with which we share a complex, mutually dependent, and beneficial relationship. Maintaining a robust microbiome includes inoculation with healthy live organisms, nutrition to support microbiome diversity, and avoidance of anti-microbial substances such as antibiotics (unless they've been deemed necessary for a specific condition), and environmental toxins.

Minimal toxicity.

Many foods are toxic, especially those contaminated by pesticides and environmental toxins. Some foods can be safe or toxic depending on the "dose." Some foods also contain "new to nature molecules," designed to alter taste and extend shelf life. Our goal is to minimize food toxicity while supporting our bodies' intrinsic detoxification processes.

Minimal immune triggers.

Many foods are perceived as danger signals by our immune cells. Exposure to these immune triggers can result in a range of immune responses from allergic reactions to upregulated inflammation, both leading to a wide range of potential problems.

Minimal simple sugars.

Simple sugars in excess are toxic and not necessary for human function. What constitutes excess depends on the "dose" of the sugar, the context of an individual's overall diet and lifestyle, and one's genetic predispositions for how blood sugar is regulated.

Low excess calories.

No human dietary strategy has as much positive effect on human longevity as caloric restriction. Likewise, calorie excess is strongly associated with obesity and most human chronic illnesses. No nutritional plan is complete without considering how to eat just enough.

A VERY SHORT PRIMER ON MACRONUTRIENTS: CARBOHYDRATES, FATS, AND PROTEIN.

These words get tossed around all the time like they mean something—macronutrients, carbohydrates, fats, protein. Of course, they mean *something*, but not by themselves. They're categories. And within the categories are a wide range of very different molecules with a wide range of functions. So, any short conversation about them is bound to be a flawed one. The nuance is important.

Still, I need to give you enough background on the macronutrients so that you understand what we're talking about, and so you can go forward making the wisest nutritional choices for yourself.

First, "macro" nutrients. Macro meaning "large" or "long." Not too complicated. But not very specific either. We call carbohydrates, fats, and proteins "macronutrients" because they tend to be larger and longer than micronutrients. That's it.

Carbohydrates.

Carbohydrates ("carbs"), literally "carbon" plus "water," are a large group of organic compounds containing carbon, hydrogen, and oxygen, otherwise known as sugars. Sugars provide a primary source of chemical bond energy we convert to usable energy within the body. We call them "simple" or "complex" based on how many sugars are linked together in a molecule. The simplest sugars in our diets, like glucose, fructose, and galactose, contain six carbon atoms. Sucrose, common table sugar, is also a simple sugar. It's composed of two sugar molecules, glucose and fructose, bonded together. Complex sugars contain a variable number of sugars linked together to form what we know as starches, fiber, and cellulose.

After ingestion, both simple and complex sugars are digested and broken down into simple sugars, each of their carbon bonds destined for use as energy. Some complex sugars from the diet will be digested by bacteria in the gut and used as energy to fuel the gut microbiome.

For our purposes, the most relevant conversation is about how much sugar is released into the blood stream after consuming carbohydrates in a meal. The glycemic index (GI) ranks carbohydrates based on their effect on post-meal blood glucose concentrations. High GI foods are easily digested, quickly absorbed, and raise blood sugar more than low GI foods which are more slowly digested and absorbed.[72]

The *glycemic load* of a meal is essentially the net amount of sugar released into the blood stream after eating. There are many contextual factors which go into the glycemic load, from the thoroughness of chewing, the capacity for good digestion and absorption, and other components of a meal that effect the rate and amount of sugar entering the blood stream, such as fiber content. This is what affects our blood sugar levels most, so it's what we care about when making dietary choices most supportive of our needs. What glycemic load is enough to meet our needs and how much is too much? What are good sugars and which ones are bad?

While we use sugar to make energy, and we know how important energy is, excess sugar can lead to big problems. A consistently high glycemic load from one meal to the next is never a good thing.

Excess sugar will be stored as fat. Adipose tissue, which stores fat, is pro-inflammatory and contributes to all kinds of problems in the body. In addition to inflammation causing systemic cellular damage, an excess of adipose tissue, especially when combined with persistently elevated blood sugar levels, contributes to "insulin resistance," a problem in which the cells of the body no longer respond normally to the glucose-uptake effects of the hormone, insulin. As a result, fasting, post-meal, and average blood sugar levels remain elevated. The excess sugar molecules in the blood attach irreversibly to cellular proteins

---

[72] See "measuring the glycemic index of foods," Glycemic Index and Glycemic Load. Linus Pauling Institute. www. Www.lpi.oregonstate.edu/mic/food-beverages/glycemic-index-glycemic-load.

throughout the body through a process called "glycation." Glycation of cellular proteins damages them and alters their function, and the resulting "advanced glycosylated end products" trigger a smoldering immune response that results in further damage and inflammation. This results in a snowballing effect of cellular damage and elevated levels of circulating inflammatory cytokines throughout the body.

Glycation of cellular proteins is what causes the well-known complications of diabetes—eye, kidney, nerve, and vascular problems—though the process begins long before diabetes is diagnosed. Elevated blood sugar and all its associated problems of inflammation and tissue damage is known as "metabolic syndrome" and is a central problem in most chronic health problems worldwide. These include obesity, fatty infiltration of the liver (a leading cause of liver failure), hypertension, elevated blood sugar, diabetes, vascular disease, heart disease, lipid abnormalities, cancer, dementia, and countless other bad outcomes.

Our focus here will be on minimizing excesses of dietary sugars, especially sources of simple sugars like fructose and glucose and highly toxic man-made sugars like high-fructose corn syrup.

Fats.

Fat has gotten a bad rap. People assume all fats are equal, and all fats are bad. Not at all true. Fats consist of a wide variety of molecules, many of them essential for human health.

Fat phobia took western culture by storm during the 1960s because of scientifically baseless claims that eating fat would both make us fat and cause heart disease. This, along with cultural notions of beauty that emphasized being skinny, became the basis for the insanely successful multi trillion-dollar weight loss and low-fat food industries that poisoned our minds with nutritional nonsense while slowly killing us with diets based on high sugar-content ultra-processed low-fat foods. This has been slow to change because our healthcare system has adapted itself to the management of the resulting chronic disease pandemic. The medical industrial complex has profited hugely from skyrocketing rates of chronic disease related to problems associated with excess dietary sugar and obesity, while failing to address the upstream causes through nutrition education. To this day, nutritional advice is delivered as a secondary measure to drugs and urgent interventions, if given at all.

Karyn Shanks MD

Fats belong to a large family of molecules known as lipids. Lipids are fatty, waxy, or oily in consistency, and insoluble in water. They include fatty acids, triglycerides, phospholipids, waxes, and steroids.[73] The lipid family are involved in a wide array of critical structural and functional aspects of the body, including:

- Support the integrity of key barriers of the body, such as skin, mucus membranes, and gut lining.
- Support both structural and functional aspects of cell membranes.
- Help regulate inflammation via eicosanoid hormones.
- Supply carbon atoms for energy production via beta-oxidation of fatty acids.
- Form the backbone of key steroid hormones, including estrogens, testosterone, and cortisol.
- Involved in the bioavailability of fat-soluble nutrients.

Lipids are essential parts of a healthy diet because, aside from cholesterol and triglycerides, the body can't make them. Dietary fats must include omega-6-fatty acids and omega-3 fatty acids. Omega-6 fatty acids are derived from vegetables, meat, poultry, and eggs. Omega-3 fatty acids are found in green leafy vegetables, nuts and seeds, soybean oils, oily fish, krill oil, algae oil, and meat obtained from animals that feed on natural grasses. The "parent" omega-3 compounds found in plants must be converted into omega-3 compounds with longer carbon chains to become biologically active. Because most people are not able to reliably make this conversion, it is best to obtain omega-3 fats in their most downstream form: pre-formed EPA and DHA from fatty wild-caught fish, krill oil, algae oil, grass-fed or wild meat, and EPA/DHA supplements obtained from fish, krill, and algae oils.

Other attributes of dietary fats important for a healthy diet include the fat-soluble micronutrients, antioxidants, and phytonutrients contained in unprocessed fatty foods and cold-pressed, extra "virgin" oils such as olive oil.

---

[73] Saba Ahmed et al. *Biochemistry, Lipids.* 2023.

Protein.

Protein provides the component amino acids needed to build, repair, and maintain all the structural aspects of your body. These include cell walls, connective tissue, muscle, bone, and blood proteins. Amino acids, the building blocks of protein, are also used to create hormones, neuropeptides, and myriad other communication molecules throughout the body, and comprise the enzymes involved in the infinitesimal chemical reactions running all the business of your body.

Proteins are critical for optimal healthy function of the body, yet most adults I've worked with are protein deficient, particularly with regards to the amount and types of protein required for *muscle protein synthesis* (MPS), the ability to build and maintain lean muscle mass. It takes some work to dial this part of your diet in, and for many it requires a return to whole foods-based healthy eating, but it's well worth the deep benefits.

Dietary proteins are digested and absorbed as their constituent amino acids and small peptide molecules. There are twenty amino acids required for optimal function of the body. Nine of these have been labeled "essential," meaning they must be accounted for in the diet because the body cannot synthesize them. The "essential" nomenclature is unfortunate because *all* the amino acids utilized by humans are essential for optimal function, and synthesis of "non-essential" amino acids is often not adequate. I consider all twenty amino acids essential to include in a complete healthy diet.

It is important to consume enough protein, as well as individual amino acids. The typical adult will make approximately 350 grams of protein per day while consuming much less than that. So, we are constantly both manufacturing and turning over protein in the body. Because we want to preserve as much lean body mass as possible, namely muscle, it is imperative to eat enough protein-containing foods to support this function on a daily basis. Muscle is regarded as the organ of longevity because muscle mass, strength, and energy metabolism are so central to living long healthy lives. So, all my recommendations about dietary protein are designed to optimize MPS, also assuming you're actively working on optimal movement and strength training of muscle, the other keys to muscle mass, strength, and energy metabolism, and living a long healthy life.

Animal proteins are more bioavailable than plant proteins and typically contain more complete amino acid profiles, including leucine, the main amino acid driver of MPS.[74] It is unclear how much more protein is needed for a vegan diet to support MPS robustly, particularly factoring in aging. While plant-focused diets, both vegan and omnivorous (containing both plants and meat), are superior sources of micronutrients, antioxidants, and phytonutrients compared to meat-focused diets, plant proteins are of lower quality compared with animal protein in terms of digestibility, amino acid availability, and biological value. However, we can make vegan diets work to optimize MPS with the careful use of food combining and protein supplements. I'll provide guidance for both plant-focused omnivorous diets containing healthy meat sources and vegan diets optimized for protein.

When we consume enough protein of sufficient quality and bioavailability to robustly support MPS, we're also supporting all other protein needs. This is vitally important because protein is necessary for normal function of all body processes that support the experiences we need—robust energy, clear head, good mood. All our potential and possibilities.

A very short primer on micronutrients.

Though we eat them in smaller quantities than macronutrients, micronutrients are also an important nutritional consideration. These include vitamins, minerals, antioxidants, and phytonutrients. While I'm separating these out for the sake of a few teaching points, micronutrients live together in nature. So, if we follow an eating plan in keeping with what nature intended for us (whole unadulterated food and so on), they will all be included.

Vitamins and minerals.

Vitamins and minerals run the body's chemistry. Sparing you the biochemistry lesson, let's just say they're all vital and they must be accounted for in the diet in some way. In my experience, the bulk of all essential vitamins and minerals can be obtained through a healthy whole foods omnivorous diet, though most people also require high quality supplementation to fill in gaps and address special needs.

---

[74] Insaf Berrazaga et al. *The Role of the Anabolic Properties of Plant- versus Animal-Based Protein Sources in Supporting Muscle mass Maintenance: A Critical Review.* Nutrients. 2019.

Antioxidants.

Oxidation is the price we pay for the miraculous chemistry of using oxygen to make energy in the body. Oxidative energy chemistry leads to the creation of high energy molecules known as "free radicals" that can damage DNA and cellular structures throughout the body. "Oxidative stress" is associated with many adverse health outcomes and is one of the primary mechanisms of aging.

*Anti*oxidants are nutrient molecules obtained from plants and animals that mitigate oxidative stress by absorbing some of the excess energy produced by free radicals. The antioxidant family includes vitamins C, A, and E; the minerals copper, zinc, and selenium; the orange, yellow, and red carotenoids; glutathione and other sulfur-rich compounds; alpha-lipoic acid; and ubiquinol (coenzyme Q-10). Some of the most antioxidant-rich foods include darkly colored berries, brassica vegetables (broccoli, cauliflower, kale, cabbage, Brussel's sprouts, watercress), dark green leafy vegetables, tomatoes, sweet potatoes, and organ meat from pastured animals. In addition, many spices are rich sources of antioxidants. The most important are cloves, peppermint, allspice, cinnamon, oregano, thyme, and sage.

Phytonutrients.

The prefix "phyto" means plant-derived, and many vitamins, minerals, and antioxidants come from plants. However, there are also important nutritive plant compounds that don't specifically fall into our other micronutrient categories. Phytonutrients comprise a wide variety of compounds used by plants for functions such as attracting pollinators, defense against insects and other pests, and protection from environmental stresses like dry conditions or ultraviolet light. In addition to benefiting the plants, they also benefit the humans who consume them in important ways due to their antioxidant effects, micronutrient content, detoxification and microbiome support, anti-inflammatory effects, and anti-cancer properties.[75]

HOW TO CHOOSE YOUR FOOD (MADE SIMPLE).

---

[75] Nicolas Monjotin et al. Clinical Evidence of the Benefits of Phytonutrients in Human Healthcare. Nutrients. 2022: 10.3390/nu1491712.

Eat only real food.

To optimize nutrient density while avoiding toxicity, eat only whole, real food, nothing manufactured or ultra-processed. This means avoiding most of the inner isles in your grocery store. A good rule of thumb is to avoid anything that comes in plastic or a box, while making most selections from produce and meat sections. It may also mean growing your own food and participating in local farmer's markets and CSAs (community supported agriculture).

Eat a wide variety of plants.

Fill your plate so it's at least two-thirds to three-quarters plants. To optimize nutrient diversity and density, choose a wide variety of colors (often described as "eating the rainbow") that are seasonal and grown locally when possible. Include dark green leafy varieties, the brassica family (broccoli, cauliflower, cabbage, kale, Brussel's sprouts, watercress), alliums (onions, shallots, garlic), dark berries, and a variety of herbs and spices daily. Most plants are easier to digest and more nutritionally bioavailable when lightly cooked (steamed, sautéed, roasted).

Whenever possible, choose vegetables, fruit, grains, and legumes that are organic and non-GMO to help maximize nutrient content and minimize important sources of toxicity.

Optimize protein intake.

After filling two-thirds to three-fourths of your plate with healthy plants, fill the rest with healthy protein.

What does "healthy" mean regarding protein? And how much is enough? We need a daily dietary protein intake that accomplishes the following:

- The protein sources contain a complete profile of biologically necessary amino acids—all twenty.
- The protein sources are highly digestible and absorbable.
- The protein is in sufficient quantity to support essential biological processes in the body, such as muscle protein synthesis (MPS), energy production, and immune function.
- Each meal also contains enough of the amino acid leucine to stimulate MPS.

How much protein is enough?

We can estimate the amount of protein necessary each day to run all the structure-function needs of the body by focusing on the amount required to maintain robust MPS. This is the amount of daily protein you need for optimal lean body mass, strength, and energy production.

Calculate your daily protein goal based on these guidelines: 0.8 grams per pound ideal body weight per day for sedentary to moderately active people; 1.0-2.0 grams per pound ideal body weight per day for highly active people.[76] Divide this daily protein total by the number of meals you'll be eating.

Once you've established your daily protein target, use a diet macronutrient tracker to help you accomplish your goal.[77] The main purpose for using a tracker is to help you learn how much of your chosen protein sources to eat at each meal.

Omnivores.

Eat only high quality, sustainable animal protein sources: pastured grass-fed beef, pastured poultry and eggs, wild-caught fish, and wild game.

Avoid all animal products mass produced from commercial sources: feedlot beef, grain-finished beef, and commercial poultry. Their diets and living conditions lead to infections, obesity, and chronic illness (yep, just like humans). Pastured, grass-fed varieties are healthier because of living conditions that allow them to move and consume nutritionally dense grasses and insects. Their flesh and organs contain higher micronutrient and phytonutrient contents and a healthier fat profile that reflect their native diets. Grain-finished beef will lose much of the omega-3 fat content produced by grass-focused diets.

---

[76] This protein intake level is necessary for ample muscle protein synthesis to maintain healthy lean muscle mass and muscle glucose utilization. It is especially important for people over the age of 35.

Karyn Shanks MD. How to Optimize Protein for Energy and Vitality. www.KarynShanksMD.com. Also see Bauer J, et al. *Evidence-based recommendations for optimal dietary protein intake in older people: a position paper from the PROT-AGE Study Group.* J Am Med Dir Assoc. 2013.

[77] MyMacros, MyFitnessPal, and Lifesum are excellent diet tracking apps: www.verywellfit.com/best-macro-tracking-apps-5096757. 2024.

Consume wild-caught fish for their high omega-3 fat content and bioavailable protein. Avoid large predator fish such as tuna and swordfish to avoid plastic and mercury toxicity.[78] Also avoid lake trout and catfish due to chemical pollutant content.[79]

To meet your daily protein requirement, you may choose to use high quality protein supplements. To optimize digestibility, absorbability, and ability to robustly stimulate MPS, choose a hydrolyzed whey protein isolate (removes the casein and lactose; converts intact whey protein into individual amino acids) derived from grass-fed cows. This can be supplemented with hydrolyzed collagen derived from grass-fed cows. Collagen will not contain a complete array of amino acids, but it will supply amino acids used for bone and connective tissue abundantly.

Vegans and vegetarians.

The best sources of plant-derived protein come from organic, non-GMO, unprocessed legumes, nuts, and seeds. To identify your total daily protein need, do the calculation above and add 10% to offset the lower bioavailability of plant-derived protein.

It is important to rotate and combine varieties of plant-sourced protein to optimize amino acid content. Use a nutrient tracker to help you monitor relative amounts of amino acids, so you include all twenty in sufficient quantity, especially those less abundant in plants but important to human health. These include lysine, leucine, and methionine.

To meet the daily protein and leucine requirements to stimulate MPS most vegans will need to supplement with high quality plant-derived protein formulas. Use a product that contains "hydrolyzed" proteins to obtain highly usable amino acids. Make sure it contains a minimum of 3-5 grams leucine per serving to stimulate MPS most robustly.

---

[78] See chart developed by the EPA for fish to avoid due to higher levels of mercury contamination. www.epa.gov/fishadvice.

[79] Epa.gov/choose-fish-and-shellfish-wisely.

Eat healthy fats at each meal.

The best sources of healthy dietary fats are:

- Olives and fresh-pressed olive oil.
- Avocados and avocado oil.
- Coconut oil, butter, milk, and yogurt.
- Pastured or wild animal products (conventional meat should be avoided), eggs, and fatty wild-caught fish.
- Organic, non-GMO nuts and seeds.

Don't be afraid of cholesterol containing foods, such as egg yolks. Consuming cholesterol in the diet signals the liver to make less cholesterol of its own, so the net result is no appreciable change in blood cholesterol, if this is a concern for you. I've seen blood levels of cholesterol go down even when people consume large amounts of cholesterol in the diet.

Avoid all vegetable oils such as corn, canola, sunflower, and safflower oils. They are easily oxidizable with exposures to light, air, and heat, and become toxic to consume.

Avoid all "hydrogenated" fats, also referred to as "trans" fats, which are chemically altered to make them more solid at room temperature. Trans fats have been banned in food manufacturing in the US, due to being toxic and pro-inflammatory. In addition, avoid exposing oils to high heat as this will hydrogenate them in your pan.

Eat complex carbohydrates.

Limit carbohydrate intake to the complex carbohydrates found in plants. These contain a wide array of micronutrients as well as important sources of fiber—a vital food source for your gut microbiome.

Avoid most grains due to their high carbohydrate content and fast release of sugar during digestion (grains = sugar). In addition, most commercially available grains are heavily contaminated by herbicides toxic to both humans and microorganisms (your precious microbiome).

Limit your grain use to whole, unprocessed, organic, non-GMO sources.

Use simple sugars (sucrose, glucose, honey, maple syrup, agave, rice syrup, and so on) very sparingly and in combination with complex carbohydrates, protein, and fat to slow digestion and absorption, keeping your glycemic load as low as possible.

Eat fermented foods.

Consuming fermented food and drink helps support the microbiome, the trillions of microorganisms (more cells than our own) that inhabit our bodies and participate in running all the important chemistry of our bodies. You can experiment with fermenting your own food or purchase commonly available sources: yogurt, kefir, kimchi, sauerkraut, kombucha, and miso.

Time your meals.

Eat just two to three meals per day, experimenting to find periods of fasting between meals that suits you. Avoid snacking between meals and maintain an overnight fast of at least twelve hours.[80] Allowing your body ample "rest" times between meals has been shown to have many important health benefits.

Avoid eating too much.

No need to overcomplicate this. Eat your fill, then stop. Don't eat when you're not hungry. Avoid eating between planned meals.

There is no other aspect of diet as well grounded in science as the relationship between excess caloric consumption and health risks. Extra calories lead to obesity and participate in the development and exacerbation of most chronic illnesses effecting humans.[81] Caloric restriction is strongly associated with increased longevity in humans.[82]

---

[80] Read more about the health benefits of intermittent fasting in my article: How to boost energy with ketosis and intermittent fasting. www.KarynShanksMD.com.

[81] Health Effects of Overweight and Obesity. CDC. 2022.

[82] The Comprehensive Assessment of Long-term Effects of Reducing Intake of Energy (CALERIE) study looks at health outcomes associated with a 25% calorie restriction in healthy adult humans.

Limit alcohol intake.

Alcohol is a toxin that must be cleared by your liver, which stresses the body.

How much is too much?

This will vary from one person to the next. Anyone with liver disease of any kind should avoid all alcohol because their ability to detoxify it is impaired. Any alcohol intake will amplify liver dysfunction and hasten the progression to liver failure. Likewise, anyone taking medications that must be cleared by the liver should avoid alcohol, because the liver's resources for detoxification are limited.

Many healthy people can tolerate alcohol consumption and benefit from small amounts of fermented beverages or "spirits." As most of us know, alcohol in excess can be highly intoxicating and is associated with a wide range of health problems including physical trauma, liver dysfunction and failure, malnutrition, sleep problems, and cognitive decline.

Avoid toxic and irritating food.

We've touched on some of this. But toxic and irritating food is such an important contributor to just about everything that ails us, I'm going to hit you with it one more time. These are the 'big four':

- Simple sugars and high fructose corn syrup.
- Processed grains.
- Food additives used as colorants and preservatives.
- Non-organic food.

Simple sugars.

Simple sugars may not be toxins in the traditional sense as they're nutritive in very small doses. The toxic effect of sugar is dose dependent, but once we reach that dose threshold—which isn't very high unless you're an endurance athlete mainlining sugar solutions on a hundred-mile run—it is as toxic as any environmental pollutant in terms of cellular damage and health devastation.

Our bodies devote an enormous amount of energy and physiological real estate to manage blood sugar levels for this very reason. As you might recall, once we consume sugar in excess of our energy needs, the rest will be stored as fat and will glycate proteins throughout the body leading to loss of function and smoldering inflammation. Ultimately, this results in obesity and all its associated health problems, diabetes, and the host of diabetic complications due to glycation injury and organ failure.

Processed grains.

Processed grain products present the same problems as sugar. They're sources of rapidly digested and absorbed sugar, excesses of calories, and have no nutritional value.

This includes all highly processed grains commonly used in cereals, crackers, baked goods, pastas, breads, and so on.

In addition, today's genetically engineered grains are higher in carbohydrate content and are extensively treated with pesticides and herbicides like glyphosate, the most ubiquitous herbicide on the planet, considered by the World Health Organization (WHO) to be a well-established carcinogen in humans, yet still extensively used worldwide.

Food additives.

Chemicals used to add color to food or to extend its shelf life are signals the food is ultra-processed or damaged, AKA not real food. Eating only real, whole, fresh food is one of our foundational tenets for optimal nourishment for the best of reasons: to provide nutrient-dense, irritant and toxin-free food to support all the energy, structure, function needs of our bodies. The colorants, preservatives, emulsifiers, stabilizers, and processes to extend shelf life are often, in themselves, toxic and immune activating food contaminants that should be avoided.

Non-organic food.

No amount of exposure to toxic pesticides and herbicides is safe. It is especially problematic to ingest these toxic substances straight into the gut, where they have direct effects on gut-derived immunity (recall how seventy percent of all immune cells reside in our gut lining), gut mucosal integrity, the gut microbiome, and are absorbed into the systemic circulation. This leads to systemic toxicity and inflammation, impaired intestinal permeability, and microbiome disruption.

The direct effects of toxic chemicals applied directly to our food are compounded by three other important ramifications to this practice.

First, it's not just humans that are affected. These toxins become widely distributed throughout our planetary ecosystem leading to extensive loss of plants, animals, insects, and microorganisms. This loss of biodiversity has had far reaching devastating consequences.

Second, plants exposed to pesticides and herbicides have lower nutrient density. This is particularly true for phytonutrient polyphenols, plant-derived defense molecules that have important health benefits in humans such as anti-inflammatory effects, antioxidation, and detoxification.[83]

Third, animals who consume plants exposed to pesticides and herbicides are affected in all the same ways as humans. Consuming meat and milk products from those animals add to human toxicity.

As much as possible, consume only organic plant foods, and beef, poultry, eggs, and milk products derived from pastured, grass-fed, organic animals.

HOW TO CHOOSE NUTRITIONAL SUPPLEMENTS.

Why do we have to have a conversation about supplements? Isn't a healthy diet good enough?

I have been assessing the nutritional needs of clients for over three decades while keeping up on the literature about nutritional medicine. In that time, it's become clear to me that no amount of healthy eating will address all nutritional needs all the time. Everyone needs *some* corrections to bolster their nutritional needs, best addressed through dietary enhancements and high-quality nutritional supplementation.

---

[83] Food for Health: Considering the Nutrient Density of Food Crops. Institute for Functional Medicine (IFM) newsletter. https://www.ifm.org/news-insights/food-for-health-considering-the-nutrient-density-of-food-crops/

Karyn Shanks MD

What are some of the reasons a healthy diet isn't enough?

- Nutrient depletion of soil (agricultural practices, over-grazing) leading to nutrient-poor food.
- Nutrient depletion of food due to food chain problems from point of origin (farm or garden) to your plate (transportation, over-processing).
- Effects of food contamination by pesticides and herbicides leading to a toxic food supply (depletion of nutrients involved in detoxification, destruction of microbiome).
- Damaged food due to rancidity, mold toxicity, other effects of food aging.
- Nutritional demands of living in a toxic environment exceeding supply.
- Mismatches between nutritional needs and supply due to genetic nutritional requirements.
- The effects of life challenges (illness, injury, pregnancy, high stress) on nutritional needs (more challenge, greater need for nutrients).
- Effects of medications on nutrition: interference with nutrient availability from food, depletion of nutrients needed for detoxification, nutrient loss in excretory products (stool, urine, sweat).

The process of identifying your unique nutritional needs begins with a thorough assessment of your functional nutrition physiology. It is important to work with someone specifically trained in nutritional biochemistry and functional nutritional medicine who has the expertise to help you with this. Physicians and nutritionists who have gone through post-graduate training in Functional Medicine nutrition will be able to help you identify and address your needs for both macronutrients and micronutrients.[84] They will also be able to help you address challenges with personalized nutritional strategies.

---

[84] Find a certified Functional Medicine practitioner in your community or to work with via telemedicine: www.ifm.org/find-a-practitioner/. Or choose a certified Integrative and Functional Nutritionist: www.ifm.org/news-insights/news-the-integrative-and-functional-nutrition-academy-announces-educational-partnership-with-the-institute-for-functional-medicine/.

I recommend functional testing of nutrient status to identify deficiencies and excesses of macronutrients and micronutrients and guide your personalized food and supplement plan. Functional test methodology is superior to simple measurement of nutrient blood levels, because it bypasses assumptions based on statistical norms. The range of "normal" nutrient blood levels for a population may grossly underestimate the needs of many individuals, because of differences in their genetics and physiological needs. Common examples of this are the testing of vitamin B12 and folate levels. There is wide variation in individual need for B12 and folate due to genetic differences, though "normal" ranges for blood levels are quite narrow. Functional testing allows us to accurately assess need based on levels of blood markers for nutrient function rather than statistically based reference ranges.

If you can't find a Functional Medicine practitioner, you can work with your conventional doctor to assess nutritional status. Have them test your 25-hydroxy vitamin D, homocysteine (a good marker for folate, B12, and B6 functional status), methylmalonic acid (marker for B12 deficiency, not folate, so can distinguish between the two when homocysteine levels are high). While incomplete, these will provide a decent spot check of your nutritional status.

In the absence of lab testing, you can also take a basic array of supplements (though lab testing is ideal). Remember, these are in addition to eating a healthy diet, *not* to make an unhealthy diet healthy.

- A high-quality multi-vitamin-mineral.[85]
- Vitamin D: 2000 IU per day.[86]
- Multi-species (lactobacilli, bifidobacteria, saccharomyces) probiotic.
- Omega-3 fatty acids: 1-2 grams (1000-2000 mg) each of EPA and DHA from fish or algae.
- Magnesium threonate (magnesium chelated to threonic acid crosses the blood-brain barrier and is superior to other forms of

---

[85] I like the "DFH Complete" series of multi-vitamin-mineral supplements from Designs for Health.

[86] Most people I test need more than this to maintain healthy blood levels of 25-hydroxy-vitamin D.

magnesium for repleting cellular magnesium): 2 grams magnesium threonate (= 145 mg magnesium) at bedtime.

- Liposomal glutathione (the "master" antioxidant and detoxicant in the human body): 200 mg per day.

HOW TO HYDRATE.

The human body consists of approximately two-thirds water. So, you could say we *are* water with bits of cellular matter thrown in. Water carries our nutrients to where they're needed, removes waste products, and comforts and cushions all our parts. Most of us need two to three quarts of clean water per day to run all the business of our bodies. Your water allotment can include herbal teas but not caffeinated beverages or alcohol.

Since the worlds' water supply is highly and almost universally contaminated, use only water that has been filtered, but not distilled.

If you are highly active or sweat excessively, you will need to replace both water and electrolytes. Electrolytes help move the water deeply into cells and tissue where it's needed, rather than just expand blood volume and make you pee more often. Having enough mineral and electrolyte-rich water in all body compartments—within blood vessels, cells, and extracellular spaces—is essential to normal function and feeling our best.

Use a high-quality electrolyte replacement that contains sodium chloride, potassium, and magnesium, but no sugars, once or twice daily.[87] You can also add ½ a teaspoon pink Himalayan Sea salt to a bottle of water to start your day.[88]

Avoid over-drinking water—more than what is needed, especially when consumed quickly and without electrolyte replacement, can dilute the body compartments, leading to dysfunctional chemistry. In the extreme, over-hydration can be fatal.

---

[87] I use ElectroPure Hydration from Designs for Health: www.DesignsforHealth.com.

[88] Salt from the Himalayan Sea may be the only source uncontaminated by microplastics.

USE FOOD AS MEDICINE.

What did we say? *We are what we eat.*

Now you know why. Food is chemistry and so are we. It's all information that talks to and shifts our genetic expression. We can use this to our advantage.

Food is at the core of *all* healing. A robust nutrient-dense whole foods diet will *prevent* most common chronic illnesses. And a robust nutrient-dense whole foods diet will go a long way to shift us out of the equilibria of illness.

We've already explored the role of dietary protein in muscle protein synthesis (MPS) and how muscle is the organ of healthy longevity. What else can we shift with food?

- Excesses of inflammation.
- Digestive disorders.
- Food sensitivities.
- Chronic pain.
- Obesity.
- Mood disorders.
- Autoimmune disorders.
- Fatigue.
- Heart and vascular disease.
- Diabetes.
- Arthritis.

On and on and on. Food is *always* part of the equation. Or should be.

USE FOOD TO HEAL INFLAMMATION.

First, let's focus on the common denominator of most chronic health problems worldwide: inflammation.

Inflammation is a very generic term used for a series of highly complex processes involving our immune cells, designed to protect us from danger. Every part of the body is involved in this protection.

What are some of the danger signals that activate inflammation?

- Microbes (bacteria, viruses, fungi, parasites).
- Allergens (pollen, toxins, food proteins).
- Toxins (mold, plants, microbes, synthetic).
- Damaged tissue (trauma, oxidation, infection).
- Persistent or high levels of "stress" activating survival biology.
- Acute trauma, shock, or distress activating survival biology.

Keep in mind that inflammation isn't bad. It's a healing response, designed to keep us safe. That said, when it goes on too long or is especially intense, it becomes a problem we need to address.

If your body hurts or you feel persistently tired, you can be sure inflammation is part of the process.

Good news. Food can be used to help shift inflammation. But for some, even the kind of healthy eating we've been discussing can trigger or worsen inflammation, so a stricter food plan must be followed. The idea is to use food to create safety, optimizing nutrient density while eliminating all possible danger signals (some unique to you)—food irritants, allergens, toxins, synthetic preservatives, damaged food, processed food, and all "new to nature" molecules. It is often referred to as an "anti-inflammatory diet," an "elimination diet," or an "autoimmune protocol (AIP) diet." In my practice, we use a plan I call "Gut-immune Restoration Intensive Nutrition (GRIN)."[89]

Follow all the recommendations listed in the "non-negotiables" we just reviewed. In addition, follow the guidelines listed below to ensure you remove all potential danger signals.

- Eliminate all grains.
- Eliminate all nuts.
- Eliminate all legumes.
- Eliminate all animal milk products.
- Eliminate all eggs.
- Eliminate all nightshades (white potatoes, eggplant, sweet and hot peppers, tomatoes).

---

[89] Karyn Shanks MD. How to Reverse Autoimmunity with Optimal Energy Nutrition (Expert Guide). www.KarynShanksMD.com.

- Eliminate simple sugars of all kinds (sucrose, glucose, cane sugar, maple syrup, agave, grain syrups, and so on).
- Eliminate all sugar substitutes and sugar alcohols.
- Eliminate all alcohol.

What's left? Include these foods frequently, if not daily:

- Fatty wild-caught fish (high in omega-3 fatty acids).
- Pastured, grass-fed only beef or poultry.
- Organ meat from pasture-raised beef or chicken, or wild game.
- Sencha or Macha ground green tea.
- Dark blue, purple, and red berries.
- Dark green leafy vegetables.
- Brassica vegetables (kale, cabbage, Brussel's sprouts, broccoli, cauliflower).
- Culinary mushrooms.
- Ginger root.
- Turmeric.
- Coconut milk products.
- Olives and olive oil.
- Avocados.

And include these in your daily supplement regimen:

- Omega-3 fatty acids from fish or algae: 2 grams each DHA and EPA daily.
- Herbal turmeric, ginger, Boswellia, black pepper combinations.[90]
- The omega-6 fatty acid, Gamma Linolenic Acid (GLA): 400 mg daily.
- Multi-species probiotics: 2-6 billion organisms daily, containing lactobacilli and bifidobacteria.
- Liposomal glutathione: 200 mg daily.[91]

---

[90] My favorite is Inflammatone from Designs for Health.

[91] I use Trifortify watermelon flavored from Researched Nutritionals.

- Liposomal alpha-lipoic acid: 100 mg daily.[92]
- L-glutamine: 5 grams 1-2 times daily to help heal gut lining.

Build your meals around all the "allowed" protein sources, healthy fats, plants, herbs, and spices. Use as much diversity as possible to maximize nutrient density. Hydrate well with filtered water and electrolyte replacement. Follow this plan as strictly as possible for a *minimum of three months*. This is the approximate length of time needed to "reset" the immune response, remove toxins, heal the gut lining to restore barrier function, and reduce inflammation to a more acceptable level. Be as strict as possible with the food plan to minimize relapse.

This food plan is critical to the fastest and most sustainable reversal of inflammation processes contributing to your illness or source of suffering. While there are many tests available to look at immunological markers for foods, toxins, and environmental sensitivities, they are far from perfect, with many false positives and negatives. The comprehensive elimination, "safe," food plan I just presented is the gold standard healing protocol for gut-immune restoration, intensification of nutrition, and reversal of systemic inflammatory and autoimmune processes to the extent which food and gut dysfunction are playing a role. This food plan will always be helpful, and for many it is curative.

USE FOOD TO SUPPORT DETOXIFICATION.

Detoxification is internal chemistry that goes on all the time. It's designed to keep us safe from the toxins and irritants that result from our bodies' operation, as well as the toxins, irritants, and medications we're exposed to from the outside world.

Because systemic toxicity is frequently a player in human disease and dysfunction, supporting detoxification is important. For those who are seeking greater resilience as they age, robust detoxification support makes us far less vulnerable to the compounding effects of dysfunction in our systems biology.

---

[92] I use C-RLA from Researched Nutritionals.

Once again, we can count on food to help us solve a world of hurt. No, I'm not talking about a seven-day "detox" or three-day juice fast! Not that these are bad, they're just not enough. And they miss the point. Detoxification goes on 24/7 and needs to be supported 24/7 if you want to achieve and live robust health.

What is detoxification?

Detoxification chemistry is a three-part process that occurs to some extent in all of our cells but is highly concentrated in the liver. Once digested and absorbed, everything we eat is transported directly to the liver for processing before circulating systemically. First, toxins transported to the liver are charged up with energy to make them "sticky." This step is highly dependent on energy and a wide range of nutrient co-factors. Next, the sticky toxins are bound to special compounds (glutathione, glucuronide, glycine, inorganic sulfate, and so forth) to make them less toxic as well as water soluble. Finally, the water soluble "bio-transformed" toxins are released into bile and blood, then eliminated from the body via the gut (stool), kidneys (urine), skin (sweat), and lungs.

There is also a detoxification process that occurs in the brain. Brain tissue shrinks while we sleep, expanding the cerebrospinal fluid (CSF) space around it. CSF circulates through this space, "sweeping" toxins and accumulated proteins out of the central nervous system, into the blood. Then they go through a biotransformation and elimination process like all other toxins.

Your essential detox primer.

- Avoid environmental toxins as much as possible. Work on what you can readily control: pesticides, herbicides, plastics, toxic food, toxic household cleaners and personal care items, industrial chemicals, and excesses of alcohol and medications.[93]
- Eat a nutrient dense diet as outlined above to provide a robust source of macro and micronutrients to run detoxification chemistry.

---

[93] More on environmental toxins and their avoidance in the *Core Resilience* steppingstone *Let Go* beginning page x.

- Stay well hydrated.
- Encourage good bile flow. Bile is used to digest fats so including healthy fat with each meal allows for regular release of bile (and the bio-transformed toxins it contains) into the gut.
- Keep bowels healthy and moving daily through adequate water intake, regular movement and exercise, dietary fiber (keep that plate heaped with plant foods!), and a healthy microbiome (fermented foods, probiotic supplements).
- Consume detoxification support nutrition daily. In addition to a nutrient dense diet, this may mean detoxification-specific supplemental nutrients, especially a B-complex with methylated forms of folate and vitamin B12, glutathione, and alpha-lipoic acid.
- Sweat, move, exercise, breathe deeply, and sleep well to assist the elimination of toxins from the body.

LAST WORDS.

You are what you eat (and what you eat eats).
Food is powerful medicine.

If you haven't already, take the leap of faith. Shift yourself in the most powerful ways. Eat in accordance with your needs. Bathe your cells in the nourishment they need to support you fully. Shift your genetic expression to download inflammation and offload a world of suffering. Take baby steps, with great kindness and patience.

As you do, hold yourself with tenderness for all the losses you've ever known that you've assuaged so brilliantly with the medicine of food, even as you choose a new direction with a new strategy that will take you straight to your potential and possibilities. Revealing your sparkly wholeness.

I PROMISE.

Here are my next three steps to shift my food and supplement strategy.
1.
2.

3.

Karyn Shanks MD

CHAPTER TWENTY-ONE
Sixth *Un*Broken Core Resilience Steppingstone:

LIBERATE.

My garden asks me to make room for the tender new plants to grow and flourish. It's not enough to compost them in the spring, water them through dry spells, then sit back to admire their abundance. I need to create space for new roots and tender sprouts to emerge. I must pull the weeds and shield them from passersby. As much as I love a disorderly garden with mad blooms and vines everywhere, this year's gorgeous chaos could be next year's demise.

NANCY'S STORY OF LETTING GO.

My client Nancy was sure she had a terrible incurable disease no one could figure out. She had been sick for years and felt doomed. I can understand why. After thousands of dollars of sophisticated medical testing from a variety of doctors and specialists, they all came to the same conclusion: "nothing" was wrong, even though she experienced persistent exhaustion, poor exertion tolerance, brain fog, muscle aches, headaches, diarrhea, and depression, an all-too-common constellation of symptoms labeled "chronic fatigue syndrome."

As Nancy told me her story, it was clear there were promising leads to pursue. She ate a "standard American diet" of highly processed foods devoid of important nutrients and filled with potential irritants and toxicity. Her sleep was poor—not only poor quality with frequent awakenings, but she spent only six hours in bed each night. She felt run ragged by commitments to family, friends, and community organizations, and starved for time to herself for rest, movement, and pursuing her own interests. In our first conversation it was clear she was overwhelmed, depleted, and exhausted.

Our first order of business? Gently create space so the new Nancy could emerge by shifting her equilibrium of suffering.

While awaiting results of our initial round of blood tests, her first prescription included:

- Shift to a healthier diet by removing potential irritants and toxins. She removed all grains, sugars, animal milk products, eggs, legumes, and nuts. She focused on eating healthy animal proteins (pastured chicken, grass-fed beef, wild-caught fish), organic vegetables and berries, and healthy fats (coconut, olive, and avocado).
- Evaluate current list of commitments and let go of the three least important to her right now.
- Set an earlier bedtime by saying "no" to television watching and social media rabbit holes.

What do you see in the three items on her list?

She let go. She liberated herself from toxins, irritants, distractions, and energy depleting activities.

What happened?

When I saw her a few weeks later, even before we discussed her lab test results, she was a new person. Yes, the initial plan was hard, especially the new food plan. But she was highly motivated, so she dove right in and stuck to it strictly. She was getting to bed earlier and clocking more hours asleep. After about a week, she noticed her brain fog was gone and her energy was increasing. She had more stamina to do things during the day. She could play with the kids and not feel like she had to sit down to recover. Her diarrhea and body aches completely resolved, she had fewer headaches, and she started feeling optimistic about her future for the first time in years. And the icing on the cake? She lost ten pounds.

WHY LETTING GO LIBERATES.

Letting go is so hard.

But here's the deal. There *are* roadblocks to our healing. Lots of them. Roadblocks we must get out of our way to rise from suffering, get unstuck, and unleash our most sparkly wholeness. Toxins, irritants, negative energy, and distractions. Loud noises, disempowering stories, and chaos. Bad food, bad friends, and bad habits. They gotta go. They're in our way. Sometimes disentangling ourselves from roadblocks is all we have to do for fresh new energy to come flooding in.

But remember our commitment to gentle, tender, and compassionate? We make letting go gentler—we "shift out of."

And more than that. We remember what letting go is really all about. It's about liberation. Mine, yours, ours. How does letting go help liberate us for healing?

- Letting go creates space for new things needed for healing.
- Letting go removes literal roadblocks to healing processes.

Nancy did both.

She created lots of new space. She let go of old commitments that depleted her energy. She got distractions out of the way for an earlier bedtime so she could sleep more. Both were huge contributions to her healing.

She also removed roadblocks to healing. Changing her diet eliminated food sensitivities and food toxins, which cause upregulation of inflammation and increased toxin exposure that injure cells, impair energy production and detoxification, and inhibit repair processes. These explain many of Nancy's symptoms, such as fatigue, exertion intolerance, pain, and brain fog, all common symptoms of persistent energy deficit.

The inflammation and toxicity caused by foods lead to direct injury of Nancy's gut lining, resulting in impaired intestinal permeability ("leaky gut") and gut dysfunction (digestion, absorption, detoxification, elimination). Both exacerbate systemic inflammation and toxicity, feeding into the vicious cycle of injury, toxicity, and energy deficit until it's stopped. We were able to stop this cycle with Nancy through a strict irritant and toxin-free "elimination" diet.[94]

So, bottom line? Yah, we may *hate* to let go sometimes, but it's one of the most powerful things we'll do to rise out of suffering and heal chronic illness. Nancy's initial care plan liberated her to do the rest of what her healing asked of her.

WHY LETTING GO IS SO HARD.

We've had this conversation before but it's worth repeating (*and* repeating) because it's so central to all the healing we'll ever do.

Letting go is hard because healing is hard. Healing is hard because we don't know another way. Or we know our old way so well, it's a tenacious mind groove keeping us stuck in a rut. Or our old way propped us up—it assuaged a world of hurt. The cookies, chocolate chips, alcohol, over-commitment, late bedtime, or social media rabbit holes. All the things we do to feel better about ourselves or feel *less* (anxiety, despair, shame, and so on). All the ways we respond to our trauma-based feelings, sensations, and energy states.

They were all smart adaptations for feeling better, genius strategies for staying alive when we knew no other ways. You get that now, don't you?

These are the reasons letting go is so hard:

- We need knowledge we don't yet have (Nancy didn't know about food irritants and toxins.).
- We're committed to well-practiced habits (tenacious mind grooves) we must change (Nancy knew she was too busy but didn't know how to change.).
- We're committed to old ways that have propped us up (assuaging hurt).

We'll keep these reasons in mind as we shift toward liberation.

---

[94] See details of the anti-inflammatory "elimination" food plan in the *Core Resilience* steppingstone, *Nourish*, on page x.

GETTING TO LIBERATION.

How do we get all the way to liberation? Not just liberation *from* the old thing that no longer serves but liberation *for* the new things that shift us, the new *us* that emerges.

Let's work with letting go in six steps, keeping in mind the reasons letting go can be so hard.

- Identify your destination. I want to feel alive. I want more energy. I want my life back.
- Identify the changes you believe will take you to your destination. I need optimal sleep. I need a nutrient dense diet. I need more time to devote to my own needs.
- Identify if there's something that serves as a roadblock to that change. I need to limit the hours I spend on my phone. I need to stop binge-watching Netflix, so I have more time for sleep. I need to ask for help with my anxiety.
- Ask yourself three questions:
    o Do I need to learn something new? (A food plan, a sleep strategy.)
    o Do I need help shifting out of an old habit?
    o Do I have difficult feelings, sensations, or energy states to reckon with as I try to change?
- Implement the letting go strategy: give it a go, see what happens.
- Hold all of it with tenderness, compassion, and curiosity.

Now, if you're like Nancy, you may not know *what* you need to change. You just want to feel better but don't have a clue how. This becomes the focus of the six steps you work through with your team of helpers. I helped Nancy identify important sources of immune irritation, toxicity, and energy depletion that I knew served as roadblocks to her healing. Nancy had to acquire new knowledge, release old well-practiced habits, and address hard feelings to let go of roadblocks to healing. She had to implement her new strategy in faith, not knowing where it would lead her.

Identify your destination.

Where do you want to be? How do you want to feel? What do you want to be capable of? What is your goal?

Say it out loud in plain language, just as you think it, feel it, know it in your bones.

I want my life back. I want my energy back. I want the energy to play with my daughter in the back yard. I want to feel like myself again. I want to climb a fourteen-thousand-foot mountain in Colorado.

Naming your destination using your own words makes this personal. And it should be. This is *your* journey. Not mine, not your doctor's, not anyone else's. You may not land exactly where you imagined. You may go much farther. There may be more to do. Either way, this is a very personal and beautiful odyssey of healing that could take you places you never imagined. In fact, I promise you it will.

This step may be hard because you're afraid. Afraid to dream. Afraid to feel disappointed yet again. That's okay. Be tender with yourself. Allow yourself to feel *whatever* you feel. But take the journey regardless.

Identify the changes you believe will take you to your destination.

What changes can you identify right now that will help you get to your destination? See if you can name three things in your own words right now.

What you need as you understand it may be as vague as:

I need to feel better. I need better sleep. I need more time. I need something to change.

Or maybe you're able to be more specific:

I need to follow that healthy food plan I know makes me feel better. I need to shut off my phone at bedtime to avoid the social media rabbit holes that keep me up too late. I need to move more and sit less.

Don't be afraid to begin *somewhere,* even if you feel you need help to go further. Start small. Don't worry about naming *all* the things you'll eventually need to change. What can you focus on right now?

Karyn Shanks MD

Identify if there's something that serves as a roadblock to that change.

What gets in the way of you implementing the change you need, if you know what that change needs to be?

I need to feel better, but I have no motivation or desire to ask for help. I need better sleep but feel too busy and stressed to figure out how. I need something to change but haven't stopped to consider what those changes might be. I'm too tired and overwhelmed to know what to do.

Sometimes there are roadblocks to our roadblocks. What are the roadblocks to the roadblocks imbedded in those examples?

- No motivation or desire to ask for help. So, what stops you from asking for help?
- Feeling busy and stressed. What small, tender, positive shift can I initiate regardless?
- Haven't stopped to analyze the problem. *So, stop. Can't? Consider why not.*

Or:

Why am I not following the food plan that makes me feel better? What keeps me on social media when I need that time to sleep? What gets in the way of moving more and sitting less?

If you have specific needs that reveal a roadblock to a roadblock to healing, literally ask what stands in the way.

If you've just gotten off track from a healthy new habit, get back on track. If you can't, there's likely a roadblock to your roadblock. The new food plan doesn't assuage painful feelings the way the old one does. The earlier bedtime takes away the social media frenzy and Netflix binge watching that soothed a world of hurt. The new movement plan is hard. Hard feels overwhelming.

Once you identify ways to improve your strategy so it better fits you, and you recognize roadblocks to your roadblocks, be very tender with yourself. Many of these have helped you in important ways even if they no longer serve you. Don't give up. Stay curious. Mobilize the support you need.

Ask yourself three questions.

These three questions will help reveal the competing commitments that serve as roadblocks to your roadblocks:

- Do I need to learn something new?
- Do I need to shift out of an old habit?
- Do I have difficult feelings, sensations, or energy states to reckon with?

What competing commitments might be revealed?

Sometimes there's not a competing commitment at all. We just need new information to support our quest.

But when there is a competing commitment that gets in the way of our goals, keeping us stuck and unable to heal, it's about safety. Those well-worn mind grooves that support old habits aren't just easy because they're what we always do, they feel safe. Those new habits aren't just more work, they're scary! And giving up old habits that soothe our difficult feelings, sensations, and energy states? That's scary too. Fear encourages us to keep things the same.

Then what?

Implement the letting go strategy.

Go for it.

What you didn't know before will soon be revealed to you. Welcome all the hiccups along the way! These are teachers, not failures. Hang in there with relentless curiosity and commitment to seeing this through.

Hold all of it with tenderness, compassion, and curiosity.

Keep in mind how all failures and outright disasters are here to teach us, not torture us. So, if this happens, shake it off, and call on all the tenderness, compassion, and curiosity you can conjure. This is what shifts us into desired change, out of suffering, into our vibrant new selves. Rolling with the punches.

WHAT IS THE TERRAIN OF LIBERATION?

Let's look more closely at our terrain of liberation. What kinds of things must we let go of to liberate ourselves? To heal, thrive, and unleash our potential and possibilities?

- Toxins and irritants.
- Negative energy and distraction.
- Disempowering stories.

LET GO OF TOXINS AND IRRITANTS.

Environmental toxins and irritants sabotage our attempts to heal. From the big challenges that derail our lives—chronic illnesses, pain, persistent fatigue, brain fog, depression, and a whole lot more. To the "normal" (*not* normal to me, mind you) low energy, poor motivation, or insomnia. Toxins and irritants are usually upstream to our symptoms, sometimes way upstream, so can be hard to see. We must look for them and remove them thoroughly.

Environmental toxins and irritants lead to cellular damage and upregulated inflammation that get in the way of all healthy biological processes in our bodies. We must get these roadblocks to healing out of our way or none of our other efforts to heal will work.

These are the 'big eight' ubiquitous toxins and irritants that challenge us all:

- Pesticides, herbicides, and industrial pollutants.
- Mold and mold toxins.
- Toxic buildings.
- Heavy metals.
- Toxic body care and cleaning products.
- Plastics.
- Toxic water.
- Toxic and irritating food (see Chapter 20 – Nourish).

There are two key components to addressing toxicity.

First, avoidance—to keep the body's burden of toxins and irritants as low as possible.

Second, we must support the body's innate detoxification and elimination processes when there is an exposure. We're designed to do this, but we need extra help when the toxic load is overwhelming or when detoxification and elimination are impaired.

We talked about bolstering innate detoxification to transform and eliminate toxins from the body in the previous chapter, *Nourish*. In this steppingstone, we will focus on avoidance.

How do we avoid the most common toxins and irritants?

Many of the 'big eight' are challenging to avoid completely. They're everywhere! I live in a largely rural state with extensive regions of working farms. I'm surrounded by farm chemicals. What do I do?

I control what I can control and make peace with the rest.

What can I control? In addition to bolstering my innate detoxification processes through a healthy diet and lifestyle, I can eliminate all the 'big eight' toxins from my home and workplace. You can do this too.

Pesticides, herbicides, and industrial pollutants.

Do your best to avoid these within your own homes, yards, and workplaces. There are always safe alternative strategies for managing pests and undesired growth of weeds. A simple online search will show you countless options.

In my area, prairie restoration versus grass is an option. Or corn gluten application as a pre-emergent to control weeds in the spring works incredibly well. I recently learned about applying a thirty percent solution of vinegar directly to unwanted weeds and the results have been spectacular. And, of course, there's good old-fashioned weeding the garden by hand. All viable options.

There's growing literature and experience with regenerative farming methods that I won't go into here, but this information is widely accessible. These methods are being used with great success from both production and ecosystem enrichment standpoints.

I fully realize most of us have no immediate recourse regarding industrial pollutants. We can be vocal activists, but this is a longstanding worldwide problem that is not going to change overnight. We can avoid excessive exposures through measures that keep pollutants out of our homes and workplaces. Removing shoes upon entering, air filtration, and water purification are all helpful.[95]

As much as possible, eat only organic food to reduce the amount of food growing chemicals you directly ingest.

Again, we control what we can.

Mold and mold toxins.

It's impossible to avoid mold entirely—it's part of our biome, in the soil, on plants, in the air.

But excesses of mold, particularly in our homes or workplaces where ventilation may not be optimal, especially for folks already hovering at very vulnerable health equilibria, can become powerful troublemakers.

There are three overarching problems associated with mold overload.

- Smoldering inflammation from powerful immune cell activation triggered by mold toxins, spores, and fungal surface proteins.
- Direct damage to DNA, cellular structures, and energy metabolism caused by mold toxins.
- The 'cell danger response' triggered by overwhelming exposure to cell danger signals from mold.

Mold avoidance includes identifying and completely remediating water damage that occurs in our homes and workplaces—preferably by professional mold remediation specialists. Or rapidly addressing a water problem within minutes or hours of onset with rapid drying and removal of all organic materials where mold can grow.

Air purification systems will reduce mold and mold toxin levels, like the high-grade IQ Air. Their "hyperHEPA" technology will remove most mold spores and toxins from the inside environment.

A robust detoxification strategy will help bind and clear mold toxins in the body. Follow the detoxification support process outlined in the *Nourish* steppingstone and work with a Functional Medicine practitioner experienced

---

[95] I prefer (and personally use in my home) the IQ Air filtration products using HyperHEPA technology that traps 99.5% of airborne particles down to a size of 0.003 microns. IQAir.com.

in diagnosing mold toxicity and can treat you with an approach that's appropriate to both your needs and the type of mold toxicity present.

Toxic buildings.

Building toxicity often occurs because of toxic chemicals, mold from water damage, and poor ventilation. This includes building materials and toxins used in the manufacture of furniture, window treatments, beds, carpets, flooring, and other building materials.

Numerous chemicals are used as flame retardants, glues, and sealants that get into our bodies. There is always a risk for absorption through lungs, skin, and mucus membranes of the mouth, nose, and sinuses that must be processed and eliminated by our detoxification systems.

Many individuals will feel unwell, some quite ill, in these buildings.

Proper ventilation, remediation of water damaged areas, air treatment, and removal of particularly toxic items is always necessary. Some folks need to avoid buildings in which they feel unwell entirely.

Heavy metals.

Heavy metals are a general term that encompasses environmental contaminants like mercury and lead. These are tricky. Where are they?

Essentially everywhere. In the land, oceans, and air masses worldwide.

Many of our exposures are from air, water, and land pollution. Even with stricter industrial regulations in the western world, heavy metals travel in large air masses from other parts of the world without the same environmental protection standards.

Heavy metals are also released from burning timber in wildfires and volcanic eruptions.

Fresh water fish and larger predator ocean fish are contaminated with high levels of mercury. You can track which fish are the most contaminated on the EPA website.[96]

Silver dental fillings contain mercury and are still commonly used in dental practice despite studies that confirm higher blood and tissue levels of mercury in dental health practitioners. The greatest risk for mercury exposure is during

---

[96] Epa.gov/report-environment/consumable-fish-and-shellfish.

Karyn Shanks MD

the placement or removal of mercury-containing dental restorations. Porcelain and BPA-free resin composite fillings are non-toxic durable alternatives (see upcoming section on plastics) to mercury amalgams you can request from your dentist.[97]

Your Functional Medicine or environmental health specialist can help you identify if heavy metal toxicity may be contributing to your chronic health problems. A simple blood or urine test may not be enough, however, unless the exposure was very recent. Because heavy metals can be sequestered in cells and tissue, it may only be possible to find them by using an oral or intravenous chelating agent prior to the test. These agents bind to metals, pulling them out of cells and tissue, so they can be measured in the blood or urine.

Toxic body care and household cleaning products.

Most body care or household cleaning products with more than three ingredients contain toxins. That's not always the case, but it's a good rule of thumb when selecting products and you're not familiar with the ingredients.

Toxic ingredients can cause a wide range of problems including damage to DNA and cellular structures that lead to shifts in function that are unhealthy. In addition to direct toxicity, they must be cleared from the body through detoxification pathways, using valuable biochemical resources that could leave the body vulnerable. Many of these toxins also activate immune cells, increasing circulating inflammatory cytokines to cause further trouble.

Water, vinegar, essential oils, baking soda, and 3% hydrogen peroxide make fine nontoxic cleaning agents and disinfectants.

Absolutely avoid phthalates and parabens (many body care products), triclosan (antibacterial soaps), aluminum (anti-perspirants), formaldehydes, and sodium hydroxide (hair products).

Check out GreenAmerica.org for more information about choosing safe body care and household cleaning products.

---

[97] Alternatives to Mercury Amalgam Fillings. IAMT (International Academy of Oral Medicine and Toxicology). 2024. Iaomt.org/for-patients/alternatives-mercury-amalgam-fillings.

Plastics.

Plastics are everywhere, *literally.*

Plastics contain breakdown products that have been linked to cancers and hormone disruption in humans which lead to impairment in reproduction, growth, and cognition.[98] These include phthalates, plasticizers found in vinyl flooring and food packaging; bisphenol A (BPA), found in bottles, can linings, dental amalgams, and dental sealants; and polybrominated diphenyl ethers (PBDEs), used as flame retardants added to furniture, mattresses, carpet pads, and car seats.

Microplastics, formed when large plastic materials are fragmented and micronized to 5 millimeters and smaller, are associated with human health problems due to their ease of ingestion and inhalation. They are known endocrine disruptors and are associated with cancer development, respiratory disorders, and cardiovascular diseases.

The manufacture of plastics introduces further toxicity through the release of carcinogenic, neurotoxic, and hormone-disruptive chemicals that permeate our entire planetary ecology and persist over long periods of time. These include vinyl chloride and dioxins (both in PVC), benzene (in polystyrene), phthalates, formaldehyde, and BPA.

How to protect ourselves from plastics:

- Avoid single-use plastics such as water bottles and shopping bags.
- Avoid the purchase and consumption of beverages in plastic bottles.
- Avoid heating food in plastic containers.
- Use non-plastic food storage containers, such as glass and stainless steel.
- Avoid facial and body cleansing products containing microplastics (these are mostly banned in many parts of the world).
- Use salt mined from high mountain water sources such as the Himalayas that do not contain microplastics.

---

[98] Geneva Environment Network. Update: Plastics and Human Health. Plastics and the Environment Series.

Karyn Shanks MD

Toxic water.

Planetary water supplies are extensively polluted, filled with carcinogens, endocrine disrupters, heavy metals, and plastics. And they taste terrible.

Ideally all water used for any purpose is filtered, including water you use for bathing.

I recommend that you install an all-house water filter to remove organic contaminants (like bacteria, algae, fungi, and viruses), heavy metals (lead, iron, arsenic, mercury), sediments (salts, soil, microplastics), and odor causing chemicals. This is not only good for you but for your plumbing and water receptacles. Installation of an all-house filtration system is a very simple process for a plumber at relatively low cost, just a few hundred dollars for both the unit and labor for installation. Filters need to be replaced every few months depending on the unit you install and the degree of water contamination in your area.

In addition, a reverse osmosis filter for your drinking water will remove all remaining metals, pollutants, and micro-organisms, and will make your water taste great.

LET GO OF NEGATIVE ENERGY AND DISTRACTION.

Recognize any of these?

- Emotionally toxic people.
- Toxic information (News: can be both negative and distracting).
- Distracted driving (Texting, talking on the phone—even hands-free. I passed a man on the highway recently using his laptop!).
- Technological distraction (social media, email, texting, gaming).
- Clutter (environmental distraction).
- Multitasking.
- Time pressure.

To get to liberation, we must let go of negative energy and distraction. Why? Because they deplete our energy, attention, and joy. They scramble our brains. They steal our time.

I've seen very sick and exhausted clients stay sick and exhausted until they tended to these aspects of their daily lives. Freedom from negative energy and excessive distraction is profoundly important to our safety and energy. They're signals to our survival-oriented brains that we're not safe. When we're persistently not safe, our brain shuts us down through the healing cycle we know as the cell danger response and survival-oriented biology that shifts us into sympathetic nervous system fight or flight, or dorsal vagal freeze responses. When persistent, it downshifts our energy.

See, letting go is all about safety. Through safety we can heal.

LET GO OF DISEMPOWERING STORIES.

The most tenacious, insidious, and tricky of all the roadblocks to our healing are the stories we tell that disempower us from our own wisdom and agency to create healing lives. From the cultural stories that define what healing means, to the familial stories about what makes us worthy, they keep us stuck. Without them standing in our way, we'd flow, we'd step so easily into our potential and possibilities.

While we've explored stories throughout this book, particularly the trauma-based stories we bump into as we create healing lives, let's reflect on them for just a moment. As storytelling creatures, we'll always work with our stories, mining them for their wisdom.

As my teacher, Gabor Maté , likes to say, "it all goes down in your mind." What does he mean? All the obstacles, "impossible" circumstances, beliefs, and assumptions we make about absolutely everything, are created in our minds. They're not objective reality. They're not reality at all. They're constructs. We manufacture all those ideas to make sense out of what we hear, what we're taught, how we perceive the world around us, everything. It all goes down in the mind. The more tenacious our stories, the more unconscious we are of them, the more they drive us and our behavior, and the higher our resistance is to evaluating and changing them, the higher the likelihood they're associated with trauma. The trauma of being hurt. The trauma of not belonging. The trauma of feeling unworthy. The trauma of losing control. You name it.

What does it sound like to have a disempowering story stand in the way of your healing?

I can't.

I don't have time.

Who am I to … (you fill in the blanks)
It's too hard.
It's too lonely.
I'm just like my mother and grandmother.
I'm stuck.
I AM my depression and anxiety.
This is who I am.
This is my genetic destiny.
I can't change this.

Endless stories. Roadblocks to healing.

Scrutinize your own obstacles to healing.

Ask: what's the story I'm telling here?

I don't have time to learn this new food plan. I can't get to bed any earlier than I do. I don't believe my thoughts have anything to do with my health. My feelings can't be making me sick. I have too much to do. I'm no more stressed than anyone else. I can't stop my sugar cravings.

Be entirely honest with yourself. And while honest, also be tender, compassionate, and curious. Because we tell stories for good reasons. We're not trying to trip ourselves up. They may no longer serve us, but they did at one time. All stories are worthy of our respect, even if it's time to change them.

Follow that question with another: what's the feeling, sensation, or energy state I'm telling my story about? Then check in with your body. What's it saying?

I'm scared. I'm lonely. I'm afraid to change. I'm afraid of letting go of control. I'm scared to try something new. I'm afraid of being left out. I'm afraid to feel. I hurt. I'm afraid to fail. I'm afraid of disappointment.

Common stories we all tell that can be roadblocks to our healing.

These are the seven disempowering stories I hear (and experience!) most often:

- Stories about our worth.
- Stories about our power and personal agency.
- Stories about time (not having enough).
- Stories about belonging.
- Stories about uncertainty of change.
- Stories about what we believe/know for sure.

- Stories about failure.

Each one of these stories has the potential to halt our progress, hijacking our creative genius to imagine a better future, to access our potential and possibilities.

Which ones do you recognize in yourself? How do they show up?

Breathe. Be very gentle with yourself. These stories served a profound purpose at one time. They may have kept you alive.

As you tell yourself the story, what's going on in your body? Check in and see if you can name a feeling, sensation, or energy state.

Then, how can you shift the story to better serve your current needs?

Keep breathing. Stay gentle.

LAST WORDS.

I often tell the story about my son's high school essay on his heroes. The assignment was to write about just one but as he told my husband and me, "I couldn't think of just one, so I wrote about my two heroes."

One was his grandfather, who survived "the troubles" in Northern Ireland to go on to become a world-famous neurosurgeon and all-round wonderful human being.

The other hero was me.

"Really? Why?" I asked, stunned.

"Because" he explained (I'm sure there was a "dumbass" in there somewhere), "look at everything you went through growing up, all the obstacles you overcame, and how much you've accomplished."

That rocked my world. It upended the most insidious, deeply embedded, and disempowering story of my life. A story I clung to because it was the story that kept me alive when I was too young to know differently. A story that kept me safe. A story I didn't know was a story, believing it was a fact of my life.

His story allowed me to reimagine my own past. Rather than unlovable, a loser, I was a savvy girl who made her way in life on her own from a very young age and did a freaking brilliant job. I was a hero.

Key to my evolution was to not condemn my old story. It helped me survive my childhood. But holding onto it (because I didn't know better, I didn't know about the storytelling brain and trauma biology back then) held me back and kept me in pain. Most importantly, while the story kept me safe, it didn't see me as I truly was or am.

So, I did what I'm now teaching you to do.

I accepted 100% responsibility for myself and my healing, releasing blame to liberate myself from the past.

I practice my new story every day, with tenderness and reverence for how I can direct my transformation.

So, remember this. No matter how hard your story is to change, practice with tenderness makes progress.

Finally, we don't just "let go" of our disempowering stories, do we? We shift them. Patiently, with baby steps, we shift into new words, better stories, our own magnificence. Into our liberation.

THREE PROMISES.

Three small steps to letting go I can start today:

1.

2.

3.

CHAPTER TWENTY-TWO
Seventh *Un*Broken Core Resilience Steppingstone:

FEEL.

I feel. I feel with abandon. I feel with fury. I feel with lightness and joy. I hold all my feelings with reverence for what they are, my truest truth. I hold all my feelings with compassion and curiosity for where they lead me, to my most authentic self, my purest wisdom, my sparkliest wholeness.

Of course we feel. We're feeling right now. We feel all the time. So, what's the big deal? Why is this a steppingstone?

I don't know about you, but I think feelings are hard. Not just hard, they're tricky as hell. What am I feeling and what is the story I'm telling *about* my feeling? They're not the same, are they?

Or how about this? How do I *feel* about my feeling? What stories do I tell about how I'm *supposed* to feel? How do I censor my feelings?

Ugh. I find this confusing. I know I'm not alone.

There's tremendous cost to our feeling confusion.

First, feelings are key parts of our neuroceptive genius. They're how we 'read the room,' read our environments, read each other. They're how we stay safe and stay connected. They tell us what's what beyond our five senses. They've kept us alive and connected throughout human history. But while feelings have helped us succeed during our evolution on this planet, we no longer trust them. No longer trusting them, we've lost their full purpose. We don't express them fully, *feel* them freely, or learn from their genius. Without the fullness of our feelings, we're limited in what we can know. We get stuck. We stay scared. We don't grow in the ways we should.

What's more, confusion about our feelings makes us sick. Feelings influence genetic expression and have a biology. They drive our behavior. Feelings are energy. When they flow and their wisdom lands, we're free. When they get stuck—when we numb them, dismiss them, or shove them down—they activate our survival biology. We get tight. We can't breathe. We can't see straight. We don't feel safe. Our internal chemistry shifts to support us toward safety. Immune cells are activated, inflammation ramps up, hormones shift to conserve vital resources. When this goes on too long, the risk for bad things happening—chronic illness, addiction, depression—goes way up. Our equilibrium of resilience is compromised. The science on this is clear and deep.[99]

So, yes, feeling *must* be one of our *Unbroken* core resilience steppingstones. Feeling, painful as it can be, confusing as it is, leads us to wisdom. Feeling helps us rise out of pain, suffering, and chronic illness. It helps us reclaim our precious wholeness so we can live who we authentically are.

We've been practicing feeling throughout this book, haven't we? As you've probably noticed, feeling is not just something we were born to do. Feeling is a skill we must learn to hone. Most of us face the arduous task of relearning *how* to feel. Feeling freely. Feeling with reverence for *what* we feel. Especially the strong feelings, the dark feelings, the feelings that make us and others uncomfortable, the feelings that most rocked our worlds as very small children or when we were vulnerable. We gave up feeling to survive, to belong, to have our most foundational needs met.

In my family we didn't do feelings. Certainly not feelings that made others uncomfortable. And especially not big feelings. Big anger, big joy, big anything. Too loud, too much. Except my dad. He got to be loud, big, and explosive. And my mom was just the opposite. Everything was always "wonderful," even when it wasn't. Which means I grew up with big-time feeling confusion. What

---

[99] Gabor Maté MD. Gabor explores the link between safety and disease in both his excellent books: *When the Body Says No: Exploring the Stress-Disease Connection,* 2011, and *The Myth of Normal: Trauma, Illness, and Healing in a Toxic Culture,* 2022.

the hell are feelings? Which ones make me good? Which ones make me bad? Which ones are real? How can I trust my own feelings?

In this steppingstone, we're going to call our feelings back and practice experiencing and looking at them for what they are. To not censor them or discriminate among them. To hold them with the reverence they deserve. To receive their wisdom. As we do, I promise to hold you and your feelings so tenderly. I promise to help *you* do the same.

Some of you may believe you don't *have* feelings, or at least not certain kinds of feelings. We don't all feel in the same ways. Some of us don't experience feelings in any of the typical ways others do. I want to assure you this chapter is still for you. There are currents of energy inside you that may not seem like ordinary feelings, but they represent how your body responds to what's going on around you all the same—*your* unique neuroceptive genius. Your body's wisdom may reveal itself as sensations, like tightness, tingling, jitteriness, agitation, or pain. Or you may notice shifts in your energy, becoming suddenly tired or energized in response to what's happening. You may feel some emotions but not others. I recently heard someone describe how they'd never felt guilt or shame and believed something was terribly wrong with them. While not typical, she learned to accept herself and acknowledged how she's still perfectly capable of the social learning that comes from feelings like guilt and shame.

FEELING AND THINKING ARE NOT THE SAME.

Our feelings are our most pure, honest, and sacred truth. Nothing about our incredible minds can hold a candle to the genius of our feelings. Nothing. Not our thoughts. Not our stories. Not our beliefs.

Our minds, smart and sophisticated and gorgeous as they are, keep us stuck ("it all goes down in the mind"). Our minds keep us sick and suffering. Our minds distort all the beautiful things about us that we keep hidden away. Our minds make deals. I'll contain my anger in exchange for being fed. Or I'll pretend to be happy in exchange for hugs. Or I'll tone down my joy, my exuberance, my light in exchange for a connection to you, so you'll take care of me. And in all that? I'll come to believe untrue things so fiercely just to stay alive.

But becoming all we were meant to, fully accessing our potential and possibilities, calls us to reclaim the wisdom of our feelings.

Let's begin our practice right now.

First, breathe. Deep inhale through your nose. Slow sighing exhale. Repeat as many times as you'd like. Allow yourself to land right here in your body.

What do you feel right now? Just say it without censoring. Don't worry about hurting my feelings or anyone else's. Blurt it out.

I hate this. I'm scared. Why are we wasting our time on this? Or *yah, sister! Bring it on!*

Whatever you feel, see if you can let it be true without judgement, censorship, or trying to "fix" it. Notice if there are stories about what's right or wrong about your feelings. Allow the stories while also allowing the feelings. This is how you feel. This is your truth. Your mind may want to *decide for you* if it's okay to feel what you feel. It's been well trained to keep you safe. But note the operational word: trained. The mind is trained. The mind can be wrong. Feelings are pure wisdom. They may be inconvenient, they may go against the grain, they may hurt like hell, but they're never wrong.

That was a beautiful start. Because first things first. To feel, you must *allow* yourself to feel. Without censorship.

Here's where we're going in this steppingstone. First, we'll review four grounding lessons to explore why feelings are so hard. Then, we'll work with three simple yet powerful practices to reclaim our feelings.

FOUR GROUNDING LESSONS TO EXPLORE WHY FEELINGS ARE SO HARD.

- We subjugate our feelings to survive.
- We subjugate our feelings to belong (to family/community/culture/planet).
- Feelings expose where we are the most vulnerable.
- We conflate our feelings with the perspectives we hold about them.

We subjugate our feelings to survive.

We know this. This is the price we paid to stay alive. I'm not overstating this. In the mind of a child or a highly vulnerable adult, safety is survival. It was a genius strategy when we needed it. Until we no longer did. Now it keeps us sick, suffering, stuck, isolated, and cut off from our truth.

We talked about how connection is a primary need of humans. We must have it to survive. Our brilliant organism knew, without having to be told, how to stay alive in utero, as pre-verbal children, and as four- and five-year-olds. We knew innately what to do to maintain our essential connections, so we'd be fed, clothed, sheltered, and loved.

Geniuses, we were. How we innately shifted the emotional currents of our bodies toward safety. The big feelings became quiet. The quiet feelings all but disappeared. We learned to make up feelings we didn't have. We dimmed our light. We became savvy at reading the feelings of others without them saying a word. We knew. We *had* to know. We were so young and vulnerable, the need so great, and the payoff so huge, we didn't know what we'd done.

Then we grew up. We asked to heal. We observed a competing need, the need to be ourselves. To be seen, heard, known, and felt for who we are, who we *truly* are. This need arose as discontent, irritability, loneliness, confusion, anxiety. Who are we? And damn it, why can't we *think* our way through this like we do everything else? Why can't we succeed at *this*? I'm a freaking doctor, for God's sake, and he's a lawyer, and we're all somebody. Why can't we figure this out? Why do we lose our shit every time we try to change?

This is the beauty of discontent, irritability, loneliness, confusion, anxiety, and losing our shit over change. Because what are they? The language of our bodies. Portals to our wisdom. These are the feelings that lead us directly to what we need to heal, uncomfortable as they may be.

They ask us to call our lost feelings back. To discover what we need. To reconnect to our authenticity.

Now, there may be more to healing than feeling. Healing-the-verb may ask you to adopt a nutrient-dense food plan, dial in your sleep, or start physical therapy to help shift your equilibrium of suffering. But first things first. Because what happens when we try to change? Right. We feel things. As we heal, we must expect our feelings to show up. They will. Those feelings are necessary to our healing. Knowing how we feel leads to knowing who we are. Knowing who we are widens the lens to knowing what we need.

Think of it this way: why is embodied awareness our path, our practice, and our prize? It's not just seeing what's in us and all around us. In fact, "seeing" is just a metaphor. What we're really interested in, what shifts us the most, is feeling. Feeling is the truest truth of what we can possibly know, undisturbed by story, perspective, belief, intellectual analysis, and censorship. Feeling is the closest we come to real lived human experience. Everything else is *description* of real lived human experience.

So, if you're set upon a path of healing, you're asking to change, to grow, to expand into yourself. You will absolutely bump into your feelings along the way, sometimes in ways you won't expect.

If we subjugated our feelings for survival, how do we reclaim them?

In reclaiming our feelings, we must feel them. In feeling them, we'll remember. In remembering, we'll experience, perhaps for the very first time, what happened to us or what should have happened but didn't. We'll experience the lack of repair. We'll understand the players. We'll feel it all. The veil will be lifted. There will be no pretending anymore. Many of our changes expose what we truly feel, what we truly need.

There's a "but" here, and it is so key. The pain and discomfort of reviewing the past through the lens of our feelings is temporary. Feelings are energy. They flow. And as we experience them in our bodies, they flow through us. They're meant to flow. They have a trajectory. The trajectory is wisdom, growth, healing, and, ultimately, freedom. These feelings may be painful and uncomfortable but they're real. And in the revelation of our truth, we're lightened.

There's more. Once we can view our pasts through a wider truer lens, we see it better. Our perspective widens. There's more data to add to our life story. This shifts us out of blame, guilt, shame, whatever the hold our past has on us. They say, "the truth will set you free." Those hard feelings, the wider lens, the shift? *Will* set you free.

Finally, what happens to the genetic expression and survival biology that kept you safe but sick when they start to flow? When you reclaim them, revere them, and widen your perspective? Right. It all shifts. Reclaiming that energy shifts you into deeper healing, moves you out of suffering.

We subjugate our feelings to belong (to family-community-culture-planet).

There's another layer to what we just explored.

Even if we were raised in families who celebrated us and our wide range of healthy normal human feelings—including the hard ones, like anger, fear, and shame—the world 'out there' is way less welcoming.

We learn this quickly, don't we? How in our schools, communities, workplaces, and relationships many of our feelings aren't safe. *We're* not safe.

But if we can go home, back to our safe havens, tell our people all about it, how unwelcome we were 'out there,' and are held in compassion and safety, validating our experiences, validating *us*, then guess what? We're okay. It's hard, but we're okay.

But for most of us, what goes on 'out there' echoes what happened 'in here.' The double whammy makes this *really* hard.

PAUSE AND BREATHE.

Practice: anger shows us what we need.

One of the things my husband and I both cherish about our relationship is that we can fight. I don't mean physically, or even cruelly, but we can freely express hard feelings. I'm not saying it's always easy. But we do it. I don't recall how or when it first happened, but I learned early in our relationship that I could get mad at him, and the sky didn't fall in. He'd listen. He didn't run away. And in our verbal tussling back and forth, we'd work things out. But more than that. We'd break new ground. We'd figure something out about ourselves or our relationship we couldn't have known otherwise. We needed the energy of what began as anger to guide us toward what we *needed* to know. Instead of separating us, which I thought it would, anger brought us together. We'd stay in the encounter until we understood one another, until we reached the new ground.

For me, this was a shocking revelation. I'd never had a safe space for anger before. In my childhood home anger came unexpectedly and with fury. The consequences were devastating. I never felt safe.

In the safety of my relationship with my husband, I could express strong feelings even before I knew *what* I felt exactly. They could bubble up (or sometimes erupt!) and I could trust he'd hold the space, and the meaning in my feelings would be revealed. My relationship became the crucible for me reconnecting to feelings I didn't know I had.

I learned two profound lessons from the emotional safety of my marriage.

First, it's *not* normal, even if it should be. Save havens for feelings, especially the "dark" emotions, like anger, rage, fear, and shame are hard to find. For me, they weren't safe. For him, they weren't allowed. And it's not just us. In many of our families, the subtext of our interactions is that "dark" emotions are not just hard, they're wrong. They're "not nice," "not acceptable," "not appropriate," "mean," "dangerous," "too loud," "too harsh." Or how about this? Not "lady-like." Or worse, "you're out of control," "you're being irrational." Gaslighting, anyone? So, of course, these feelings feel scary. In many of our homes it wasn't safe to authentically feel.

The second lesson has been how vulnerable I feel expressing these feelings. After over three decades of marriage, it's still hard. But that vulnerability has always revealed the most authentic me and what I need.

I want that for you.

Anger in its full expression has powerful energy and velocity. It's designed that way, to cut through all the crap, all our resistance, all the ways our families-communities-culture want to silence us, to show us what we need. By showing us what we need, anger leads us back to ourselves. When anger's call to action is ignored, when we continue to subjugate ourselves to the control of others, ignore our needs, and allow unacceptable circumstances to persist, it will take a terrible toll. Rather than show us our truth about fairness, justice, boundaries, and needs—our *worth*—it escalates. It makes us sick.

Suppressed anger will escalate to resentment, frustration, rage, hatred, explosive behavior, or devastating isolation. And the science is clear. When unexpressed anger persists, it will make us sick. Fatigue, depression, anxiety, headaches, insomnia, chronic pain, heart disease, autoimmune disorders, and more are experiences of the equilibrium of suppressed anger. It saps our energy, our health, and our resilience.

Let's practice. We'll work with anger first. Why? Because anger is special. It's the emotion we're the most afraid of and shamed by. It's the emotion we've been the most bullied about. And it's the emotion that, through our distorted relationship to, makes us the sickest, keeps us the most stuck.

First, breathe. Activate your safety circuit: breath, hands, heart, feet, mind.

I'm right here. I'm safe. I hold all my feelings in safety. I hold myself in compassion. I remain curious.

Ask yourself, what makes me feel angry?

If the first answer is "nothing," ask again. In *this* world? In *this* life? See if you can come up with a little something. Or a big something. Whatever it is, welcome it. Your anger, in its authentic wisdom, is dang gorgeous.

Invite the anger in. Hold. Don't try to change or fix it. Resist judging it. If you find yourself judging or censoring, ask your judge to step aside for a moment. And remember, you don't have to share your feelings with anyone else. Give it a safe space within *you* to exist. This is you. This is how you feel. It's sacred. It needs to be heard. Anger, itself, is not dangerous. It's what people *do* with it that can be dangerous. Holding it in and pushing it down is dangerous.

As you hold, tap into your strong sturdy core. Anger will arise from this core to show you where there are energy, boundary, and fairness violations, or other unmet needs that inevitably occur for all of us. Understand it as a call for reflection and action. It doesn't have to be destructive.

If your anger could speak, what would it say? Don't hold back.

Ask your anger:

- What's the truth I need to know right now?
- What's not working? What needs aren't being met?
- Where do my boundaries need strengthening? Where do I need to say "no?"
- What feelings are beneath the anger? Fear, sadness, shame?

Yes, these are big questions. You can choose just one. When you have more time, work with the others. Allow anger to be your teacher.

Then, move your body. Anger is energizing. It's a call to action. But we've been taught to mistrust it, so it confuses us. Move—walk, run, do yoga, chore hard. Step into a power pose. Engage with anger in a constructive way letting its energy move through you rather than get stuck or escalate. Sometimes I can't access my feelings until I'm moving. Their energy must rise first, then I can experience them.

Feelings expose where we are the most vulnerable.

What is vulnerability? Yes, it's that icky, scary, alone feeling of exposing our tender feelings. It's the feeling of putting ourselves in harm's way. The uncertainty of the new arena we've never stepped into before. Like the new yoga class, friend group, or creative venture. Like the difficult conversation we'd rather avoid, the apology we need to make, or the request for our time we need to say no to. We could fall flat. Everyone will see it. Yikes.

The social scientist Brené Brown, who studies human vulnerability, describes it as "uncertainty, risk, and emotional exposure." But the flip side of vulnerability, if we're willing to brave it, is everything we long for in human emotional experience. As Brown puts it, "Vulnerability is the birthplace of love, belonging, joy, courage, empathy, and creativity."[100]

Feeling is scary. It can be overwhelming. But the payoff is huge. This applies to all feelings. We can feel vulnerable in all of them.

So. Simple guidelines we know so well:

- Activate your safety circuit: breath, hands, heart, feet, mind.
- Gently shift into the uncomfortable feelings, holding them with reverence, compassion, and curiosity.
- Practice feeling your feelings alone at first, then with others.
- Move your body to mobilize feelings or to shake off their excessive energy.
- Write your feelings in a private journal—writing is another way to access and clarify feelings.

This is why change, even intentional habit change, can make us feel vulnerable. Because change makes us *feel*. Let's explore another technique for helping us navigate the discomfort of habit change.

---

[100] Brené Brown. Daring Greatly: How the Courage to Be Vulnerable Transforms the Way We Live, Love, Parent, and Lead. 2012.

PAUSE AND BREATHE.

Deprivation: what to do with the pain of habit change.

The hardest part of change is that it's, well, *hard*. Why? It makes us feel *vulnerable*.

Change asks us to learn new things, try new things, step out of our comfortable groove, and do hard work with uncertain outcomes. On paper, that doesn't sound too bad, does it? Easy peasy.

But what else happens when we try to change? That we sometimes don't expect? Feelings we didn't know we had sneak out, sometimes explode out, just as we implement our new choices. Sometimes they knock us flat. The choices seem impossible. Because many of the habits we want to change weren't choices in the beginning, were they? They were the glue that held us together. All the feelings we fed, soothed, numbed, medicated, and assuaged now land. More than land, they demand! *Pay attention to me now. Heal me now.*

Sometimes we don't know what's at stake until we implement the change. Because the "choice" of the old habit that soothed and settled us wasn't done consciously. Or its familiarity felt so safe, dependable, like an old friend. But asking to heal invites consciousness in. When we become curious, we learn the function the old habit served. Like the sugar that soothed our dissatisfaction, the alcohol that made us feel braver, the overwork that made us feel successful.

So. Good news, bad news. The good news is you get to feel. And what you feel you can heal. Bad news is you *have to* feel. To heal, you have no choice but to feel. It's a conundrum, isn't it?

Change is never easy. Especially when it's uncomfortable. But once the choice is made, we can make it sacred. We make the discomfort sacred. Because it *is* sacred. You and your growth are sacred. And more than that. Change, itself, the struggle, the feelings, the challenges, consciously made, consciously tended to, is sacred. Because it's *the crucible* for our growth. In that growth is healing, freedom, access to our potential and possibilities.

One way I like to make change sacred is to work directly with the discomfort of deprivation. Deprivation takes many forms, but it's often the word we use to describe the pain of change. We want the old thing, behavior, substance, or habit back. We feel deprived without it. We crave it. We long for what it did for us. How can we transform our pain and discomfort into something sacred?

To shift the experience of deprivation into something sacred, we have to feel it. How? Implement the change. Sometimes we don't know how deprived we'll feel until we do it. When the old habit is taken away, we get to fully experience what it did for us. We feel the pain, the discomfort, the deprivation. Its power hits us between the eyes. *Now* we can heal.

Seeding the gap.

I want us to work with a technique that helps us repurpose the gaping hole (that's how it feels sometimes, doesn't it?) left by the habit we've given up. There's a lot of space and energy in that hole we can commit to something else. Something we need. Something we desire. This practice is borrowed from Rod Stryker, the founder of Para yoga, who calls this technique "seeding the gap."[101] I've taken the liberty over the years of making it my own so it's accessible to anyone trying to create change, even though it hurts. This practice honors how sacred our pain of change is. How sacred our habits and unmet needs are.

---

[101] Rod Stryker. The Four Desires: Creating a Life of Purpose, Happiness, Prosperity, and Freedom. 2011.

It goes like this.

First, make the decision for change. Consider an example most of us know well. Let's give up sugar.

When I first started using this practice, I decided to give up my Ghirardelli chocolate chip habit. Why? I was already a low sugar girl, but those chocolate chips? They soothed a world of pain at what I used to call "the witching hour." This was when I arrived home in the afternoon after picking my kids up from school and was catapulted into juggling *everything* all at once. Kids, kids' snacks, kids' conversations, kids' homework, dogs, dogs' kisses, dogs' walks, dinner prep, and all the things a mom or dad must do at that time. Hence, *chocolate!!*

Maybe giving up chocolate was a cruel thing to do to myself but, heck, an apple or cup of berries would be a better nutritional choice, you know? So, I decided to give up my chocolate. You would have thought my world had just fallen apart. How was it that I was sobbing over a few chocolate chips? How was it that a few chocolate chips could keep me glued together? You know, though, don't you? It's what we've been talking about all along.

Enter "seeding the gap."

I walk in the house at witching hour so happy to have been reunited with my children. But then it happens. The overwhelm rises. Before I know it, I start walking toward the pantry like a zombie. I spy the bag of chocolate chips sitting there on the shelf literally calling to me. But I stop. I take three slow conscious breaths. I can do this. I can breathe. I can pause. The chips can wait for three breaths. My future can wait. In those breaths, in that pause, for just this moment, I can hold whatever it is I'm feeling. My eyes are closed and I'm all in this. There's my gap, that breath, that pause. Now, (quickly before it's too late!) I "seed" that gap. I seed the gap with my sacred intention. To feel my feelings. To honor my body. To honor myself and the overwhelm I feel as everything converged all at once, as everyone needs me, as I feel responsible for all of it and doing it all well. I call in my new future. One in which *my* needs matter, *I* matter, I ask for what I need.

Had I not given up my chocolate habit and not felt the feelings? I wouldn't have known their depth. I wouldn't have felt the pain and overwhelm and confusion. I wouldn't have asked the questions, "Is there a better way to manage all this?" "How do I need help here?" "How can I be gentler with myself?" "How do I get my needs met?"

Okay, you try it.

- Choose a habit you'd like to change. Perhaps make it small at first (those "small" habits can be surprisingly powerful, like my chocolate chips!).
- Implement. Stop the thing. Start the thing. Maybe it's both.
- Feel. Is it 'easy peasy?' You're done. Or is it 'whoa?' Seed the gap.

Keep practicing.

We conflate our feelings with the perspectives we hold about them.

Feelings are portals to the closest we can ever get to our truth—what our minds can't do, our brains can't do, our guides and mentors can't do. Feelings wordlessly express our truth through the sensations, currents of energy, and impulses of our bodies. Sometimes there aren't words even if we try to find them. We feel tightness in the chest, burning in the gut, and constriction in our throats. Our heads drop low, and we can't move. Or we're antsy and agitated. We must move, must hug, must tell, must hide under the covers.

Part of our development is to associate our feelings (and their sensations, energy currents, and impulses within our bodies) with words and meaning. This is programmed by our families-communities-culture. There are good and bad feelings. Feelings that get our needs met and feelings that are ignored. We learn to strategize our feelings for safety. We learn to associate our feelings with specific experiences. We developed perspectives about our feelings. *Anger is bad. Shame is my fault. Happiness makes others feel good. Fear means I'm unsafe. Your anger is dangerous.*

To use feelings as portals to our wisdom, it's important to distinguish between feelings and our perspectives about them. The reason is simple. Feelings are true. They exist in present time. We can't argue with a feeling. We feel what we feel, whatever it is—anger, fear, shame, joy. But what we make our feelings mean (right or wrong, good or bad, safe or unsafe, and so on) are *perspectives*. They're *not* true. Our minds make them up. They may be a close approximation to our truth, but they can also keep us suffering and stuck.

How do we distinguish feelings from perspectives?

I think this is tricky. We often feel, then describe our feelings with a perspective. Or we don't think we feel because there's no perspective, but there are sensations and energy currents present in our bodies. There's tightness in the chest, a queasy stomach, or constriction in the throat. There's a sudden loss of energy, our heads drop low, or we have to sit down. We don't have words, though the feeling is there.

Sometimes when we're asked how we feel, we don't know. We don't have the words. But our bodies know. If we check in with our bodies, we'll notice the sensations and energy currents that represent our feelings. They inform us about our feelings without words, without perspectives.

There's an upside to this confusion. We can scrutinize our perspectives, the stories we tell about our feelings. We can question them and learn from them. We can identify what we need. And we can practice embodied present moment awareness to reconnect to what we feel. In this way, our perspectives become portals too.

What's the difference between a feeling and a perspective (keep in mind we often conflate perspectives *as* our feelings).

First, consider some foundational feelings and their variations, keeping in mind feelings are highly layered and nuanced. They often defy simple words.

- *Love* (tenderness, compassion, empathy).
- *Joy* (content, fulfilled, happy).
- *Gratitude* (appreciation, thankful, touched).
- *Courage* (brave, empowered, confident).

- *Awe* (curious, excited, amazed).
- *Fear* (scared, anxious, dread).
- *Anger* (rage, hatred, mad).
- *Sadness* (lonely, grief, sorrow).
- *Shame* (self-loathing, disgust, revulsion).
- *Confusion* (bewildered, befuddled, flustered).

Now consider common perspectives, stories we tell about these feelings.

- *Love:* connection, attachment, belonging.
- *Joy:* worthy, approval, loved.
- *Gratitude:* support, indebted, relieved.
- *Courage:* strong, fearless, capable.
- *Awe:* stunned, amazed, disbelief.
- *Fear:* overwhelmed, threatened, unsafe.
- *Anger:* resentful, frustrated, annoyed.
- *Sadness:* unhappy, abandoned, betrayed.
- *Shame:* guilt, worthless, humiliated.
- *Confused:* idiotic, lost, stupid.

Some of these perspectives are healthy. Our needs are met. Like how we understand the love we feel for a close friend as "connection" or the awe we experience looking at a sunset as "amazing." There's no confusion or distortion of the experience represented by the story. The perspective doesn't keep us stuck.

But sometimes our perspectives are not just incorrect but *add to* our confusion and pain. They distort the feelings. Like me telling myself I'm an "idiot" because I've misplaced my keys. Or how so many of us conflate feeling afraid with being "unsafe."

Because what does calling myself an "idiot" or telling myself I'm "unsafe" do?

They tell a false story. Losing my keys is confusion or forgetfulness. Nothing more. Same with feeling afraid. While feeling afraid could mean I'm not safe, most of the time it does not. It's perfectly normal and healthy to feel scared when we're taking big risks with uncertain outcomes, or when we're exposing our vulnerability.

Why is a false story a problem? It's a problem when we believe it. We tell it over and over. It keeps us stuck in the same old assumptions, the same old stories.

We feel how we feel. But our perspective about the feeling may be wrong. Then what happens? We have feelings about our incorrect story! This compounds our suffering. See, our perspectives are what get us in trouble. If we can learn to bypass the story, recognize it for what it is, and 'feel all the feels' we're much better off. We may still hurt, but won't spend years, or a lifetime, hijacked by a story that's not true.

For example:

- The shame (feeling) we feel in our bodies that we misconstrue as our worthlessness (perspective), rather than someone's incorrect story about us.
- The anger (feeling) we feel in our bodies but believe is bad (perspective), makes *us* bad (perspective), rather than showing us our unmet needs.
- The confusion (feeling) we feel in our bodies that we think means we're stupid (perspective), rather than a perfectly capable brain that's trying to process too much all at once.
- The fear (feeling) we feel in our bodies that we understand as being unsafe (perspective), rather than a normal response to uncertainty.

PAUSE AND BREATHE.

Feeling is a practice.

Feeling is a verb. We can practice feeling. And like any language of living, loving, and healing, we *must* practice. Deciphering feelings is a skill, communicating feelings is a skill, differentiating feelings from stories is a skill. And beyond all that, relearning and reclaiming feelings is a skill. When we don't know what we're feeling, checking in with the body to notice what's there—the sensations and energy states—is a skill. And finally, holding all that with compassion and curiosity is a skill.

So. You know how we do this, right? One feeling at a time. One moment at a time. One breath, one pause at a time. With so many opportunities to feel, we can slowly, patiently get our reps in and make progress we can measure, progress we can feel.

Consider these to be general guidelines for your feeling practice rather than specific instructions for how to do it. I'm less interested in the specific details of how you go about it and more interested in you doing it.

First and foremost: No feeling is ever wrong. Never, ever, ever. Period. Meditate on this every day. If you don't believe it, can't believe it, that's just a perspective. Not a perspective you were born with, but a perspective you were given, which you adopted, which keeps you locked into your own suffering, locked into the perspective of your own suffering. You need a breakthrough. Keep meditating.

Set aside time every day to check in with your feelings. Like working on any skill, you have to get your reps in and practice every day. Make this a sacred habit. It can be part of your self-reflection, meditation, creative, or walking time. Check in with what's happening in your body. What feelings, sensations, or currents of energy are there? Can you welcome what's there without trying to change or fix or censor? Can you hold what you find with compassion and curiosity?

Create a container of compassion and safety for your feelings. A huge part of this is what we just talked about—the consistency of showing up every day, of practice. When you show up every day, you're saying, "I hear you, I see you, I feel you, you matter to me." Literally say this to the parts of you feeling the feelings. Like children, lovers, friends. You're showing up. Nothing can be more compassionate or safe.

Beyond the showing up, use your words. Say to your sadness, fear, shame, or anger, "You are welcome here with me, I hold you with compassion, you are safe with me."

Ask for help from a feeling professional. Feelings, especially the hard feelings, can feel so scary. We need help holding them, help exploring them, and help extricating ourselves from our perspectives about them that keep us suffering. Work with a therapist trained in "trauma-informed" therapies.[102]

Share your feelings with those you trust. I think we're meant to heal in relationship just as we're meant to live in relationship to others. Risky as it may seem, share your feelings with people you trust. If you're not used to doing this, just dip your little toe in the water at first. Share a little tidbit of something. Connect to your feeling and share it as authentically as you can. Then allow yourself to experience the outcome of that. Not everyone will get you. But some folks *will* get you, in fact, they'll be so grateful you shared with them and more than a little relieved to learn they're not the only ones to feel like they do!

Stay curious about your feelings. Remember what curiosity does? It opens space for learning something new while loosening the grip of your well-practiced perspectives. Curiosity doesn't say outright, "you're wrong." But it invites a new story, a new angle, more data to widen your perspective.

Don't let anyone tell you how you feel (or that your feelings are wrong). Just don't. Only you can possibly know how you feel (and even that's hard!). Repeat your new mantra: *My feelings are never, ever, ever wrong.*

---

[102] Healing professionals trained in trauma-informed therapies will often use language like "trauma-informed" so you recognize them. Some highly effective trauma-informed approaches are Compassionate Inquiry, Internal Family Systems, and Somatic Experiencing. Talk therapy or strategies to bypass feelings will not work.

It's okay to not know how you feel. Sometimes it's hard. You may have disconnected from certain feelings to keep yourself safe. Or they're showing up as sensations and energy states within your body. Don't worry—you're neither defective nor lost. This is the value of checking in daily. You get to know the subtle ways your body can speak your truth. A little tightness or energy loss can speak volumes about what's not working for you. Whereas lightness, joy, or an upshift in energy is giving you the green light.

Use movement and writing to help you access your feelings. Movement helps you manage the intensity of feelings. The running, stomping, or meandering amongst the trees helps you shake off the excess energy feelings can bring. Sometimes noticing myself stomping around is my first signal that what I'm feeling is more intense than I thought. Writing invites feelings into your consciousness and can provide a safe place for you and your feelings to land.

Be tender and patient with your feelings. Which is to say, be tender and patient with yourself. You matter. Your feelings matter. We're bringing you and your feelings back together because you're one hundred percent a match made in heaven.

Always ask, "is this a feeling or a perspective about a feeling?" It makes a difference, doesn't it? Because our feelings carry our truth while our perspectives about our feelings carry someone else's truth. Our perspectives have kept us suffering and stuck. By scrutinizing them through a wider lens, they can liberate us. But we're not wholesale discarding them, are we? Because we are grateful for how our closely held perspectives kept us alive. Though many of these perspectives no longer serve, they are signatures of our genius.

LAST WORDS.

I hope by now you realize how wise you truly are. How your untapped potential isn't a deficit, it's already there inside you. Currents of wisdom flowing, ready to show you everything. All the truth you ever need to know. Yes, you are all that. All you need to do is pay attention. First with the simplest observer's mind. Then with curiosity for what you see, compassion for what you feel, and reverence for what a freaking miracle it all is, what a freaking miracle *you* are.

Thank you for taking this courageous journey with me.

THREE PROMISES.

Three small practices I can start right now, then come back to every day, to help me know, revere, and trust my feelings. So tenderly.

1.
2.
3.

CHAPTER TWENTY-THREE
Eighth *Un*Broken Core Resilience Steppingstone:

LOVE.

Always love, right? Always love. In everything we do. Even as we hold our hardest, darkest feelings, we do it out of love. Love isn't all soft and blissful. Love isn't just what makes us feel good. Love can be the hardest damned thing of all.

I once broached the tender subject of self-love with my client Molly. She surprised me with her quick declaration, "I *hate* that word." "Love?" I asked. "Yes," she replied, "love, self-love, all the loves." She explained, "I don't trust them. I don't believe in them. I don't *understand* them." Though an exceptionally loving person, she had a complicated childhood that lacked love. She never felt safe or cared for as a child and struggled to do so as an adult. She struggled to love *herself.* I asked her what word she preferred. "Compassion?" "Nope." "Tenderness?" "Definitely not." "Okay, how about reverence? You know, for the sacred being you are." "Okay," she said thoughtfully, "I can do reverence. I revere all life. I believe we are all Divine."

She reminded me how complicated our relationship to love is. So tainted by commercialism, insincerity, and countless superficial notions of love—so *not* Divine—the word has lost its sacred meaning. So, though love is everything, it helps to contemplate love by using words that are less misused. Molly's word was reverence. I love it.

And it's true, isn't it? How *much* there is to revere when we consider the incredible attributes of the human organism. So much genius built right in us. From the moment we're born. When we have no words. When we're innocent and naïve, with undeveloped brains. How we *know*. How our bodies know. How we survive. How every nuance of who we become makes perfect sense. How we can evolve into conscious, caring, sophisticated people regardless of what happened to us. To deeply reflect on ourselves, as we are together here. To see what we never could before, focusing on parts of ourselves we never had, then expanding our lens beyond ourselves. To understand ourselves in a whole new way, in the context of our families-communities-culture. To ask the questions that take us to growth and healing, our potential and possibilities unleashed. *We do that.* What's not to revere?

So, with the deepest heart-felt reverence for all of us, let's shift into love.

I'm going to use the word "love" a lot in this chapter, as I have throughout this book. But I invite you to insert the word you're most comfortable with. Here are some suggestions: reverence, compassion, devotion, appreciation, tenderness, respect, okayness, awesomeness. Meet yourself where you're at. Create your own love language. What other words speak to you?

In this *Unbroken* core resilience steppingstone, we'll explore two primary perspectives that I think are most important to the work we're doing: safety and transcendence.

Safety, because as humans we must feel safe to thrive. Love in its best iterations will always lead us toward safety. If it doesn't, it's not love.

Transcendence, because love is the energy that connects us to everyone else. Through our actions, love is the light we beam to lovers-friends-families-communities-culture-planet that transcends our self-interest, to serve us all.

We need both. We need safety to become ourselves and rise beyond ourselves. We need safety to receive and experience love. To trust love. To love ourselves. We need transcendence to connect to our people-communities-culture-planet most deeply. In ways that ask, what do you need, what do my people need?

Safety deepens and strengthens our experience of love, our trust in love. Transcendence helps us spread the safety, spread the love.

It makes perfect sense that after everything we've talked about in this book about safety and connection, love would be so inextricably linked to safety.

Love, *real* love, *unconditional* love, *is* safety. Because it *feels* safe. It *holds* us in safety. It helps us trust and receive love. Unconditional love says, "I see you exactly as you are, I accept you exactly as you are, I love all iterations of you."

Transcendent love zeroes in on how we most need to feel and experience safety. What brings us most to love.

Think about those who love us. *Really* love us. Those we know without question love us, not just those who *say* they do. How they literally rise above their own self-interest to do so. How they show up for us when we need them, even when it's inconvenient, even in the middle of the night, even when it's hard and involves sacrifice. They're curious about us. They listen to us and make it clear we matter to them. They hold us in absolute connection and safety just as we are. That's transcendent love. The very best versions of parenting are examples of transcendent love.

For thirty years I've watched my husband up close as he's interacted with our sons. I've seen him hang on "with every last neuron," as I've often described it, exhausted after a long workday, listening and counseling in ways to make sure they feel seen and heard—to feel safe—no matter what it takes to do so. He loves them with transcendent love. It's magnificent. They will always carry that love inside them.

The love of both safety and transcendence are verbs. They're all about action, what we *do* for love. Not what we say and not necessarily what we feel. While we feel all kinds of things in love—joy, peace, calm, excitement, sadness, grief, and so on—feelings by themselves don't lead us to safety or transcendence.

For our purposes here, we'll shift into love in very practical ways. By making love a practice, we get better at it. We make it a growth process, a healing practice. Our practice includes self-connection and reverence through compassion and curiosity. These bring us to safety. Safety becomes the foundation for transcendent love, when we can go beyond our own interests to see, hear, know, and experience the safety needs of others.

If, like my client Molly, we didn't receive unconditional love as we were growing up, we may feel confused about love. We may not know how to show it or express it or how to recognize it when it shows up. But we can learn. That's the good news here: if we're awake, aware, and willing, we can learn. And as we get our love-the-verb reps in, we'll get good at it. We'll learn to love ourselves, our people, and to practice transcendent love.

As we practice love-the-verb, we'll direct it toward ourselves, and we'll direct it toward others. In both, we connect and create safety.

Throughout our practices we'll be on the lookout for false love. How will we know? Ask the questions: Do I feel safe in this love? Do I feel seen? Do I matter? If the answer is "no" to these questions, it's not love. Period.

I once had a friend who effusively expressed "love" to everyone around her. Her friends, her students, me. "I love you, I love you so much," she'd proclaim with big hugs to everyone who passed her by, always with a huge smile on her face. It was warm. People appeared to appreciate her effusiveness. But I was always wary. I'd ask myself, "is it *me*?" Was I just an old fuddy duddy who couldn't receive love? Over time, I learned her words were often not supported with actions. She'd say, "I love you," then not show up when it mattered or follow through on her promises. Eventually I leveled with myself. As she professed her love one day, I acknowledged "she's full of shit." I realized her overtures were about her, not me. Likely not about anyone else either. My body knew all along though it took my mind awhile to catch up. I would override my feelings with logic, like how could I mistrust this person everyone else seems to adore? Adored by everyone or not, I was barking up the wrong tree. It wasn't really love. It wasn't safe. It wasn't transcendent.

We'll be working with love in our active, living, breathing bodies. Like balancing challenging lives within our sturdy cores, love is physical. We'll practice love within our sacred centers of love, compassion, empathy, and wisdom. Can you guess? Yes! Our hearts.

Let's begin right now.

Stand tall, feet against the ground, hip distance apart. Place hands over your heart. Breathe deeply. Sigh. Notice your breath, your feet against the ground, and your hands on your heart. You're activating one of your primary safety circuits, breath-hands-heart-feet-mind. Rest here for a moment without trying to change or fix anything. Allow yourself to breathe and sigh, hold yourself with compassion for whatever you are feeling right now. Every part of you. Just hold. Rest.

Say to yourself, "I hold you and all your parts, all your iterations, right here in my heart. You are welcome here. I can hold you and all your feelings with compassion and reverence. I'm right here. You are safe with me."

That was our first love (or insert your own word) practice. We used our bodies, activated a primary safety circuit, and spoke our powerful words. How did it feel? Was it doable?

There's no wrong answer to that question. While I hope you said things like, "warm," "safe," "loved," "relaxed," or "reassured," this practice may be opening a completely new way of relating to yourself. It may feel awkward. You may not have felt as safe as you deserved in your important relationships. This makes it hard to fully experience a practice that is self-reverent. That's okay. There's nothing to fix. With practice, you will one hundred percent shift into the safety, compassion, and connection you deserve. Stay with me. Stay with the practice.

Can we try one more thing?

Remember the empathy practice we used in the first steppingstone, *Be Present*? Empathy is a self-reverence practice.

Back to Molly for just a sec. In the same session in which she chose reverence as her love language, we tried to figure out how she could practice it with herself. Not surprising, it was hard for her, given the complicated relationship she had with love. So, I asked her to simply think about someone she loves. She instantly thought of her grandson Will. She had no trouble identifying her feelings for him as deep unconditional love that filled her entire chest. She described it as the most sacred connection she's ever experienced with anyone. So, that's where we began her self-reverence practice. By recalling her love for Will and tuning into how it felt in her body. That's all. Not even trying to direct it toward herself. But to simply feel the sensation of love inhabiting her own body and acknowledge: this is what unconditional love feels like, this is in my own heart, this is real.

Your turn.

Consider someone you love unconditionally. Bring them to mind. Notice what you feel in your body. Hold it. Feel how tangible it is, how it has a location, how it moves. Sink into the experience, holding it for as long as you can.

LOVE IS SAFETY.

Love can only bring safety if it tells the truth. *Our* truth. We all get that now, yes? Love is truth. It's not all flowy and glowy. It's not what's prescribed for us. Love, love-the-verb, is hard. It's especially hard for those of us who didn't learn about love when we were very young. But even if you did, even if you were loved beyond measure, even if you knew it, felt it, and had it demonstrated for you in countless powerful ways, it wasn't all perfect, was it? Not from your parents. Certainly not from the families-communities-culture you landed in. Not all the time. So, this lesson applies to us all.

When we're teeny-weeny babies, safety is in connection that holds and soothes and feeds and sees us, that shows us who we are. As adults, it's in authenticity and self-acceptance. The road to that safety is love. Self-love. Or, like Molly, self-reverence.

So, for this part of our steppingstone, let's work with self-love as it leads us to safety. As it holds us in our truth. We can't always count on it from others, can we? We must teach ourselves how to show up for *ourselves* in tenderness, compassion, gentleness, reverence, and the deepest respect for who we are, where we've been, and how we kept ourselves safe when we didn't have a clue what we were doing, how savvy we were, how magnificent we are. In love. In so much love.

Richard Schwartz, PhD, psychotherapist and founder of the "Internal Family Systems" (IFS) approach to trauma therapy, describes us as having "no bad parts."[103] All the parts of us that show up do so because they helped us survive and thrive. Even the parts that make us uncomfortable. Even the parts we're not proud of. Even the parts that hurt others. They were all necessary. All to be revered for how they helped us survive.

In this context, what's our work to merge love, safety, and truth?

Tell the truth, yes. But before we can tell the truth, we must understand a foundational truth about ourselves. If there are no bad parts, and if we develop parts to adapt to our circumstances, to survive and create safety in our early years and into our adulthood, what work must we do before we're capable of telling the truth about ourselves?

We must see ourselves and our parts through that lens—the lens of love, the lens of truth, the lens of wider understanding. A lens of faith, but also a lens that accounts for how we understand the human organism from the sciences of early childhood development, neurobiology, and trauma psychology.[104] When we look at ourselves through these lenses, we can see no bad parts. Every part served a vital function to keep us safe and connected, to get our

---

[103] Richard Schwartz PhD. *No Bad Parts: Healing Trauma and Restoring Wholeness with the Internal Family Systems Model.* 2021. Excellent read about this highly practical psychotherapeutic model for lay people. Can be used as a manual for self-care.

[104] Insert references here.

primary needs met. More than that, as we see ourselves through these lenses, we are amazed by the spectacular genius of our parts. So, no matter what the parts are—jealous parts, parts that don't tell the truth, shy parts, angry parts, bragging parts, shut down parts, addicted parts—they all participated in our survival. And to do all that in service of us, what do they deserve? Yes. Reverence. Appreciation. Tenderness. Compassion. Love. All of it. Even if our parts' strategies need upgrades, they served us well at one time.

This is our work to get to self-love. Self-love tells us the truth, perhaps for the very first time. It takes us to safety. Love. Truth. Safety. That's the connection.

Since words aren't always enough, we're going to have to experience self-love. We'll have to feel. We'll have to experience our feelings through the lens that understands the genius and beauty of all our parts. Beyond words, our brains need proof to believe truth, to feel safe. When we show up, do the hard work of feeling, the hard work of shifting our perspectives, of giving ourselves credit instead of grief, that's our proof.

LOVE IS SAFETY PRACTICE.

We've been working with safety throughout this book. Let's take a moment to circle back in a different way.

In safety we find our truth. When we're safe we can receive love.

Sit or stand comfortably. Notice your breath without trying to change or fix it. Check in with your body. What feelings, sensations, or energy states do you notice?

Activate your safety circuit: breath, hands, heart, feet, mind.

Ask your body—your feelings, sensations, or energy states—what do you have to say? Listen without trying to understand or fix or apply logic. If your mind steps in, gently ask it to give you space.

Be in your body. Notice what's there.

Then ask: what do you need? Listen. Stay curious. Hold yourself with tenderness. Hold any answers that come with tenderness.

Continue to ask. What do you need to feel seen, heard, to know you matter? How can I earn your trust? What proof do you need?

Circle back with your questions every day. Remind your body that you're there. Bring your proof.

ASK FOR HELP WITH SAFETY.

Love and safety are hard. Confusing. Overwhelming. Lonely. Sometimes we need help.

Love and safety are powerful in relationships. But how do we find it, trust it, and hold it for ourselves when we're scared?

Please don't hesitate to ask for help sorting this out. You already know how excited I am about the uniquely therapeutic practices of Compassionate Inquiry (CI) and Internal Family Systems (IFS) as avenues to establishing safety and returning to wholeness. Use their directories to find certified practitioners and participants in their professional programs to work with in-person or remotely via telehealth visits.[105]

TRANSCENDENT LOVE: LOVE BEYOND SELF.

Do you have someone in your life who loves you beyond measure and makes that clear to you in tangible ways you can understand? Someone that you feel safe with? And in that safety and all the ways they show up, you know with your whole being that you and your needs matter to them? Do they seek out knowing what your needs are? And then show up? And show up? In ways specifically designed for *you*? Day or night? According to *your* needs, not theirs?

That's transcendent love.

If you've been blessed to have that kind of love, how does it make you feel?

Yes, safe. So many adjectives but in the end, transcendent love is the safest. And in that safety, we connect more deeply. We're safe to connect, safe to be vulnerable, safe to be exactly who we are. We belong in a sturdier, more meaningful way than all our other belongings.

Transcendent love circles back. We get what we give. Transcendent love leads to safety in others. Safety leads to deeper connection. In deeper

---

[105] www.CompassionateInquiry.com/practitioners.

www.ifs-institute.com/practitioners.

connection, *we're* safer. Our families-communities-culture-planet are safer. Transcendent love leads to everything worth anything for the entire planet.

The life's work of the great psychologist Abraham Maslow depicts the "circling back" of transcendent love. His original work, encapsulated in his "Maslow's Hierarchy of Needs," which many of us are familiar with from Psychology 101, represents human development as a pyramid. The base of the pyramid includes physiological needs such as food, water, sleep, and shelter, followed closely with other aspects of personal safety, indicating that once survival and safety needs are met, we're supported and available for higher levels of human experience depicted at the top of the pyramid. The pinnacle of his original model is what he called "self-actualization," characterized by the attainment of personal growth, creative expression, and self-fulfillment—all self-benefitting attributes.

Maslow's Hierarchy of Needs

Self-Actualization
Personal Growth, Peak Experiences, Self-Fulfillment

Self-Esteem
Dignity, Respect, Achievement, Independence

Love & Belonging
Friendships, Intimacy, Family, Connection

Safety
Security, Health, Personal Well-Being

Physiological
Food, Water, Sleep, Shelter

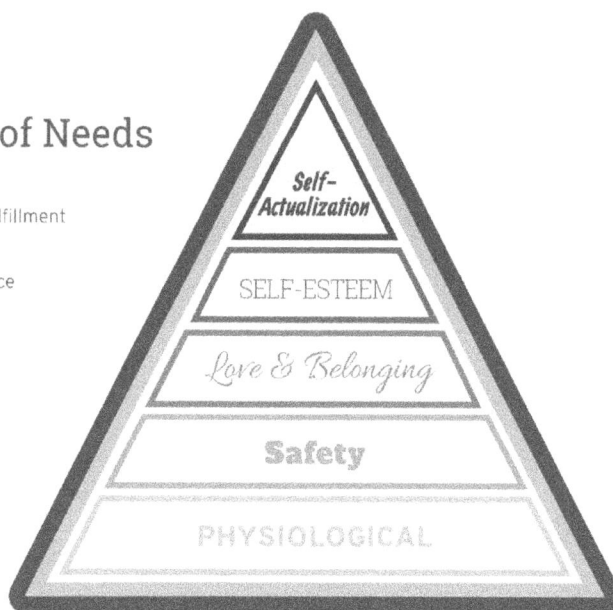

Shortly before his death, Maslow wrote that his popular model of human development was incomplete, having neglected the powerful human attribute of altruism. He suggested an additional level at the top of his pyramid, superseding self-actualization: self-transcendence.

> *"The fully developed (and very fortunate) human being working under the best conditions tends to be motivated by values which transcend his self. They are not selfish anymore in the old sense of that term. Beauty is not within one's skin nor is justice or order ... It*

is equally outside and inside: therefore, it has transcended the geographical limitations of the self."[106]

Maslow's *Evolved* Hierarchy of Needs

Self-Transcendence
"All is One" Consciousness
Selfless acts of Unconditional Love, Kindness, and Mercy

Self-Actualization
Personal Growth, Peak Experiences, Self-Fulfillment

Self-Esteem
Dignity, Respect, Achievement, Independence

Love & Belonging
Friendships, Intimacy, Family, Connection

Safety
Security, Health, Personal Well-Being

Physiological
Food, Water, Sleep, Shelter

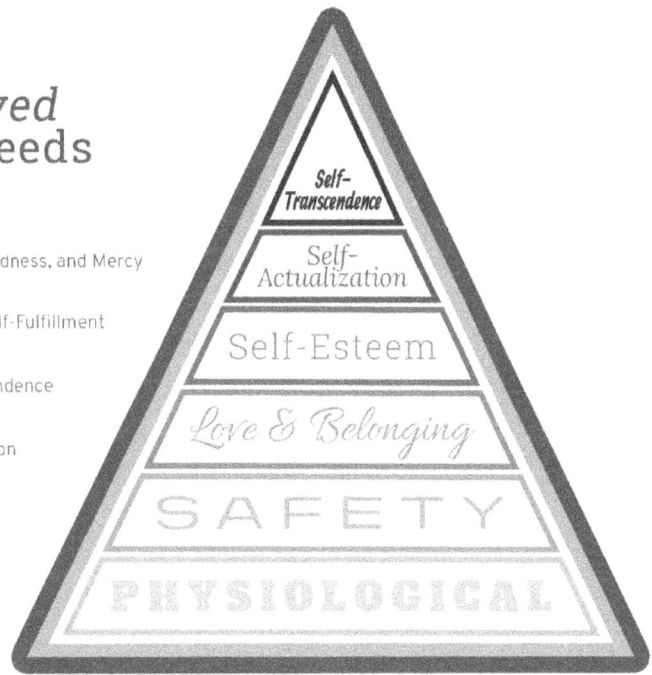

Rising to the top of Maslow's evolved pyramid, one can continue to reach a deeper level of wisdom, transcending oneself to help create safety and connection for others, including the collective human population (all-is-one consciousness). Self-transcendence is expressed by actively considering the needs of others and caring for family-community-culture-planet in ways that serve their needs beyond oneself.

I would take Maslow's theory further by saying that recipients of transcendent love rise in safety. The transcendence of one raises the safety of another, which expands their potential, deepening their lived experience and wisdom as humans. Maslow's pyramid simplifies the trajectory of human development. But it's really a circle, not a one-way bottom-to-top process.

Which is to say what we all surely know by now. Love is safety. Love creates a circle of safety. Love elevates everyone.

---

[106] Maslow, 1969a, pp. 3-4. From Koltko-Rivera Mark E. Rediscovering the Later Version of Maslow's Hierarchy of Needs: Self-Transcendence and Opportunities for Theory, Research, and Unification. Review of General Psychology. 2006. DOI: 10.1037/1089-2680.10.4.302.

HOW DO WE GET TO TRANSCENDENT LOVE?

Let's land in transcendent love right now.

Name one person you love beyond measure.

Without overthinking, name three simple things you can do for that person that responds to their needs and helps them feel safe.

If you don't have an immediate answer, consider that you may not know what their safety needs are. So, what can you do? Yes, ask them. Then, come back to the question: what three things can I do to respond to my loved one's needs? To help them feel safe?

Can you commit to doing these three things every day? Without asking for anything in return? Perhaps without telling them what you are doing?

That's transcendent love.

See? Not rocket-science. Not an esoteric practice.

Transcendent love arises from our own strength. Our sturdiness. Our ability to be fully present to ourselves as well as the needs of others. When we ask our loved ones what they need, we're standing in our strength, sturdiness, and presence to do so.

Which is perhaps the most important lesson about transcendent love. It doesn't ask us to be exceptional or to live on a mountaintop. It doesn't require a level of sophistication most of us don't already have. It's a verb. It's simple. We're all capable of it. It takes practice. That's all. And in that practice, we get our reps in. We get good at it. It's transcendent because we consider and respond to others' real needs, not because we're extraordinary in some way to know what their needs are. We *asked*. We do it from our ordinary everyday bodies, from the version of us we've curated through all our growth practices.

We don't leave our bodies to show up in transcendent love, do we? We maintain our own safety, keeping our boundaries strong to protect our energy. We remain fully conscious of our *own* needs, so our acts of transcendent love are not done out of obligation or expectation. We don't abandon ourselves to perform them.

With the intention to love people-communities-culture-world-planet, transcendent love asks, "what do you most need, how do you feel most safe, what do you need to grow, how can I help support you in fulfilling that need in the most relevant way to you?" It's always motivated by what *they* need for growth and safety, even while it strengthens growth and safety for everyone.

If you want to learn how to help the loved ones, family, communities, culture, world, and planetary individuals and collectives you care about, simply ask what they need.

So. Your transcendent love practice: *Ask*. Then, act. Stay in your body. Practice this every day.

LAST WORDS.

Love is connection, truth, and safety. That's all we'll every need.

How do we return the world to connection and safety?

We start with ourselves, gently, relentlessly, compassionately working our steppingstones, dialing in our personal terrain of healing. Learning, growing, becoming sturdier every day.

From that strength, we reach out to others. Not out of obligation but because we care and have made a conscious choice to do so. More than reach out, we ask: what do you need to feel safe?

Then, very gently, with deep compassion for ourselves and everyone else, we step into love. One question, one small step, one act of love at a time.

THREE PROMISES.

Where do I start? With three small things. Promises I make and come back to every day. I'm getting my reps in. Reps for love. Reps for safety. Reps for connection. I breathe and stay in my body as I do.

1.
2.
3.

CHAPTER TWENTY-FOUR
Ninth *Un*Broken Core Resilience Steppingstone:

LIVE YOUR PURPOSE.

I live and love with all my being. I ask: Who am I at my core?
What do I love? What do I need? At the end of the day, what inspires
me, what emboldens me, what sparks my joy? That's my purpose.

We don't find our purpose, we *live* it.

We don't curate our purpose to align with what our families-communities-culture expect from us or reward us for. That's *not* the purpose we're talking about here.

Let's work with a notion of purpose that aligns with who we authentically are and what we do that arises from *that*. We'll call it *true* purpose.

True purpose is not in the external things where we're taught to look for it—our jobs, families, or accomplishments.

We may live our true purpose through our jobs, families, and many of our accomplishments, but they themselves are not our true purpose.

True purpose is never 'out there,' at all. It's inside us. It's in who we are and how we live that arises from that.

In this way, true purpose is a verb that we live from our most authentic being.

Karyn Shanks MD

True purpose is never passive, though it's usually not loud or splashy either. It won't make headlines or attract zillions of followers. Purpose lived at its deepest and most meaningful can be so quiet. Yet its alignment with who we authentically are is so beautiful, so resonant, so satisfying.

True purpose is in the creation of a life: how we grapple, caretake, struggle, chore, rest, play, connect, *all* the things we do, done with the clear conscious intention to be ourselves. It's the thread of meaning in everything we do that is our reason for living, our reason for waking up each day, our reason for being.

So, *True Purpose = Authenticity.*

But let's take that further.

True Purpose = Authenticity + Divinity + Being + Bells on.

That's more like it.

In this *Unbroken* steppingstone, we explore how to live our truest, most authentic life. Express our truest, most authentic selves. Be completely in our wholeness. That's what true purpose asks of us. How do we live *that*? How do we live our truest truth? Our most authentic life?

If true purpose is already there inside us, our task is to shed what hides it. It's in remembering who we are: *Already whole.*

What must be shed to reveal who we authentically are, to live our true purpose more fully?

- Accomplishments that don't feel like they fit but make us "successful."
- Attributes that are expected of us, even though they're not who we are: we're "nice," we're "good," we're quiet, we're loud, we're aggressive, we're meek, and so on.
- The ways we say "yes" to fit in or "no" to avoid risks.
- Habits that numb or distract us from our true feelings.
- Hypervigilance, perfectionism, or over-work that exhaust us.
- Avoiding stillness, quiet, listening.
- Holding back our true thoughts and feelings to "fit in" or avoid rejection.
- Narratives borrowed from family-community-culture that aren't our own and don't align with our personal values.

What would you add to that list? What hides who you authentically are? How do we shed these things that hide our true selves?

It's not easy. We must come at it with our questions and relentless curiosity. Who are we at our core of cores, our heart of hearts? What makes us shine and sparkle? How do we reconcile that shine and sparkle with the narratives for success and good behavior we were born into?

HEART AND SOUL QUESTIONS.

If true purpose is not external—not something outside us, not something we strive for like a big job or massive book contract—but rather it's internal—something that arises from our most authentic precious being—how do we access it? How do we talk about it?

Just like our bodies, our minds, *us*, our true purpose is multidimensional and dynamic. It changes from one day to the next. It evolves. It takes on character and nuance over time. It grows up. It expands. It defies being sized up. Our true purpose will always be a journey of discovery of who we are at our core of cores, our heart of hearts, and how we live from that.

So, to discuss our purpose, to access it, and to define it for ourselves, we'll ask questions. Instead of focusing on the big things we can be, we'll focus on big questions that lead us to who we are. We'll call them *heart and soul* questions. Because where do we land when we connect to our most authentic precious being? I'd say that's our heart and soul.

Because we and our purpose grow, we'll ask our questions every day. We'll experience the evolution every time we ask.

So, our heart and soul questions:

- Who am I at my core of cores, my heart of hearts?
- What do I most need at my core of cores, my heart of hearts?
- What do I love at my core of cores, my heart of hearts?
- What brings me joy from my core of cores, my heart of hearts?

We're going to work through each one of these questions. Write your answers down or say them out loud. I like to write because it accesses deeper levels of my inner truth. I learn things when I write I wouldn't otherwise. But you do what works best for you.

Karyn Shanks MD

Before each question, we'll get quiet, get our minds out of our way, and tap into the deep inner wisdom within our bodies (our heart and soul) the ways we've been practicing through this entire book. You'll know what to do.

As we ask our questions, I want you to ask then let go. Don't think. Gently ask your mind to step aside. Stay in your body. Quietly listen. Feel how the questions land. What comes up for you in words, images, sensations, feelings, or shifts in your energy? These are the "answers" we're looking for. I assure you the wise inner part of you is listening and *something* will arise within you as you ask. Perhaps not now, but at some time. As you continue to ask, which I hope you do, your answers will come. The more you ask, the more your body will trust you. The more your body trusts you, the more of your answers will be revealed. But don't force them. Heart and soul answers will arrive when they're ready. We all receive our answers at all kinds of crazy times and all kinds of ways. What's key is you are available to hear them through your daily practice of getting quiet, asking, and staying curious.

As you ask and answer these soul questions, see if you can let go of the ultimate question, "what is my purpose?" After our soul question practice, we'll connect the dots. We're trying to get as close as possible to an answer that is as true as possible for today, that touches our authenticity, and that is devoid of all the external factors that have influenced what we've thought our purpose was (success, the big job, and so on).

I'm going to share with you some of the answers my clients and I have gotten as we've done this practice. That said, please don't compare your experience to ours. Some of us have been asking soul questions for a very long time, while for others of us this practice is new. You may find this practice to be quite easy, but if you're new to present moment embodied awareness or tapping into your own inner wisdom you may not. Wherever you are at and whatever happens for you is completely excellent and as it should be—you're getting your reps in. With practice, this will become second nature to you.

We'll circle back to these questions daily. This is key to this practice because one of our foundational premises is how purpose is as dynamic as we are and changes every day. Daily check-ins also make your intentions known. You're available to receive.

Finally, you can drop questions in even if you have no time to stop for the answers. I like to do this just before I go to sleep at night. I briefly ask, hold the questions in my body, then drop off to sleep. It always feels like I'm using myself as a question box. Like I have a little slit on the top of my head, I'm plopping my questions in on a little slip of paper, then walking away. Someone will read them and get back to me.

WHO AM I AT MY CORE OF CORES, MY HEART OF HEARTS?

The ultimate existential question, yes? And like most existential questions there aren't concrete answers, rather whispers and glimmers. Who we are is more about energy, feelings, and experiences. We flow. And when we can't flow, when we're stuck, or numb, or distracted, we can't access who we are. So, we ask. And we ask. And we keep asking.

Sit or stand comfortably and quietly. Gently drop into your body. Notice your breath without trying to change it. Notice any feelings or sensations present in your body without trying to change or fix them. Rest here for a moment.

Continuing to breathe, soften your body. Soften your face, soften your jaw, soften your neck. Breathe. Soften your shoulders, soften your arms, soften your belly. Soften your hips, your pelvis, your legs. Soften your skin. Enjoy the softening, the relaxation, the rest.

Ask: Who am I at my core of cores, my heart of hearts?

Let your question go. Stay in your body. Breathe.

If an answer comes, any answer at all, record it immediately. It may be a word, a string of words, a sentence, or a string of sentences. It may be an image, a sensation somewhere in your body, or a shift in your energy. It may be unexpected or seem strange. Don't ignore any of it. Record it all.

If an answer doesn't come or you feel your mind coming online, let it go. You've asked and your answer will come.

Some client answers:

I am love.

I am weird (she loved that one!).

I am an artist.

I'm confused.

Sometimes the answers aren't words, but rather images, sensations, and feelings.

One of my answers was a combination of sensation and words. The sensation was swirling warm glowing energy running through the core of my body. It felt like love. So, my answer to the heart and soul question was "I am love."

WHAT DO I MOST NEED AT MY CORE OF CORES, MY HEART OF HEARTS?

What we need, *really* need, at our core of cores, heart of hearts, is a signature of who we are. It speaks to what we identify as what uniquely supports us and our authentic truth.

Drop back into your body, letting the previous question and answer go. Breathe. Soften. Rest here for a moment, aware of the feelings and sensations in your body, without trying to change or fix them. Enjoy the rest.

Ask: What do I most need at my core of cores, my heart of hearts?

Let your question go. Stay in your body. Breathe.

Notice any words, images, sensations, feelings, or shifts in your energy that arise. Record what comes. Again, let it be unexpected, strange, whatever it needs to be.

Client answers:

To be heard.

To heal.

To have more fun.

To trust life.

To leave my husband.

More help with the chores.

For me just now: Sleep, rest, play, fun, fuzzy puppies (seriously!). Yah, I need all of those!

WHAT DO I LOVE AT MY CORE OF CORES, MY HEART OF HEARTS?

If love is reverence and reverence is acknowledgement of our Divinity, then love is authenticity, love is true purpose.

All the people, places, and things we most love and the memories of that love we carry within us, remind us of who we are and who we can be in the experience of love. When we hold the energy of that love in our awareness, we create a beacon, calling upon all the people, places, and things we want to love. In this way, we *create* our true purpose.

Drop back into your body. Let go of the previous questions and answers. Notice your breath. Check in with your body. Notice the feelings or sensations in your body without trying to change or fix them. Bring your mind back from the

previous experiences and rest here. Take several deep cleansing breaths. Sigh out
loud if you need to. Soften.

Ask: What do I love at my core of cores, my heart of hearts?

Let the question go. Stay in your body. Breathe.

Record any words, memories, images, sensations, feelings, or shifts in your energy that come.

Client answers:

My children.

Walks in the woods.

Throwing pots.

My dogs.

Waking up after an awesome night of sleep.

My garden in bloom.

Fall.

My comfy bed.

For me recently it was a whole string of words and sentences: I love sitting right here feeling the aliveness of my body through sensations and feelings, I love Nature, I love my husband and boys and fuzzy puppies, I love the beauty and vulnerability and courage of my clients, I love learning and growth and exploring ... It was a flood of emotionally charged things, all that I love.

Note about this question: In the *Love* steppingstone we explored how problematic the word "love" can be for many of us. It can be difficult to simply tell the truth versus inserting answers reflecting what we were taught we "should" love. Even the people we love beyond measure, we may not *feel* love for them every single moment. If we're exhausted and mad at our partner or frustrated with our kids, would it be completely honest to name them as we ask what we love? Do you get what I'm saying? We're after answers from our bodies here, not our heads. Let whatever is true for you in this moment be true, knowing it may not be your *whole* truth.

WHAT BRINGS ME JOY FROM MY CORE OF CORES, MY HEART OF HEARTS?

What gets us out of our minds and their limiting beliefs? Our "smart" brains who know it all, our critics who watch us like hawks, our myriad distractions?

Or something else? What helps us become completely who we are, in our most unfettered, unadulterated, sparkly wholeness? And our most embodied, most real, most aligned with our true human purpose upon this planet?

Joy.

What else could we call it? Lightheartedness. Free-spiritedness. Playfulness. Exuberance. Aliveness. Connected to our essential lifeforce.

It's what our children were born knowing. Joy is pure light. It's everything worth anything.

Drop back into your body. Breathe. Rest. Soften. Notice the feelings and sensations there without trying to change or fix them. Breathe and sigh, letting go of the previous questions.

Ask: What brings me joy from my core of cores, my heart of hearts?

Record any words, images, memories, sensations, feelings, or shifts in energy that arise.

There are times when we can't access joy. That's okay. More than okay, it's utterly human. If you can't access joy right now, what *can* you tap into? Simply notice what's there in sensations, feelings, or energy states without trying to change or fix them. We don't want to "fix" anything, we want to understand the language of our bodies. Hold onto what's true for you with absolute reverence. This is all part of your true purpose, your authenticity, your Divinity.

We all respond to words so differently, don't we? Like my client Molly preferring "reverence" over "love." Words like "fun" and "play" can be just as problematic. As the culture of doers doing, what the hell is play if not laziness? You get my meaning. Use the word that has the least friction for you right now.

And finally ...

WHAT IS MY TRUE PURPOSE?

Keep in mind, true purpose is energy. It moves, it's dynamic. It inhabits our bodies. It flows in present time. It's not a thing; we can't capture or stop it. We can scarcely name it. But we feel it's presence when we're joyful, reverent, and filled with love, all those moments when we're the most tuned into present moment embodied awareness, and the excitement of being alive.

We also connect to our purpose when we're sad, scared, alone, but feeling what we feel with reverence for our authentic experience. We're aware of it when we are the most who we are, without self-consciousness, without concern for how others receive us, and when we're in full recognition of our needs. We get close to it with regularly asking our heart and soul questions.

What we're going to do now is string together the answers to our heart and soul questions to create a true purpose statement that gets as close as we can to defining our true purpose for this day, this moment. Your true purpose statement may not look like any notion of purpose you've ever had. You may also notice, as you continue to participate in this practice, that your true purpose statement will morph and change. Over time, you'll see how it evolves. Through this practice of paying exquisite attention to who you are, you'll experience how your purpose shifts, how alive and nuanced and beautiful it is.

Once your true purpose statement is created, consider: How does it land? What do you notice in your body as you say or write it? How resonant does it feel inside you? Does your true purpose statement name your life's true purpose with clarity? How does it differ from your previous notions of what your purpose is?

My true purpose statement for today: I am love. I need sleep, rest, play, fun, and fuzzy puppies to support me. I love sitting right here feeling the sensations and feelings in my body. I love Nature. I love my husband and boys and fuzzy puppies. I love the beauty and vulnerability and courage of my clients. I love learning and growth and exploring.

Does this feel like my true purpose? Does it authentically express who I am at my core of cores and heart of hearts?

Yes, it does. It looks different from one day to the next, but the essence is similar. It's not always as lengthy or effusive as this one but it always reflects what I most love and what brings me the most joy. My true purpose statements show me how I live in alignment with my true purpose. And they encourage me to keep living this way.

On the days when I'm exhausted and overwhelmed and perhaps feel little love or warmth or fuzziness for anything (full disclosure!), it's more my answers to "what do I need" that define my true purpose for that day.

What's your first crack at a true purpose statement?

WHAT IS MY NEXT STEP TO LIVING MY PURPOSE?

How do we live in ways that are more aligned with our true purpose?

First, we ask, right? In our asking we start to shift.

What is my next step to living my true purpose?

Asking keeps us growing and deepening our purpose practice.

Asking for a "next step" (rather than sweeping life overhauls) keeps us tender and compassionate in our commitment to growth. It's the microdoses of care that shift us the most.

So, as an old pro, drop back into your body. Breathe. Notice any sensations or feelings you find without trying to change or fix anything. Rest here for a moment in this sanctuary of your body.

Ask: What is my next step in living my true purpose?

Breathe. Let the question go. Notice what arises. What words, images, memories, sensations, feelings, or shifts in energy come? Record them.

If your body's response to this question provides you with clear guidance about what your next step is, is there a way to make that next step happen?

Finally, keep asking. One step becomes a thousand steps becomes a life of true purpose.

LAST WORDS.

Where does our true purpose practice take us?

It comes full circle, doesn't it? Everything we've worked on through our nine *Unbroken* core resilience steppingstones has connected to, grown from, and fed into all the others. That's how it is and how it was always meant to be. Our beautifully complex terrain of healing flows, makes us *us*, leads us to our potential and possibilities. The promise of the exquisite relationship between our genes and everything we do. And if all we ever aspire to is to be ourselves? We've nailed it.

So, bravo. Incredibly well done. That you're here at all is so rare, so beautiful. You are stunning as you shine and sparkle, courageously living this healing life.

THREE PROMISES.

May I suggest?

I promise to breathe and stay in my body. I promise to hold myself with the utmost tenderness for everything I experience. I promise to commit showing up as much as I'm capable of at this moment.

Your turn:

1.

2.

3.

Last Words to the Wise

We're works in progress, aren't we? That's all we'll ever be, but that's enough. The equilibrium of progress is *bad ass*. It means we're brave. We're showing up. We're dismantling the cultural legacy of disconnection we were born into. We're rising out of pain, suffering, illness, and feeling stuck, shifting into an equilibrium of flow, resilience, and who we were meant to be. One small but fierce step at a time.

Now you know what you've known all along. The wisdom is in you. It's not rocket science and it's not magic either. It's how we're made, from the Earth, of her complexity and genius, with potential and possibility built right into us that we're claiming as our own and directing to our own advantage.

The first three *Unbroken* core resilience steppingstones—*Be Present, Balance,* and *Rest*—are like personal superpowers bolstering you for all the rest. Setting you up for success. You're tapping deeply into yourself, decoding the language of your body while unlocking the critical pathways to your energy, your flow, your expansion out of suffering. That's right, your healing.

The remaining *Unbroken* core resilience steppingstones—*Move, Nourish, Liberate, Feel, Love*, and *Live Your Purpose*—well, they're superpowers too. They help you settle into yourself more deeply and know yourself more authentically, while personally directing your healing, your flow, your *life.*

Remember, you can't *not* heal. You can't *not* flow. You can't *not* be one hell of a glorious miracle. No matter how unconscious you are of your own magnificence, that's what you are. But to know your magnificence? To understand your genius? To realize your potential and possibilities? You'll flow so hard, straight into your zone. Reconnecting to yourself, you'll expand into that gorgeous sparkly wholeness that is you. That has been you all along, just waiting for you to remember.

In that spirit, let's remember together one more time. Hands over heart, let your heart know you're there. Quietly breathe. Become your witness. Hold whatever you notice with compassion. Invite what's there to emerge with your relentless curiosity.

That's all your gorgeous sparkly wholeness needs to reveal itself. To be seen, heard, felt, and held, *to matter. You* matter.

Love,

Karyn

Resources and Reading Suggestions

SECTION ONE: WE BELONG.

Stephen W Porges. *Polyvagal Theory: A Science of Safety*. Front Integr Neurosci. 2022.

Rachel Yehuda and Amy Lehrner. *Intergenerational transmission of trauma effects: putative role of epigenetic mechanisms.* World Psychiatry. 2018.

Convention on Biological Diversity (CBD). *Biodiversity—The Web of Life.* 2020.

WWF (World Wide Fund for Nature). *Living Planet Report 2020—Bending the curve of biodiversity loss.*

Jeff Tollerfson. *Why deforestation and extinctions make pandemics more likely.* Nature. August 2020.

World Health Organization (WHO). *Biodiversity and Infectious Diseases Questions & Answers.*

WWF. *10 Things you can do to help save our planet.* 2021.

Greenmatch. *70 ways to save the earth.* 2021.

The Nature Conservancy. *Can the Earth Be Saved?* 2020.

United Nations. *The Paris Agreement.* 2015.

David Fideler. *Restoring the Soul of the World: Our Living Bond with Nature's Intelligence.* 2014.

Graham Lawton. *Rescue plan for nature: how to fix the biodiversity crisis.* New Scientist. 2021.

Gabor Maté. *When the Body Says No: Exploring the Stress-Disease Connection.* 2003.

Neeta Mehta PhD. *Mind-body dualism: A critique from a Health Perspective.* Mens Sana Monographs. 2011.

Jonathan Westphal. *Descartes and the Discovery of the Mind-Body Problem.* The MIT Press Reader. 2019.

Matthew Desmond. *In order to understand the brutality of American capitalism**Error! Bookmark not defined.**, you have to start on the plantation.* The 1619 Project. The New York Times Magazine. August 14, 2019.

Gabor Maté. *The Myth of Normal: Trauma, Illness, and Healing in a Toxic Culture.* 2022.

American Heart Association (AHA). *2022 Heart Disease and Stroke Statistical Update Fact Sheet Global Burden of Disease.* 2022.

Centers for Disease Control and Prevention (CDC). *Health Care Expenditures in the United States, 2020-2021.*

J. R. Hampton, et al. *Relative Contributions of History-Taking, Physical Exam, and Laboratory Investigation to Diagnosis and Management of Medical Outpatients.* British Medical Journal. 31 May 1975.

Justin Jagosh et al. *The importance of physician listening from the patients' perspective: Enhancing diagnosis, healing, and the doctor-patient relationship.* Patient Education and Counseling. 2011.

Wendell Potter. *Big Insurance 2022: Revenues reached $1.25 trillion thanks to sucking billions out of the pharmacy supply chain—and taxpayers' pockets.* 2023.

R E Jordan. *Covid-19: risk factors for severe disease and death. BMJ.* 2020.

SECTION TWO: WE FLOW.

Stephen Kotler. *The Rise of Superman: Decoding the Science of Ultimate Human Performance.* 2014.

A.H. Almaas. *Diamond Heart: Elements of the Real in Man.* Second edition, 2000.

Karyn Shanks MD. *Heal: A Nine-Stage Roadmap to Recover Energy, Reverse Chronic Illness, and Claim the Potential of a Vibrant New You.* 2019.

Suresh I. S. Rattan, Marios Kyriazi, editors. *The Science of Hormesis in Health and Longevity.* 2018.

Deepak Chopra MD, Rudolph Tanzi PhD. *Super Genes: Unlock the Astonishing Power of Your DNA for Optimum Health and Well-Being.* 2015.

Siddhartha Mukherjee. *The Gene: An Intimate History.* 2016.

Mark P Mattson. *Hormesis Defined.* Ageing Res Rev. 2008.

Kelly McGonigal PhD. *The Upside of Stress.* 2016.

Alia J Crum et al. *Rethinking stress: The role of mindsets in determining the stress response.* Journal of Personality and Social Psychology. 2013.

Alia J Crum et al. *Optimizing Stress: An Integrated Intervention for Regulating Stress Responses.* Emotion. 2020.

Karin Roelofs. *Freeze for action: neurobiological mechanisms in animal and human freezing.* Philos Trans R Soc Lond B Biol Sci. 2017.

Norman Doidge MD. *The Brain that Changes Itself: Stories of Personal Triumph from the Frontiers of Brain Science.* 2007.

Norman Doidge MD. *The Brain's Way of Healing: Remarkable Discoveries and Recoveries from the Frontiers of Neuroplasticity.* 2015.

Kenneth R Pelletier. *Change Your Genes, Change Your Life: Creating Optimal Health with the New Science of Epigenetics.* 2018.

Rachel Yehuda et al. *Holocaust Exposure Induced Intergenerational Effects on FKBP5 Methylation.* Biol Psychiatry. 2016.

Nagy A Youssef. *The Effects of Trauma, with or without PTSD, on the Transgenerational DNA Methylation Alterations in Human Offsprings.* Brain Sci. 2018.

Leonard A Wisneski. *The Scientific Basis of Integrative Medicine, 2nd edition.* 2009.

The Institute for Functional Medicine. *What is Functional Medicine?* ifm.org/functional-medicine/.

Karyn Shanks. *What is Functional Medicine?* www.KarynShanksMD.com/what-is-functional-medicine. 2017.

Stephen W Porges. *Polyvagal Theory: A Science of Safety.* Frontiers Integrative Neuroscience. 2022.

Deborah A Dana. *Anchored: How to Befriend Your Nervous System Using Polyvagal Theory.* 2021.

Robert K Naviaux. *Perspective: Cell danger response Biology—The new science that connects environmental health with mitochondria and the rising tide of chronic illness.* Mitochondrion. 2020.

Neil Nathan. *Toxic: Heal Your Body from Mold Toxicity, Lyme Disease, Multiple Chemical Sensitivities, and Chronic Environmental Illness.* 2018.

Victor J. Strecher. *Life on Purpose: How Living for What Matters Most Changes Everything.* 2016.

NPR. *Take the ACE Quiz—And Learn What It Does and Doesn't Mean.* 2015.

SECTION THREE: WE RISE.

Amy Cuddy. *Presence: Bringing your boldest self to your biggest challenges.* 2015.

Amy Cuddy. *Your body language may shape who you are.* TED talk. 2012.

Kelly McGonigal PhD. *The Science of Compassion: A Modern Approach for Cultivating Empathy, Love, and Connection.* 2016.

Bronnie Ware. *Top Five Regrets of the Dying: A Life Transformed by the Dearly Departing.* 2019.

Tania Singer, Olga Klimecki. *Empathy and compassion.* Current Biology. 2014.

Compassionate Inquiry (CI) Practitioners. www.CompassionateInquiry.com/practitioners. 2024.

Karyn Shanks MD. *Compassionate Inquiry.* 2022.

Zaya Benazzo and Maurizio Benazzo. *The Wisdom of Trauma.* 2021.

Richard Schwartz PhD. *No Bad Parts: Healing Trauma and Restoring Wholeness with the Internal Family Systems Model.* 2021.

James Nester. *Breath: The New Science of a Lost Art.* 2021.

Kelly Howell. *Meditate Me App.*

The Best Meditation Apps. The New York Times/Wirecutter. 2023.

Rod Stryker. *The Four Desires: Creating a Life of Purpose, Happiness, Prosperity, and Freedom.* 2011.

Eyal Ophir et al. *Cognitive Control in Media Multitaskers. PNAS.* 2009.

Edita Poljac, et al. *New Perspectives on Human Multitasking.* Psychological Research. 2018.

Karyn Shanks MD. *Simplicity: The Fine Art of Doing Just One Thing.* www.KarynShanksMD.com. 2017.

American Psychological Association. *Driven to Distraction: Driving and Cell Phones Don't Mix.* 2006.

The National Safety Council. *Distracted Driver Research: Learn, Share, and Help End This Deadly Epidemic.* 2017:

The University of Utah. *Drivers on Cell Phones Are as Bad as Drunks.* 2016.

D. L. Strayer et al. *A Comparison of the Cell Phone Driver and the Drunk Driver.* Human Factors. 2006.

Deane Alban. *Seven Ways Multitasking Hurts Brain Health and Performance.* Be Brain Fit. 2024.

Marie Kondo. *The Life-Changing Magic of Tidying Up: The Japanese Art of Decluttering and Organizing.* 2014.

Karyn Shanks MD. *Simple Is Better: The 'Rule of Threes.* www.KarynShanksMD.com. 2017.

Ben Johnson. *Using the Rule of Three for Learning.* Edutopia: George Lucas Educational Foundation. 2016.

Bessel van der Kolk, MD. *The Body Keeps the Score: Brain, Mind, and Body in the Healing of Trauma.* 2014.

James S. Gordon, MD. *The Transformation: Discovering Wholeness and Healing After Trauma.* 2019.

Tricia Hersey. *Rest is Resistance: A Manifesto.* 2022.

Catherine Price. *How to Break Up with Your Phone: The 30-Day Plan to Take Back Your Life.* 2018.

Arianna Huffington. *The Sleep Revolution: Transforming Your Life, One Night at a Time.* 2017.

Colten HR, Altevogt BM, editors. *Sleep Disorders and Sleep Deprivation: An Unmet Public Health Problem.* Institute of Medicine (US) Committee on Sleep Medicine and Research; Washington (DC): National Academies Press (US). 2006.

Xie L. et al. *Sleep Drives Metabolite Clearance from the Adult Brain.* Science. 2013.

Andrew Mendelsohn and James Larrick. *Sleep Facilitates Clearance of Metabolites from the Brain: Glymphatic Function in Aging and Neurodegenerative Diseases.* Rejuvenation Research. 2013.

Till Roenneberg and Martha Merrow. *The Circadian Clock and Human Health.* Current Biology. 2016.

Bjorn Rasch and Jan Born. *About Sleep's Role in Memory.* Physiol Rev. 2013.

Kate Porcheret PhD et al. *Psychological Effect of an Analogue Traumatic Event Reduced by Sleep Deprivation.* Sleep. 2015.

Mindy Engle-Friedman. *The Effects of Sleep Loss on Capacity and Effort.* Sleep Science. 2014.

National Sleep Foundation. *Shift Work Disorder.* 2023.

Christian Benedict et al. *Gut Microbiota and Glucometabolic Alterations in Response to Recurrent Partial Sleep Deprivation in Normal-Weight Young Individuals.* Molecular Metabolism. 2016.

Jason R. Anderson. *A Preliminary Examination of Gut Microbiota, Sleep, and Cognitive Flexibility in Healthy Older Adults.* Sleep Medicine. 2017.

Max Hirshkowitz PhD et al. *National Sleep Foundation's Sleep Time Duration Recommendations: Methodology and Results Summary.* Sleep Health. 2015.

Huber Reto et al. *Exposure to Pulsed High-Frequency Electromagnetic Field During Waking Affects Human Sleep EEG.* NeuroReport. 2000.

Sheldon Cohen et al. *Sleep habits and susceptibility to the common cold.* Arch Intern Med. 2009.

The National Institute for Play: nifplay.org. Compendium of current research articles on the benefits of play.

Norman Cousins. *Anatomy of an Illness: As Perceived by the Patient.* First edition. 1979.

Katy Bowman. *Move Your DNA,* 2015.

John Durant. *The Paleo Manifesto: Ancient Wisdom for Lifelong Health. 2014.*

Aviroop Biswas et al. *Sedentary Time and Its Association with Risk for Disease Incidence, Mortality, and Hospitalization in Adults: A Systematic Review and Meta-analysis.* Ann Intern Med. 2015.

Ashish Sharma MD et al. *Exercise for Mental Health.* Prim Care Companion J Clin Psychiatry. 2006.

Katy Bowman. *Don't Just Sit There.* 2015.

Kelly Starrett and Juliet Starrett. *Built to Move: The Ten Essential Habits to Help You Move Freely and Live Fully.* 2023.

Kelly Starrett and Glen Cordoza. *Becoming a Supple Leopard 2nd Edition: The Ultimate Guide to Resolving Pain, Preventing Injury, and Optimizing Athletic Performance.* 2015.

Acknowledgements

I have so many teachers and wisdom bearers to thank.

First, my clients. The bold woman who walked into the room for our first encounter when I was a new physician, handing me a book she believed I needed to read so I could help her, not carte blanch accepting my own knowledge. The countless courageous folks who knew they needed something they hadn't gotten before but saw something in me that told them I was someone they could trust. All whom, beyond how they taught me to help them, helped *me* become courageous myself. I saw how they stepped away from institutions, cultural dictums, and 'the way things are,' when their needs were unmet, pursuing other avenues. You showed me how it's done, how to step away from what doesn't serve, to seek something *somewhere* we may not know exists. Through all that, you shaped me into the kind of doctor who could see how things are, not just what conveniently fits the paradigm. You trusted me to hold the certainty of science, the wild chaos of humanity, and the unique people you are, all at the very same time. I am beyond grateful to you all.

My teachers and mentors. There have been many of you. Some up close, many more from afar. Particularly pertinent to this book are the mentors who have helped me understand trauma—what it is, how it feels, how it shapes who we are, how it shows up in our bodies (*all* of our bodies), and most importantly, how to hold our wounded parts with the tenderness and compassion they deserve to restore the safety we need to heal. Thank you, Gabor Maté MD, for your encyclopedic mind and ability to distill trauma into the simple ideas that help us understand ourselves with greater clarity while leading us to safety. I am grateful for your year-long intensive professional Compassionate Inquiry training program that challenged me beyond words while preparing me to work with clients more deeply.

Karyn Shanks MD

Thank you to my editor, William Boggess. You made this book zing. I'm awed by how deeply you sank into this material and relentlessly questioned my ideas down to the finest detail. You expanded my vocabulary while teaching me the power of economizing words. And someone finally taught me where all those pesky commas go! Thank you from the bottom of my heart. You are a total rock star.

Finally, thank you to the friends and family who have supported and believed in me. Thank you, Sean and Aidan, for knowing my story but keeping me humble, never missing an opportunity to find something about me worthy of humor. Thank you, Jasper, Pax, and Nutmeg, for making me laugh and soothing me with pets and kisses. And, Brian, thank you for your unshakable belief in me and what I'm capable of, and supporting me with whatever I say I need without questioning it (not saying you shouldn't sometimes!).

Finally, thank you to all the intrepid explorers who show up here, now and in the future. Know that I see how courageous you are. Thank you.

Author's Bio

Karyn Shanks MD is a physician, author, and pioneer in the field of root-cause healing, with over forty years of experience helping clients recover their lives from chronic, complex illness. She is board-certified in both Internal Medicine and Functional Medicine, and a founding diplomat of the American Board of Integrative and Holistic Medicine. She is also trained in trauma-informed psychotherapy through Dr. Gabor Maté's Compassionate Inquiry Professional Training Program.

Karyn brings together the sciences of directable human potential—epigenetics, neuroplasticity, core functional systems biology, and transformational psychology—with the deep wisdom of lived experience, spiritual inquiry, and narrative transformation. Her work centers on the belief that people are not broken, but wise and whole, and that sustainable healing begins with reclaiming that truth. Her private practice, teaching, and writing are deeply influenced by her own journey through illness and recovery.

Karyn is the founder of the Unbroken Academy, an online educational platform for healing through story, self-trust, and embodied resilience. She is the author of two previous books—*Heal: A Nine-Stage Roadmap to Recover Energy, Reverse Chronic Illness, and Claim the Potential of a Vibrant New You* and *The Wisdom of COVID-19*. Her voice is known for its clarity, warmth, and fierce compassion.

Through her work, writing, and lived wisdom, Karyn is trusted by both patients and professionals alike—as a guide, mentor, and visionary voice in a new healing paradigm. Karyn is also an author, teacher, wife, mother of two sons, dog lover, and avid enthusiast of nature.

Website: www.KarynShanksMD.com

Instagram: @karynshanksmd

Facebook: <u>Karyn Shanks MD</u>

Index

Karyn Shanks MD

Karyn Shanks MD

www.ingramcontent.com/pod-product-compliance
Lightning Source LLC
Chambersburg PA
CBHW051323020426

42333CB00032B/3458